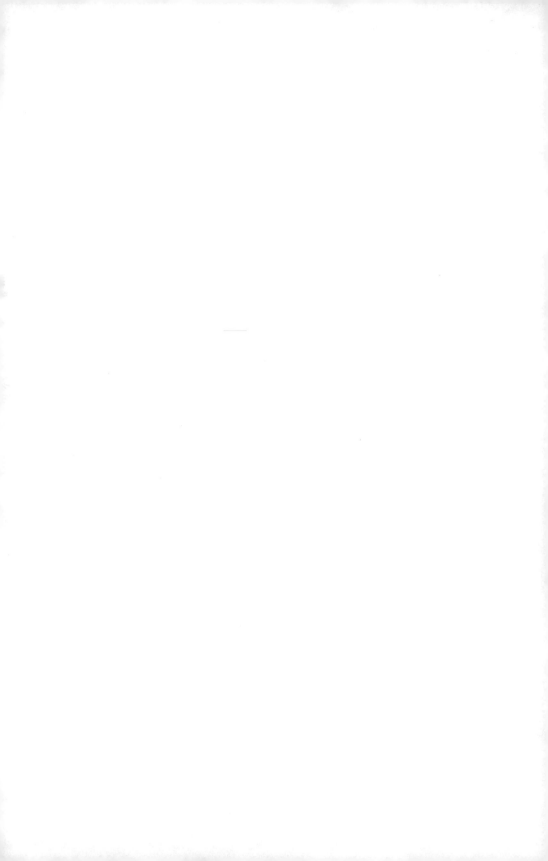

DRGs

Their Design and Development

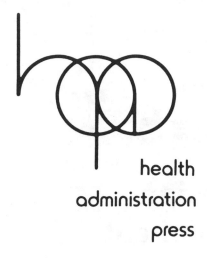

health
administration
press

DRGs

Their Design and Development

Robert B. Fetter, Senior Editor
David A. Brand, Editor
Dianne Gamache, Editor

Health Administration Press
Ann Arbor, Michigan 1991

95 94 93 92 91   5 4 3 2 1

Library of Congress Cataloging-in-Publication Data

DRGs : their design and development / Robert B. Fetter,
senior editor. Donald A. Brand, editor. Dianne E. Gamache, editor.
    p.   cm.
   Includes bibliographical references.
   Includes index.
   ISBN 0-910701-60-1 (hardbound : alk. paper)
   1. Diagnosis related groups. I. Fetter, Robert B. II. Brand, Donald A.
III. Gamache, Dianne E.
   [DNLM: 1. Diagnostic Related Groups. WX 157 D7785]
RA971.32.D74 1991   338.4'336211—dc20
DNLM/DLC for Library of Congress   90-4872 CIP

The paper used in this publication meets the minimum requirements of American National Standard for Information Sciences—Permanence of Paper for Printed Library Materials, ANSI Z39.48-1984.   ∞™

Health Administration Press
A division of the Foundation of the
   American College of Healthcare Executives
1021 East Huron Street
Ann Arbor, Michigan 48104-9990
(313) 764-1380

Contents

Part I   The DRG Patient Classification System

Part II   Use of DRGs for Managing Hospital Resources

List of Figures

List of Tables

List of Appendixes

Contributors

Richard F. Averill is director of product development, 3M Health Information Systems. He has extensive experience in health care consulting, systems programming and analysis, operations research, and statistics. Mr. Averill has been a leader in the application of case-mix technology to problems in health care. He has directed many large-scale projects in hospital reimbursement, management planning, and quality assurance. He is one of the developers of the diagnosis-related groups (DRGs) patient classification scheme and was instrumental in the design and implementation of the prospective reimbursement system in New Jersey.

William A. Bauman, M.D., vice-president of medical affairs at Danbury Hospital, attended Harvard University and received his medical degree from the College of Physicians and Surgeons, Columbia University. After internship in internal medicine he completed residencies in pediatric pathology and pediatrics at Babies Hospital. He did graduate work in biostatistics at Columbia University. As a board-certified pediatrician he practiced and spent much of his career in the advancement of computer technology in medicine. He has been an officer in organizations and committees related to information technology in medicine and is currently responsible for medical/administrative activities at Danbury Hospital. His investigative work and publications have focused on the use of information technology to help quantitate and manage the delivery of health care.

Ian R. Chandler is a recipient of a National Research Service Award, with which he is pursuing both an M.D. and a Ph.D. in operations research at Yale University.

Leo M. Cooney, Jr., M.D., is the Humana Foundation Professor of Geriatric Medicine, School of Medicine, Yale University. Dr. Cooney directs the program in geriatric medicine at the school. He is particularly interested in the most effective methods of delivering care to the frail elderly. He is medical director of the Continuing Care Unit, a rehabilitation unit at

Yale–New Haven Hospital, and also medical director of discharge planning and utilization review at the hospital. He has worked on developing predictors of the need for placement of elderly persons in nursing homes, and on better matching resources to patient needs for the institutionalized elderly.

Donna Diers, R.N., M.S.N., is professor of nursing in the graduate program, School of Nursing, Yale University. Formerly dean of the school, she is a member of the Institute of Medicine and the National Academy of Sciences; the author of numerous publications in nursing research and health services delivery and policy; and editor of *Image*, the national journal of Sigma Theta Tau, nursing's honorary society. She teaches courses in health policy and management, nursing and policy, and clinical research methods, and has a special interest in alternative systems of care.

Charles C. Duncan, M.D., is associate professor of surgery/neurosurgery and pediatrics at the School of Medicine, Yale University, and is chief of pediatric neurosurgery at Yale–New Haven Hospital. He is director of the Health Systems Management Group in the School of Medicine.

Paul W. Eggers, Ph.D., is chief of the Program Evaluation Branch in the Office of Research, Health Care Financing Administration. His research interests include health care utilization by Medicare beneficiaries, methods of assessing quality of care, and trends in the end-stage renal disease program.

Audrey L. Fetter, M.B.A., M.P.H., was vice-president for administration at Bridgeport Hospital in Bridgeport, Connecticut, until her retirement in 1989. She received her M.B.A. from Indiana University and an M.P.H. in hospital administration from Yale University. Before joining Bridgeport Hospital in 1981, she served at the Hospital at Parker Hill in Boston and at Scottsdale Memorial Hospital in Scottsdale, Arizona. The work reported in Chapter 7 was drawn from her master's essay at Yale.

Daniel H. Freeman, Jr., Ph.D., is professor of community and family medicine (biostatistics) at Dartmouth Medical School and adjunct professor of mathematics and computer science, Dartmouth College. Dr. Freeman is also director of the New Hampshire State Cancer Registry. He has been an associate professor of biostatistics at the School of Medicine, Yale University, and an Indo-American Fellow at the Indian Statistical Institute, Calcutta, India. His research interests are clinical trials, cancer research, survey sampling, and categorical data analysis. Dr. Freeman received the B.A. and M.A. degrees in mathematics from Boston

University and the Ph.D. degree in biostatistics from the University of North Carolina.

Jean L. Freeman, Ph.D., is assistant professor of community and family medicine at Dartmouth Medical School. Before that appointment, she was a research scientist with the Health Systems Management Group, School of Organization and Management, Yale University. She has collaborated on numerous studies involving the development and application of product-line management systems in health care institutions. Currently, she designs and directs research projects that evaluate the utilization and costs of hospital care. Dr. Freeman received degrees in mathematics (B.A., Mount Holyoke College; M.A., Boston University) and in epidemiology and public health (Ph.D., Yale University).

Louis Gottlieb, M.D., F.A.C.P., is an internist and director of emergency services at St. Mary's Hospital, Waterbury, Connecticut; assistant clinical professor of medicine at Yale University; and associate clinical professor of medicine at the School of Medicine, University of Connecticut. He graduated cum laude from the University of Bologna and served his internship and residency in medicine at St. Mary's Hospital. His interests in research are new pharmacologic strategies in treatment of alcohol withdrawal states, and he is developing clinical algorithms for the care and management of common ambulatory medical problems.

Timothy F. Greene, M.B.A., is an economist in the Institutional Studies Branch, Division of Reimbursement and Economic Studies, Office of Reimbursement and Economic Studies, Office of Research and Demonstrations, Health Care Financing Administration. His research interests include the impact of Medicare prospective payment on non-Medicare payers and the evaluation of patient classification systems.

Stuart Guterman is senior health policy analyst with the Prospective Payment Assessment Commission. Previously he served as chief of the Institutional Studies Branch in the Division of Reimbursement and Economic Studies, Office of Research, Health Care Financing Administration (HCFA), where he supervised HCFA's efforts to evaluate the Medicare Prospective Payment System (PPS) for the congressionally mandated annual report on the impact of the PPS.

Edward A. Harms received his Ph.D. in physics from Rensselaer Polytechnic Institute in 1969. Since then he has been actively involved in the application of computers to scientific and business problems. He is currently president of his own consulting firm and director of the Institute for Personal Computers in Business at Fairfield University.

John S. Hughes, M.D., received his undergraduate and M.D. degrees from the University of North Carolina. He was an intern and junior resident in internal medicine at Ohio State University Hospitals, and did his senior residency at Yale-New Haven Hospital. He was a Robert Wood Johnson Clinical Scholar at the School of Medicine, Yale University, and subsequently practiced general internal medicine at the Fair Haven Community Clinic in New Haven. Dr. Hughes joined the full-time faculty at the Yale School of Medicine in 1983, and currently serves as the director of the Medical Primary Care Center at Yale-New Haven Hospital. He has been a participant in DRG refinement projects at the Health Systems Management Group since 1980.

Michael J. Kalison, J.D., is a graduate of the Wharton School of Economics and the Law School of the University of Pennsylvania. After a clerkship on the Supreme Court of New Jersey under Associate Justice Nathan L. Jacobs, Mr. Kalison served with the Division of Rate Counsel, Department of the Public Advocate, primarily in the financial, utility, and health payer areas. Thereafter, he was engaged by the New Jersey State Department of Health to develop a prospective payment system based on patient case mix. Currently, Mr. Kalison is a partner in the law firm of Manger, Kalison, Murphy & McBride. He has been a frequent national lecturer on financial and corporate issues affecting hospitals, with articles published on these subjects. He has consulted to the staffs of congressional committees and key members of Congress.

Philip J. Leaf, Ph.D., is an Associate Professor in the Departments of Epidemiology and Public Health, Sociology, Psychiatry, and the Institution for Social and Policy Studies of Yale University. He is co-director of an NIMH-sponsored training program in mental health service system research and Chairman of the Mental Health Section of the American Public Health Association.

Jeffrey L. Lichtenstein, M.D., is a graduate of Franklin & Marshall College. He graduated with honors from the University of Tennessee School of Medicine and was an intern and resident in internal medicine at the New York Hospital—Cornell Medical Center and Memorial Sloan Kettering Cancer Center and completed his postdoctoral fellowship in gastroenterology at Yale-New Haven Hospital. At Yale he was also a Robert Wood Johnson Clinical Scholar. Dr. Lichtenstein has served on the faculty of Columbia University in New York, Ben-Gurion University in Israel, and Yale University. He maintains an active role in research and teaching at Yale. Dr. Lichtenstein is a diplomate of the American Board of Internal Medicine and certified in the subspecialty of gastroenterology. He is a contributor to many medical journals and is on the editorial board of the *Journal of Clinical Gastro-enterology.*

Christopher M. Murtaugh, Ph.D., worked on the development of Patient Dependency Groups while a doctoral student at the Health Systems Management Group. He has been at the National Center for Health Services Research since graduating from Yale. Mr. Murtaugh's research interests include the financing and delivery of nursing home services and the relationship between acute and long-term care.

Robert C. Newbold has been a computer programmer and analyst since his graduation from Stanford University with a degree in mathematics in 1974. From 1982 to 1986, as a member of Yale's Health Systems Management Group, he worked on research projects for the United States, French, Portuguese, and Australian governments. While at Yale he designed and wrote a software package to do hospital cost analysis; he has also written DRG and Ambulatory Visit Group (AVG) grouping programs. Mr. Newbold currently writes data base management software for the Iris Health Information Systems Corporation in New Haven, Connecticut.

George R. Palmer, M.E.C., Ph.D., is professor of health administration in the School of Health Administration, the University of New South Wales. During 1987 he was visiting professor in the School of Organization and Management, Yale University. He is a fellow of the Australian College of Health Service Administrators and an honorary fellow of the Royal Australian College of Medical Administrators. He has been a consultant to the governments of the states of Victoria and South Australia and to the Australian federal government for the analysis of hospital case mix with use of DRGs. Professor Palmer's research interests include international comparison of hospital bed utilization based on DRGs, the economic evaluation of hospitals by case-mix measures, and the analysis of rational health policies.

Hayoung Park is an assistant professor, Department of Preventive Medicine, Catholic University Medical College, Seoul, South Korea. While at Yale, she was involved in studies concerning the development of cost accounting, budgeting, and management information systems in hospitals for the Australian and Irish governments, and has collaborated on the study refining DRGs to improve intragroup homogeneity in resource utilization. Her research interests also include the impact of payment policies on efficiency in health services delivery. She received a Ph.D. in operations research and management science from Yale University, and an M.S. and a B.S. in industrial engineering from Seoul National University in Korea.

Carol S. Portlock, M.D., is an associate attending physician at Memorial–Sloan Kettering Cancer Center. She is a clinical investigator with research interests in the lymphomas and melanoma.

Gerald Riley is a research analyst in the Division of Beneficiary Studies, Office of Research, Health Care Financing Administration. His current research topics include Medicare utilization in the last year of life by cause of death, modifications in health maintenance organization reimbursement, and the impact of prospective payment on beneficiaries.

Jean-Marie Rodrigues is currently professor of public health at the Saint-Etienne Medical School. He obtained his degrees in medicine and health economics at the University of Nancy, and in biostatistics at the University of Strasbourg. He was formerly director of the French DRG Project and has been in charge of the regulation of the standardized medical record summary and the new French classification of procedures. He has also collaborated with the Health Systems Management Group at Yale University on the adaptation of the DRGs and the cost model to the French GHM and cost-accounting system. Professor Rodrigues is presently the chairman of a coordinated medical research program of the Council of Europe on the computerization of medical data and DRG use to improve the quality and efficiency of hospital information systems. He is also World Health Organization temporary adviser for DRGs in Europe. His main research interest is efficiency and equity in health services.

Karen C. Schneider is a consultant on health care issues in New Haven, Connecticut. She has coordinated health care studies in the areas of quality of patient care, hospital management, ambulatory patient classification, and long-term care reimbursement. She recently managed a project at Yale to refine DRGs for Medicare payment based on secondary diagnoses.

Helen L. Smits, M.D., is the director of the John Dempsey Hospital at the University of Connecticut Health Center and a professor of community medicine at the university's medical school. From 1981 to 1985 she was an associate professor in the Department of Medicine and the Department of Public Health at Yale University. She served during the Carter Administration as director of the Health Standards and Quality Bureau in the Health Care Financing Administration.

Sherry A. Terrell is chief of the Noninstitutional Studies Branch, Division of Reimbursement and Economic Studies, Office of Research and Demonstrations, Health Care Financing Administration.

John D. Thompson is professor emeritus of public health in the School of Medicine and the School of Nursing, Yale University. His major research has been in health systems analysis and, with Dr. Robert B. Fetter, he was one of the originators of the diagnosis-related group (DRG) system of management and planning. His present interests include the refinement and enhancement of the DRG management system: first, the application of DRGs in strategic planning for hospitals and populations served by hospitals, with use of product-line decisions for effectiveness measures; second, the interface between the DRG system and various health professions, specifically concerning nursing intensity and quality of patient care. His experience includes work on the history of hospital architecture and the early use of statistics in health care (the late nineteenth century).

Acknowledgments

Over the years since this work began in 1967, a very large number of people have been involved in one aspect or another. It would be impossible to acknowledge everyone and for this, I apologize. It is important, however, to single out some who made significant contributions and are not represented in this book as authors or contributors.

Ronald E. Mills worked virtually from the beginning as a systems designer and programmer, providing all of our initial technical support. Youngsoo Shin made substantial contributions to the clinical dimensions of the first complete version of DRGs. Donald C. Riedel motivated the utilization review applications of DRGs. Alfonso Esposito served as project officer of the DRG work supported by the Social Security Administration. Royal Crystal was project officer for our work with the PSRO program in utilizaiton review. Harry Savitt was our project officer for the recently completed DRG refinement project which is described here. Stephen Jencks, Julian Pettengill, and James Vertrees served as advisors during the development of the current version of DRGs.

Over the years numerous graduate students helped us on our various projects. A large number pf PSRO directors and support personnel made important contributions. Support was provided by many hospital administrators and physicians. In our international work, many contributions toward improvements in the DRGs were made by our collaborators in Australia, England, Finland, France, Ireland, the Netherlands, Norway, Portugal, Spain, Sweden, and Wales.

Earlier versions of this book were provided with editorial assistance by Rita E. Watson and Joyce Shanahan Rivers. Finally, we extend our deep appreciation to Marla Demusis and, especially, to Ann Palmeri, who made the greatest contribution of all by making our work easier.

Introduction

This book presents an overview of the design and development of the diagnosis-related groups (DRGs) together with a variety of DRG applications. Included also are extensions of the concept of product definition in health care to ambulatory and long-term care services.

This original work was begun in 1967 at Yale University as a joint effort by Professor Robert B. Fetter of the Department of Administrative Sciences and Professor John D. Thompson of the Department of Epidemiology and Public Health of the School of Medicine. In 1969, work was consolidated by the founding of the Center for the Study of Health Services. With the founding of the School of Organization and Management at Yale in 1975 and with the support of the Henry J. Kaiser Family Foundation, the Health Systems Management Group (HSMG) was established in 1977. This latter entity, with Professor Fetter as director, has carried out all DRG-related work at Yale. With the retirement in 1989 of Professor Fetter, the School of Organization and Management has terminated HSMG, but the group is attempting to continue under a new organization in the Yale School of Medicine.

This book includes selected material from a large number of publications, case studies, lectures, working papers, and other documents produced by the Center for the Study of Health Services and the Health Systems Management Group.

The book is organized in five sections, covering (1) the DRG patient classification system, (2) the use of DRGs for managing hospital resources, (3) the use of DRGs for financing patient care, (4) international use of DRGs, and (5) DRG analogues for ambulatory care and long-term care.

PART I: THE DRG PATIENT CLASSIFICATION SYSTEM

Part I reviews the development and design of DRGs, from their conception in the late 1960s to the current HSMG project refining DRGs with severity measures. The version of DRGs developed in 1981 is composed of 467 patient groupings, and is a classification system for describing inpatients according to similar patterns of resource use.

Chapter 1 offers an insight into the impetus behind DRG creation and the major obstacles encountered by its originators. DRGs were created not for payment purposes, but rather as a tool of management, allowing the activities in a hospital to be measured, evaluated, and to some extent "controlled." Identifying the "products" of a hospital required developing an underlying structure and the appropriate technology by which to measure and understand the data. The steps involved in the building and rebuilding of the DRG model and its extension to hospital management are presented.

Chapter 2 outlines the process of DRG development and the basic characteristic structure. As the function of DRGs was to relate case mix to resource intensity, it was necessary to develop groups of clinically similar patients with similar resource intensity. The resulting process integrated physician judgment with statistical analysis. The DRGs were based on four characteristics thought necessary to meet the requirements of practicality and meaningfulness: routinely collected information, manageable numbers, similarity in resource intensity, and clinical coherence. The four-tier structure of the current Medicare version of DRGs is illustrated.

Chapter 3 updates DRG development, with a look at a project currently refining DRGs with severity measures. Because the original system did not distinguish between patients with major multiple comorbidities and complications (CCs) and those with a relatively minor CC, it has been criticized for not adequately accounting for differences in levels of severity that affect resource consumption. The goal of the project was to provide sets of CCs that represent different levels of resource use while maintaining the basic structure and characteristics of the current DRGs. The project has resulted in a refinement model for DRGs with up to a four-level adjustment for case complexity for each basic diagnostic or procedural group.

PART II: USE OF DRGs FOR MANAGING HOSPITAL RESOURCES

Part II focuses on the essence of DRGs—their application to hospital management. DRGs, as a common unit of measure of hospital performance, allow for a new approach to hospital management and accounting, an approach that focuses on the final products of a hospital—the bundle of services provided to individual patients.

Chapter 4 introduces the concept of product-line management, which, in viewing hospital services along product lines, integrates the physician into the organizational structure. Product-line management is based on an industrial matrix model that incorporates the work of both managers and engineers in the production of highly complex products. Applied to the hospital setting, the matrix model allows both the efficient production of goods and services and their effective utilization by physicians in the bundle of services provided to an individual patient.

Chapter 5 describes the DRG accounting system, which, in identifying costs, permits the appropriate assignment of responsibility to those who provide patient care. The case-mix cost-accounting approach focuses on the cost of treating a particular type of patient rather than on the aggregate cost of support services. Cost identification requires a breaking down of costs to the level of detail necessary to meet the needs of a particular hospital. The cost model follows an eight-step process in breaking down costs from aggregate levels, those in the general ledger, to specific levels, those incurred in treating individual patients. The end result is a cost for each DRG as well as the individual services utilized in treating the DRG. The detailed cost and patient information allows managers to assess where, and to what extent, money is being lost and made in the different areas of the hospital and to compare hospital performance both internally and externally.

Chapter 6 describes a project conducted by the HSMG to associate use of nursing resources with DRGs. Data were assembled from a variety of hospitals in the United States and were analyzed in depth both by case and by day of stay within each case. In addition, a normative study of nursing use by DRG was conducted. The results provide a basis for predicting the amount of routine nursing care required for a patient in a particular DRG.

Chapter 7 summarizes a case study illustrating the breaking down of costs in a hospital department as a means of quantifying management and medical practices and comparing their cost effects. Variance analysis is utilized to break down resource costs into three cost-influencing variables (case mix, physician utilization, and operating efficiency) across three different levels (departmental, micro-costing, and DRG). The study identifies the factors that account for cost variations—complex interactions of inflation, management efficiency, clinical practices, and patient mix.

PART III: USE OF DRGs FOR FINANCING PATIENT CARE

Part III covers the use of DRGs in prospective payment systems, focusing on the design and impact of the federal DRG-based Prospective Payment System (PPS) for Medicare hospital reimbursements.

Chapter 8 describes the first DRG payment system, the "New Jersey Experiment" in 1980, and compares it with the federal DRG scheme implemented three years later. The overall objective of the federal system was to stem the growth in hospital costs while ensuring quality health care. The achievement of this objective in the first years of PPS, in regard to hospital utilization, is assessed.

Chapter 9 assesses the initial impact of the federal Prospective Payment System on the various groups in the health care sector—hospitals, payers of inpatient hospital services, providers of health care, and Medicare beneficiaries—as well as on Medicare expenditures. While the impact of PPS is felt most directly by hospitals, the entire industry has experienced significant effects. The impact of PPS suggests a changing role for the hospital and a shift in economic control.

PART IV: INTERNATIONAL USE OF DRGs

Part IV discusses the manner in which DRGs have been extended and are being further developed internationally. The concept behind DRGs, the identification of a product upon which to measure and evaluate performance, lends itself to many areas of application outside the United States for inpatient hospital care.

Chapter 10 presents the use of DRGs internationally, particularly in eight European countries and in Australia. The chapter includes a discussion of the problems presented by the use of various coding systems for diagnoses and procedures, the introduction of a minimum basic data set in Europe, and results of the Yale DRG projects in Europe and Australia. Details of these projects in France, England and Wales, Australia, and Portugal are presented.

Chapter 11 presents a series of international comparisons of hospital utilization and performance based on the data made available by the projects described in Chapter 10. Variations in length of stay across a range of DRGs and countries are presented and their implications assessed. Finally, characteristics of hospital utilization in the United States and Australia are compared. These show discharge rates per 10,000 of population for selected DRGs in the United States and three states in Australia.

PART V: DRG ANALOGUES FOR AMBULATORY CARE AND LONG-TERM CARE

While ultimately one would like to describe an episode of illness in terms of the resources required for its diagnosis and treatment regardless of the setting, it will first be necessary to identify care processes in each principal setting. "Ambulatory visit groups" (AVGs) were developed to describe the product of ambulatory care, while "patient dependency groups" (PDGs) are concerned with requirements for care in long-term care settings.

Chapter 12 introduces ambulatory visit groups, or AVGs, which define the "products" of outpatient care in a manner analogous to that of the DRG definitions of inpatient care. AVGs were developed by Yale's HSMG to serve as a unit of analysis for management in measuring and evaluating economic performance and as a potential basis for an outpatient prospective payment system. All patient encounters are classified into one of 570 AVGs, based on an outpatient visit and defined by principal diagnosis, procedure, and status of visit.

Chapter 13 reviews a HSMG project that developed a classification system for long-term care patients. The system is based on nursing care requirements and classifies a patient into one of five patient dependency groups (PDGs) defined on the basis of activity of daily living. PDGs capture differences in the care required by most of the residents in nursing homes.

Robert B. Fetter

Part I

The DRG Patient Classification System

1

Background

Robert B. Fetter

Diagnosis-related groups (DRGs) are often associated with Medicare's prospective payment system (PPS) for hospitals, but they were initially developed for other purposes. The original goal of DRGs was to facilitate hospital management by providing a system that would allow the measurement and evaluation of hospital performance.

Attempts at applying industrial concepts to hospitals date back to the early 1900s. Advances in technology and skyrocketing health care costs provided the means and the necessity to recommence such efforts. The DRG approach to managing hospital services differs from the traditional in that the focus is on the final "product" of the hospital—the bundle of goods and services provided to a patient with a particular illness—rather than on the individual services as ends in themselves. This change of focus allows for consideration of the effective utilization of services as well as efficiency in the production of services.

The first section of this chapter describes the motivations underlying the DRG classification scheme. The second section explains how DRGs, as a hospital management tool, were extended to hospital payment schemes. Health care operates in a market unlike that in most industries. Health consumers have limited access to value and quality information and, for the most part, are not the payers for the services they receive. By establishing a rate of payment for a DRG, one may keep production costs closer to the limits that would have been established in an open market.

The third section takes note of the inherent difficulties in identifying the specific products that institutions provide. These difficulties stem from variability in disease definitions and codes. Since variability is inevitable, the task of product identification becomes that of discovering a way to predict the variability. If variability can be predicted, the process can be managed.

The fourth section describes the development of the organ-system approach to DRG classification, upon which the present version is based. The basic structure is divided into three levels: the first level describes organ systems, the second level distinguishes between surgical and medical procedures, and the third level describes a hierarchy of procedures and medical problems and other indicators that differentiate process. The classification of diagnoses into relatively cohesive groups allows for an analysis of differences in resource utilization, both expected and unexpected. The discovery of causes for instability in the process is the essential first step in improving quality of care and enhancing cost effectiveness.

The final section reemphasizes the purpose for which patients are grouped—to allow administrators to manage their hospitals more effectively. DRG-based product-line management and case-mix accounting systems provide managers with a basis for measurement and evaluation of hospital performance.

THE ORIGIN OF DRGs

Utilization Review and Quality Assurance

In 1967 a group of physicians at our local university hospital asked for help with a problem in utilization review. At the time, two years after the advent of the Medicare program, all hospitals were required to operate a program of utilization review and quality assurance as a condition for receiving Medicare funds. The physicians asked whether industrial methods of cost and quality control could be adapted and applied to the hospital industry. Thus began a 20-year process, which continues today, of measuring hospital production as a means of evaluating what takes place in a hospital.

This process centers on measurement and evaluation of activity in an institution as a means of evaluating performance. The ability to evaluate allows managers in industry to do their jobs: to understand the multidimensional relationships between the cost of producing goods and services and the quality of that production. In engineering, measurement is necessary to understanding.

The problem that had to be addressed first was simply how to measure productive activity in a hospital. Hospital production is not the same as production in a factory, where there are clear standards and criteria pertaining to the utilization of materials, labor, and equipment. In manufacturing, design quality, production quality, and performance are continually subject to monitoring, measurement, feedback, and adaptation of the processes of production. The physicians at the local hospital were asking us, in effect, how to begin a process of measurement and evaluation that would serve to improve the processes and would obtain, simultaneously, efficiency and effectiveness in the utilization of resources.

A means of measuring performance allows for the development of a system to understand, to predict, and ultimately to control. *Managerial control* refers to understanding and mastering the process rather than restraining it.

The Need for Product Definition in a Hospital

The idea of applying industrial concepts to hospitals was not new in the 1960s. The idea had been presented throughout the century, but had not met with wide support. As a result, it was rare to find "blueprints" or specifications in hospital departments underlying production of the important services.

In the early 1900s, Eugene Codman, a surgeon at the Massachusetts General Hospital in Boston, attempted to interest hospitals in focusing on patient care processes rather than on support services. In an address to the Philadelphia County Medical Society in 1913, Codman stated:

> It would be supposed that in the annual reports of hospitals some account of their products would be found. To a certain extent this is true, but often much of the material in an annual report is but a mere account of money subscribed and the proportionate amounts which are spent on the different departments....
> Really the whole hospital problem rests on this one question: What happens to the cases?...
> We must formulate some method of hospital report showing as nearly as possible what are the results of the treatment obtained at different institutions. This report must be made out and published by each hospital in a uniform manner, so that comparison will be possible. With such a report as a starting-point, those interested can begin to ask questions as to management and efficiency.[1]

Codman urged hospitals to focus not on hospital services but on the individual cases—the object of the institution. He suggested the formulation of a method comparing the treatment of patients among different institutions so that questions could begin to be asked regarding management and efficiency.

Dr. Codman was not popular among health care professionals. In 1916 he was asked to resign from the Department of Surgery at the Massachusetts General Hospital and from the faculty of the Harvard Medical School. Codman then opened his own hospital to practice what he called his "end result system." Physicians were required to describe in detail the care of their patients (including the mistakes), to record all costs, and to follow up on the patients who left the hospital. He attracted few physicians, but they were all very good.

In the preface to his book on ailments of the shoulder, Dr. Codman included a classification matrix, similar to DRGs, which organized treatments by different parts of the body.[2] In the early 1920s, Codman was unable to carry out his plan. It was extremely difficult to establish a system of control in the absence of a functioning system for measurement.

In 1969, the year of Yale's first serious attempt at patient classification, we also lacked a basic system for interpreting clinical data. A two-year digression was necessary to develop the technology that would allow us to analyze hundreds of thousands of patient records that were available to us.[3] This technology enabled us in the early 1970s to look both statistically and clinically at these records and to discern relatively homogeneous processes of care.

We initially convened a panel of physicians and asked them to describe care processes in terms of their important elements. The result was many thousands of different types of patients.[4] At some level every patient is unique, just as every item produced by a factory is unique. Nevertheless, the issue is to identify the similarities rather than to point out the differences. What needs to be discovered is the glue that holds things together—the underlying structure that enables one to measure and evaluate the activities that take place in a hospital.

The problem is to identify the ordinary, the usual, the routine, and then, applying the techniques of statistical process control, to filter out and examine the aberrant cases in order to understand the causes of the aberrations.

The Cost/Quality Model

Cost and quality issues, from an engineering perspective, are simplified in Figure 1-1 to illustrate the "choices" that must be made in regard to cost and quality. Cost is represented on the vertical axis and quality on the horizontal axis.

Moving to the right signifies an increase in technical excellence. Achieving technical superiority in any process is often understood to mean spending more money—to hire more highly skilled labor and management, or to buy better equipment, stronger materials, and the like. At some point, however, there is a limit to increasing technical excellence through increased spending.

The efficient production frontier illustrated by the "cost" curve in the graph represents the maximum amount of technical superiority available given a range of costs. The curve is a frontier in the sense that there

Figure 1-1: Cost and Quality—The Efficient Production Frontier

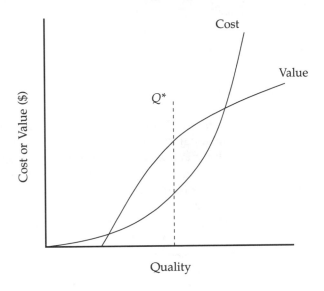

are no points to the right of the curve; only a future breakthrough in technology could drive the curve farther out.

The "cost" curve represents the cost/quality relationship at the frontier. The same quality can always be produced at a higher cost, at a point to the northwest of the curve, and quite often is. The objective of the engineer—the designer of products and processes—in any production process is to get as close as possible to the "frontier." Where on the line to situate one's institution requires a choice, a preference for higher technology, based on different levels of cost and quality. And in increasing quality where should additional resources be invested—in better material, more advanced equipment, or more highly skilled staff?

Part of the general solution to this problem depends on the market for the product—the use people have for the product being sold and therefore the value associated with the product, as illustrated by the "value" curve in Figure 1-1. The product or process designer seeks to establish optimal quality (Q^*), the quality at that point at which value exceeds cost to the greatest degree. As will be discussed later, the health care market is in a sense distorted, in that consumers often do not pay directly for the services nor do they have a means of objectively determining quality among providers. The technical solution to this question is simply to spend more money and increase technical excellence to its limit regardless of benefit. In a world of limited resources, however, such an approach is no longer feasible.

EXTENSION OF DRGs TO REIMBURSEMENT

The Need to Simulate an Open Market

A common misconception about DRGs is that they were created as a payment mechanism for hospital reimbursements. DRGs were created rather to serve as a tool for management in running a hospital. The federal government, seeing the potential of prospective payment schemes in better understanding and restraining soaring health care costs, supported DRG research and utilized the payment scheme for its purposes.

In the late 1960s and early 1970s it was difficult to secure support for a project aimed at defining hospital products. Most people in the hospital business found this notion, at best, uninteresting; the information that was being sought was not what they wanted to know. Since hospitals were reimbursed for whatever their costs might be, there was little incentive to investigate cost and quality trade-offs.

We received funding from the Social Security Administration, which, in 1974 and 1975, was investigating methods of health care cost containment. In the office of the director of research we discussed the ability of case-based payments to achieve the Medicare law's mandate to pay hospitals the cost of producing the required services.

The administration sought the simplest regulatory mechanism that could substitute for the absence of an open market (a market based on cost and quality information) in health care. The notion of a regulatory method to ensure a minimum level of performance stems from the lack of a market establishing value among providers. Health consumers not only do not have the information upon which to assess value and quality but, in most cases, do not pay directly for the services they receive. This lack of information and absence of incentive to minimize costs distorts the market forces that operate more effectively in other industries. DRGs could establish a rate of payment that would discourage hospitals from producing at a higher cost than an open market would tolerate (region A in Figure 1-2).

In order to insure, however, that any cap on revenue would not result in low quality of output, some kind of peer-review mechanism would need to be established with the responsibility of assuring a minimum level of quality. Peer review would identify providers who attempted to produce in region B on the graph, which represents services

Figure 1-2: Rate Setting—Its Effect on the Market

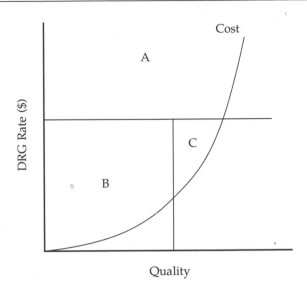

of a lower quality than would be acceptable if information were available. Most providers would actually operate in region C, a condition analogous to that of a marketplace limiting the scope and cost of operations. This is the idea behind DRG-based prospective payment systems.

Defining the Products of a Hospital[5]

The major function of a hospital is to provide the diagnostic and therapeutic services required by physicians in the clinical management of their patients. In doing so, the hospital also makes available certain hotel and social services. Unlike many other kinds of enterprises, a hospital actually consists of two separate, separable production functions illustrated in Figure 1-3.

The first function is to convert raw materials (labor, supplies, equipment) into standard outputs (meals, clean linens, laboratory procedures, medications). These outputs do not constitute the real business of the hospital's care for patients but are really intermediate products. Unfortunately, in the traditional organizational structure of a hospital, the line organization consists of layers of administration that end up managing the various service departments. The implication is that somehow by managing these departments you will end up managing the institution.

Figure 1-3: Defining the Products of a Hospital

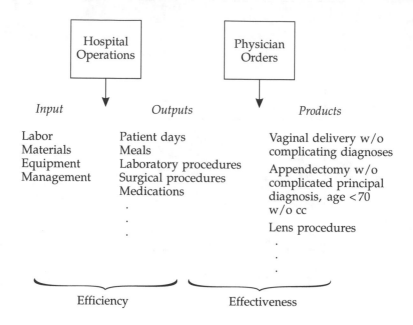

The second function, and the main line business of the institution, is to accept, one at a time, human beings who have a problem, a disease, or a disorder, and to evaluate and treat, through physicians and other professionals, the problem and the patient. Under the direction of these professionals, the institution provides a set of goods and services deemed appropriate to the diagnosis and treatment of the illness. It is this bundle of "things" that we define as the product of the hospital.

The labor, supplies, and equipment used in a hospital are similar to what appears in the bill of materials for a chair or a jet engine in the manufacturing environment—arms, legs, rails, cushions, nails, pegs, screws, and so forth. Although there are obvious differences between a health care institution and a chair factory, T. Levitt has pointed out the importance of the analogy:

> So many things go wrong because companies fail to adequately define what they sell. Companies in so-called service industries generally think of themselves as offering services rather than manufacturing products; hence they fail to think and act as comprehensively as do manufacturing companies concerned with the efficient, low-cost production of customer-satisfying products.[6]

The main problem in managing a hospital is to separate issues of *efficiency* in the production of intermediate products from issues of *effectiveness* in the utilization of these intermediate products. To manage an institution competently, the issues and measures of differential efficiency and differential effectiveness must be clearly separated. It is quite important to produce each lab test efficiently in the sense of utilizing a standard set of inputs for each output. If, however, the test is not used effectively or is ordered inappropriately, it is a waste of resources no matter how efficiently produced. It is our assertion that about 80 to 90 percent of the observable differences in hospital performances are a function of differential effectiveness in utilizing services; the differences have little to do with the relative efficiency with which the intermediate products are produced.

To focus simply on the intermediate products is to miss the point of the enterprise, which is treating patients who have illnesses. The effective utilization of a hospital's resources is primarily a function of its ability to treat specific kinds of illnesses.

In order to evaluate and compare hospital performance and provide relevant feedback on it, it is necessary to identify the specific products that these institutions provide. If classes of patients with the same clinical attributes and similar processes of care are identified, then the framework with which to aggregate patients into case types is established.

MAJOR OBSTACLES

The Effort to Reduce Variability

To make the method work, it is essential to identify the cost of delivering services and to let managers know where they stand with respect to the estimated cost established. It is necessary to define an episode of illness in a manner that permits a reasonably accurate prediction of the goods and services to be delivered. In attempting to do so, we encountered three major obstacles:

— Not all diseases are equally well understood. Some diseases physicians find easy to define; for others, it is difficult even to reach agreement on a label.

— There are fundamental differences in the treatment of diseases that make accounting for the treatment very difficult. Some diseases physicians know very well and there is consensus, at least locally, as to how they ought to be treated. The treatment of many diseases, however, varies among physicians. Significant barriers exist to defining norms in the practice of medicine for a given type of illness.

— There are difficulties in the coding of illnesses, that is, in the descriptive labels used. If we look at ICD-9-CM codes, for example, there are areas, from the point of view of the process of care, that are significantly overidentified (for example, there are 39 different ways to describe a cataract). In other areas (for example, cerebrovascular accidents) one label is used to describe patients receiving a broad spectrum of treatment regimens.

The DRG classification system was developed in spite of these obstacles. It is important to remember that in any system variability is bound to occur. Variability in the utilization of goods and services in treating a given illness is not itself the problem. The problem is to establish a mechanism for predicting the variability. If the variability can be predicted, the process can be managed. The problem of analyzing resource consumption in a hospital therefore centers on discovering the illnesses for which stability in the utilization of resources, at least at the institutional level, can be determined.

Guidelines for Grouping Diagnoses

Stable patterns of resource utilization had to be discovered through the use of standard, commonly collected review data. We therefore chose to use the Uniform Hospital Discharge Data Set.[7] Practical utility was a second requirement of the classification: a given case type had to occur with enough frequency to merit formation of a separate group. In addition to requiring statistical stability of resource utilization within a class, we recognized the need to ensure that patients in a given class constituted a clinically coherent group. Otherwise, physicians would reject the classification.

In sum, the four characteristics that guided us through the first four versions of the DRGs[8] were:

— Class definitions based on information routinely collected on hospital abstracts

— Manageable number of classes

— Similar patterns of resource intensity within a given class

— Similar types of patients in a given class from a clinical perspective

DRGs have been revised in response to changes in disease and procedure coding schemes, new conceptual models of health service utilization, and feedback from the health care community regarding both clinical interpretability and statistical evaluations of resource use.

VERSION 4 OF THE DRG CLASSIFICATION: AN ORGAN-SYSTEMS APPROACH

Developing the DRG Structure

The DRG classification scheme used an organ-systems approach for the first time in the current version. This approach divided the classification process into two major steps. The first step considered the diagnosis. ICD-9-CM codes representing diseases or disorders that could serve as a patient's principal diagnosis (that is, codes representing illnesses that would bring patients to acute care hospitals) were organized by medical specialties or organ-system involvement. This resulted in a set of 23 mutually exclusive and exhaustive categories that were called "major diagnostic categories" (MDCs) (see Table 2-1). The 23 MDCs included about 10,000 individual ICD-9-CM diagnosis codes.

The second step in the process of classification involved identifying from the surgical code books those procedure codes requiring acute care hospital surgical facilities. A patient undergoing such a procedure was classified into one of 22 "surgical MDCs" based on the organ system inferred from the principal diagnosis (one MDC, 20, does not include patients undergoing procedures). Any record of patient care in an acute care hospital, by virtue of its diagnoses and procedural codes, can be placed into one of these 45 classes.

The third step consisted of examining the process of care by considering all variables available in the hospital discharge abstract. This involved taking all the records of patients in a given MDC who had surgery, submitting them to a statistical clustering algorithm to establish common patterns of resource consumption, and handing them over to a group of clinicians who would determine the fundamental clinical organizing principles underlying the results.

The final step was to investigate diagnoses which represent problems that would influence the treatment process other than the fundamental problem that brought the patient to the hospital. This exercise was done with 1979 data, which were less than complete with regard to coding of additional diagnoses. Most of our hypotheses of what ought to make a difference could not be supported in the data. We came up with some clusters of secondary conditions that were important. For the most part, however, we had to rely upon generic identification of secondary problems. When all else failed, we used age. Age is not the best indicator of state of health since there obviously are healthy old people and unhealthy young people, but at the time we were forced to use it. Because of the improvement in coding of patient health, including comorbidities and complications, Medicare has recently dropped age as a variable in DRG classification.

The result of our efforts is a set of product definitions, exemplified by a diagram of the current structure of MDCs in general (Figure 1-4) and a diagram of MDC 5, for the circulatory system, in particular (Figure 1-5). It is important to look at the diagnosis and procedure codes that describe each of these classes because the names alone are not always descriptive.

The first level describes organ systems; the second level distinguishes between surgical and medical procedures; and the third level describes a hierarchy of procedures, a hierarchy of medical problems, and, finally, other indicators that differentiate processes of care.

Identifying Instability in Resource Consumption

This diagnostic and procedural information allows for discovery of some rather significant differences. For example, in a cardiac valve operation with a pump, whether the catheterization is being done in the same episode (DRG 104) or was done previously (DRG 105) makes a difference; it indicates a different kind of patient. Sometimes a generic variable, such as the presence of a significant complication or comorbidity, had to be used to identify a more seriously ill and more expensive patient.

We identified, for each of the 23 MDCs, the diagnostic and procedure codes and classes that were expected to be relatively stable, at least at the institutional level, in their utilization of resources. Of course, this does not mean that every patient follows precisely the same pattern of resource utilization; variability should be expected and accounted for. It is necessary to be able to predict and thus control the consumption of resources as a function of the types and volumes of patients expected to be served. Such process stability is a natural consequence of an understood and managed process.

It is to be expected that for any hospital, the process of care for a given illness will exhibit a stable and predictable pattern. That is, in the sense of statistical process control, the process will be "in control."[9]

Observations that do not belong to the central stable process need to be identified. It is relatively easy to separate these observations from the main mass statistically and then to search for the cause or causes of the instability. Was it an error in treatment, an unexpected response of the patient to therapy, delays in the diagnostic process, an error in recording? Such cases do not fit the pattern and need to be reviewed.

The discovery of causes for instability in the process is the essential first step in improving quality of care while, at the same time, enhancing

Figure 1-4: Structure of DRG Classification within Major Diagnostic Categories*

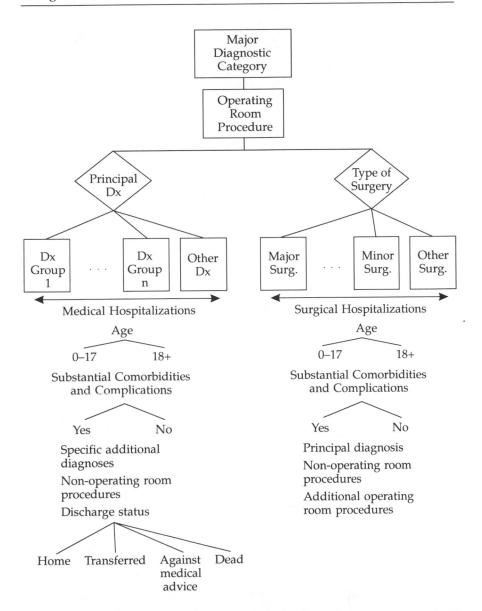

*Structure according to the fourth revision of the DRGs.

Source: Robert B. Fetter, Jean L. Freeman, and Harry L. Savitt, "DRG Refinement with Diagnostic Specific Comorbidities and Complications: A Synthesis of Current Approaches to Patient Classification," final report of cooperative agreements nos. 15-C-98930/1-01 and 17-C-98930/1-0251 between the Health Care Financing Administration (HCFA) and Yale University, January 1989.

Figure 1-5: Major Diagnostic Category 5—Diseases and Disorders of the Circulatory System

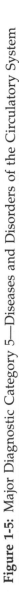

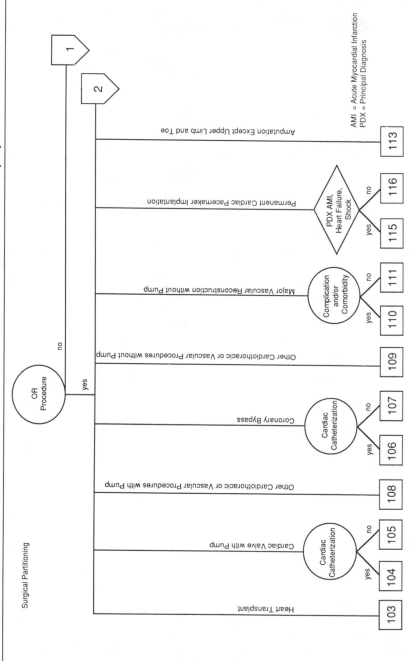

Surgical Partitioning

OR Procedure

no

yes

1

2

Heart Transplant — 103

Cardiac Valve with Pump — Cardiac Catheterization
- yes — 104
- no — 105

Other Cardiothoracic or Vascular Procedures with Pump — 108

Coronary Bypass — Cardiac Catheterization
- yes — 106
- no — 107

Other Cardiothoracic or Vascular Procedures without Pump — 109

Major Vascular Reconstruction without Pump — Complication and/or Comorbidity
- yes — 110
- no — 111

Permanent Cardiac Pacemaker Implantation — PDX AMI, Heart Failure, Shock
- yes — 115
- no — 116

Amputation Except Upper Limb and Toe — 113

AMI = Acute Myocardial Infarction
PDX = Principal Diagnosis

Continued

Surgical Partitioning (cont')

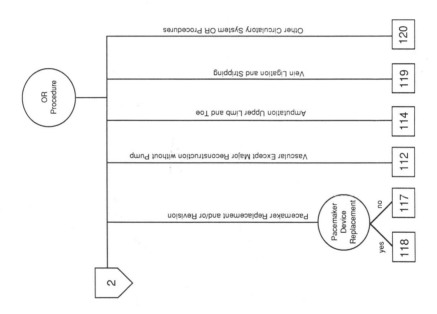

Figure 1-5: Continued

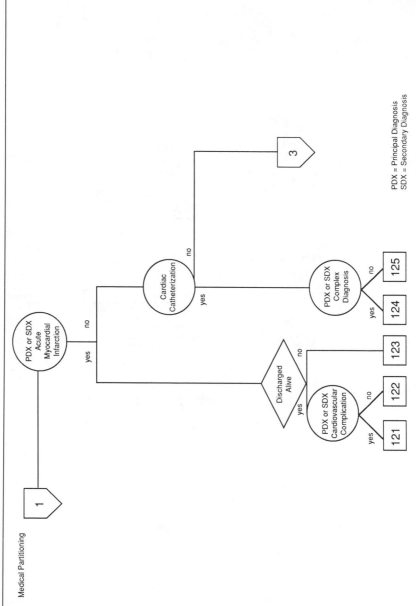

Medical Partitioning

PDX = Principal Diagnosis
SDX = Secondary Diagnosis

Background   *19*

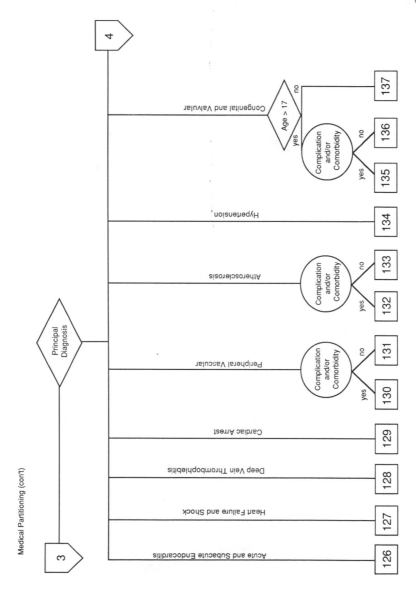

Medical Partitioning (cont')

Continued

Figure 1-5: Continued

Medical Partitioning (con't)

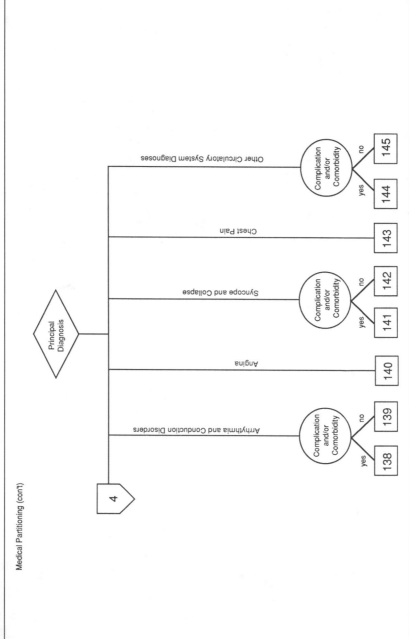

Source: *DRG Definitions Manual*, Fourth Revision (New Haven, CT: Health Systems International, 1987).

its cost effectiveness. The purpose of the system is to facilitate the separation of the expected from the unexpected and to discover the causes of that unexpected instability in the statistical pattern. Even if a stable, well-defined process exists at an institution, all patients will not necessarily fall into that one clearly defined distribution.

The concept of the payment system is to pay one price for the "normal" cases and to pay a different price for the remainder or "outlier" cases. That is a persistent problem with the Medicare system since its method of outlier identification is based upon budgetary limits. As a result, many cases that are not normal are being paid for as if they were, especially in more technically sophisticated institutions.

The basic idea of management by DRG is to represent resource consumption by identifiable, relatively homogeneous processes at the institutional level in order to separate cases judged relatively effective in terms of resource utilization from cases that, for one reason or another, are perceived as having been treated less effectively. The latter need to be reviewed and the treatment judged appropriate or inappropriate on the merits of the individual case. This type of review is possible only when a certain level of precision in identifying different processes is reached.

MANAGEMENT BY DRG

The purpose of grouping patients was to allow managers to run their institutions more effectively by establishing a "product" as a basis for measurement and evaluation. The advent of the Prospective Payment System assisted this effort by making DRG data readily available to administrators. DRGs have created a profound change in the management style of hospitals, encouraging administrators to view the use and cost of hospital services along product lines based on individual DRGs or groups of clinically similar DRGs.

DRGs allow cost and resource information to be collected at many levels. The use and purpose of DRG analysis will vary among hospitals according to their individual needs. Implementing the product-line approach requires a new organizational structure for the hospitals' medical and administrative staffs.

A clinical matrix structure captures the concept of product-line management in operational terms; department heads oversee the conversion of inputs for a given product line while the physicians manage the bundling of these intermediate outputs. A matrix can be developed to assign responsibility and accountability to those responsible for providing patient care, with management being responsible for the efficient delivery of intermediate products and physicians being responsible for their effective utilization.

In defining a product, DRGs facilitate the use of product-based (case-based) cost-accounting systems analogous to those used in industry to measure resource costs and utilization. Costs can be compared across DRGs, intermediate services, DRG clusters, time periods, and institutions. Variance analysis reveals the sources of the cost differences resulting from changes in:

— Factor prices (labor, material)

— Volume (number of patients treated)

— Case mix (types of patients treated)

— Efficiency (use of input factors)

— Treatment effectiveness (variations in physician practice)

Reports can also be designed that allow hospital managers to examine variations between budgeted and actual costs from year to year. DRG analysis can be extended to other areas of hospital production: product selection and design, process selection, facility location, and quality control.

The analysis addresses simultaneously the administrative concerns of department managers and the clinical concerns of the providers. This combination should allow for a constructive dialogue between management and clinician.

Monitoring and accountability by product lines is critical in light of DRG-based hospital payment. Under this system, it is clearly important, for the financial viability of the hospital, to have accurate information pertaining to the costs of treating different types of cases. As administrators and physicians become more familiar with DRGs and DRG applications in hospital management, the benefits of DRGs, both for containing costs and for increasing quality, can be realized.

REFERENCES

1. E. A. Codman, "The Product of a Hospital," *Surgery, Gynecology, and Obstetrics* 18 (1914): 491–96.
2. E. A. Codman, preface to *The Shoulder* (Boston: T. Todd Company, 1934).
3. R. E. Mills, R. B. Fetter, D. C. Riedel, and R. Averill, "AUTOGRP, An Interactive Computer System for the Analysis of Health Care Data," *Medical Care* 14, no. 7 (1976): 603–15.
4. R. B. Fetter, "Financing Health Care: Discussion," *The Recognition of Systems in Health Services*, Operations Research Society of America Health Applications Section (1969): 209–21.

5. R. B. Fetter and J. L. Freeman, "Diagnosis Related Groups: Product Line Management Within Hospitals," *Academy of Management Review* 11, no. 1 (1986): 41–54.
6. T. Levitt, "Product Line Approach to Services," *Harvard Business Review* (September–October 1972): 41–52.
7. National Center for Health Statistics, *Uniform Hospital Discharge Data Set: Minimum Data Set*, report of the National Committee on Vital and Health Statistics, Department of Health, Education, and Welfare publication no. (PHS) 80-1157, U.S. Public Health Service (Washington, D.C.: U.S. Government Printing Office, April 1980).
8. A fifth version of the DRGs that introduces a more refined accounting for severity of illness has been developed. See Chapter 3.
9. H. Gitlow, S. Gitlow, R. Oppenheim, and A. Oppenheim. *Tools and Methods for the Improvement of Quality.* (Homewood, IL: Richard D. Irwin, Inc., 1989).

SELECTED BIBLIOGRAPHY

Averill, R. F., and Kalison, M. J. "Are National DRG Rates the Best Choice for PPS?" *Healthcare Financial Management* 39, no. 8 (August 1985): 62–66.
———. "The Challenge of 'Real' Competition in Medicare." *Health Affairs* 5, no. 3 (1986): 47–57.
———. "The Next Step: Introducing Competitive Pricing into PPS." *Healthcare Financial Management* 40, no. 8 (August 1986): 58–62.
———. "Part 2, Responding to PPS: Development and Interpretation of the Diagnosis Related Groups (DRGs)." *Healthcare Financial Management* 38, no. 2 (1984): 72–84.
———. "A Positive First Step: Prospective Payment by DRG." *Healthcare Financial Management* 37, no. 2 (1983): 12–22.
———. "Present and Future: Predictions for the Healthcare Industry." *Healthcare Financial Management* 40, no. 3 (March 1986): 50–54.
Averill, R. F.; Kalison, M. J.; Sparrow, D. A.; and Owens, T. R. "How Hospital Managers Should Respond to PPS." *Healthcare Financial Management* 38, no. 3 (1984): 72–86.
Catterall, J.; Fetter, R. B.; and Scott, T. "Doing It with DRGs." *The Health Service Journal* (September 1988): 1089–91.
Fetter, R. B. "Cost Models and DRGs: An International Comparison." *Australian Health* 8, no. 2 (1985): 116–25.
———. *Development of an Ambulatory Patient Classification System.* Final report, Health Care Financing Administration grant nos. 18-P-98361/1-01 and 18-C-98361/1-02. New Haven, CT: Health Systems Management Group, School of Organization and Management, Yale University, December 1987.
———. *Development, Testing and Evaluation of a Prospective, Case-Payment Reimbursement System.* Final report, Social Security Administration, Health Care Financing Administration contract no. 600-75-0180. New Haven, CT: Health Systems Management Group, School of Organization and Management, Yale University, January 1981.
———. *Diagnosis Related Groups (DRGs) and Nursing Resources.* Final report, Health Care Financing Administration grant no. 15-C-98500/1-01-02. New Haven, CT: Health Systems Management Group, School of Organization and Management, Yale University, November 1987.

————. "Diagnosis Related Groups: The Product of the Hospital." *Clinical Research* 32, no. 3 (1984): 336–40.

————. "DRGs—Fact and Fiction." *Australian Health Review* 8, no. 2 (1985): 104–15.

————. "DRGs in Europe and Australia." *Business and Health* 3, no. 5 (1986): 58–59.

————. "Els DRGs i la Seva Experiencia en el mon." *Annals De Medicina* 74, no. 6 (1988): 30–34.

————. "Les DRGs, le PMSI, et l'expérience DRG dans le monde." *Journal d'économie médicale* 4, no. 5 (1986): 265–73.

————. *The New ICD-9-CM Diagnosis Related Groups Classification Scheme.* Health Care Financing Administration (HCFA) grants and contracts report; HCFA publication no. 03167. Washington, D.C.: Health Care Financing Administration, U.S. Department of Health and Human Services, September 1984.

————. *Resource Utilization Groups: Validation and Refinement of a Case Mix System for Long Term Care Reimbursement.* Final report, Health Care Financing Administration grant no. 18-C-98499/1-01. New Haven, CT: Health Systems Management Group, School of Organization and Management, Yale University, December 1986.

Fetter, R.B.; Averill, R. F.; Lichtenstein, J. L.; and Freeman, J. L. "Ambulatory Visit Groups: A Framework for Measuring Productivity in Ambulatory Care." *Health Services Research* 19, no. 4 (1984): 415–37.

Fetter, R. B., and Freeman, J. L. "A Product Oriented Approach to Productivity Improvements in Health Care." Chapter 11 (149–73) of *Health Care: An International Perspective,* ed. John M. Virgo. Edwardsville, IL: International Economics and Management Institute, 1984.

————. "Diagnosis Related Groups: Product Line Management within Hospitals." *Academy of Management Review* 11, no. 1 (1986): 41–54.

Fetter, R. B.; Freeman, J. L.; and Mullin, R. "DRGs: How They Evolved and Are Changing the Way Hospitals Are Managed." *Pathologist* 39, no. 6 (1985): 17–21.

Fetter, R. B.; Riedel, D. C.; and Thompson, J. D. "The Application of Diagnostic Specific Cost Profiles to Cost and Reimbursement Control in Hospitals." *Journal of Medical Systems* 1, no. 2 (1977): 137–49.

Fetter, R. B.; Shin, Y.; Freeman, J. L.; Averill, R. F.; and Thompson, J. D. "Case Mix Definition by Diagnostic Related Groups." *Medical Care* 18, no. 2, Supplement (1980): 1–53.

Fetter, R. B.; Thompson, J. D.; and Mills, R. E. "A System for Cost and Reimbursement Control in Hospitals." *Yale Journal of Biology and Medicine* 49 (1976): 123–36.

Freeman, J. L.; Fetter, R. B.; Newbold, R. C.; and Rodrigues, J. M. "Hospital Utilization before and after the Implementation of DRGs for Hospital Payment: United States, 1979–1984." *Journal of Management in Medicine* 1, no. 4 (1987): 309–23.

Freeman, J. L.; Fetter, R. B.; Newbold, R. C.; Rodrigues, J. M.; and Gautier, D. "Development and Adaptation of a Hospital Cost and Budgeting Model for Cross-National Use." *Journal of Management in Medicine* 1, no. 1 (1986): 38–57.

Freeman, J. L., and McMahon, L. F. "Diagnosis Related Groups: A Fundamental Change in Health Care Financing—Part 2: How Patients are Classified." *PA Drug Update* 4, no. 6 (1984): 17–20.

Hughes, J. S.; Lichtenstein, J.; Magno, L.; and Fetter, R. B. "Improving DRGs: Use of Procedure Codes for Assisted Respiration to Adjust for Complexity of Illness." *Medical Care,* forthcoming.

Kalison, M. J., and Averill, R.F. "Building Capital into Prospective Payment." *Business and Health* (June 1985): 34–37.

———. "Part 1, Defining the Hospital Product—The Response to PPS: Inside, Outside, Over Time." *Healthcare Financial Management* 38, no. 1 (1984): 78–88.

———. "Part 5, Responding to PPS—Responding Over Time: Regulation vs. Contract." *Healthcare Financial Management* 38, no. 5 (1984): 104–12.

———. "Regulation vs. Contract: The Future of Capital under PPS." *Healthcare Financial Management* monograph series, 1984.

Kalison, M. J.; Averill, R. F.; and Webb, R. J. "Part 4, Responding to PPS—The Outside Response." *Healthcare Financial Management* 38, no. 4 (1984): 92–100.

McMahon, L. F. "The Development of Diagnosis Related Groups." In *DRGS and Health Care: The Management of Case Mix.* London: King Edward's Hospital Fund for London, 1987.

———. "Diagnosis Related Group Hospital Reimbursement: A Fundamental Change in Third Party Payment—Part 3: Rules and Regulations." *PA Drug Update* 4, no. 6 (1984): 40–42.

———. "Diagnosis Related Group Hospital Reimbursement: A Fundamental Change in Third Party Payment—Part 4: Impact on Physician Assistants." *PA Drug Update* 4, no. 7 (1984): 45–46.

———. "Diagnosis Related Group Hospital Reimbursement: A Fundamental Change in Third Party Payment—Part 5: Impact on Prospective Payment, the Future." *PA Drug Update* 4, no. 8 (1984): 31–33.

———. "Diagnosis-Related Group Prospective Payment Effects on Medical Quality Assurance." *Evaluation and the Health Professions* 7, no. 1 (1984): 25–41.

———. "Diagnosis Related Groups: A Fundamental Change in Health Care Financing—Part 1: The Birth of DRGs." *PA Drug Update* 4, no. 5 (1984): 38–40.

———. "Diagnosis Related Groups, Part 1: How the New System Works." *Hospital Therapy* 10, no. 1 (1985): 45–52.

———. "Diagnosis Related Groups, Part 2: Impact on Hospitals." *Hospital Therapy* 10, no. 2 (1985): 62–64.

———. "Diagnostic Related Groups—Past and Future." *Infection Control* 9, no. 10 (1988): 471–74.

———. "Physicians and the Hospital: An Expanded Managerial Role Expected with Diagnosis Related Group Based Hospital Reimbursement." *Connecticut Medicine* 48, no. 3 (1984): 167–70.

McMahon, L.F.; Fetter, R. B.; Freeman, J. L.; and Thompson, J. D. "Hospital Matrix Management and Diagnosis Related Group Based Prospective Payment." *Hospital and Health Services Administration* 31, no. 1 (January–February 1986): 62–74.

McMahon, L. F., and Billi, J. E. "The Measurement of Severity of Illness and the Medicare Prospective Payment System: State of the Art and Future Directions." *Journal of General Internal Medicine* 3, no. 5 (1988): 482–90.

McMahon, L. F., and Newbold, R. C. "Variation in Resource Use within Diagnosis Related Groups: The Effect of Severity of Illness and Physician Practice." *Medical Care* 24, no. 5 (1986): 388–97.

McMahon, L. F.; Shapiro, L. R.; Weissfeld, L. A.; and Billi, J. E. "Prior Hospitalization Characteristics of DRG Outlier versus Inlier Patients." *Medical Care* 26, no. 4 (1988): 423–29.

McMahon, L. F., and Smits, H. L. "Can the Medicare Prospective Payment System Survive the ICD-9-CM Disease Classification System: A Challenge to Physicians." *Annals of Internal Medicine* 104, no. 4 (1986): 562–66.

Mills, R. E.; Fetter, R. B.; Riedel, D. C.; and Averill, R. F. "AUTOGRP: An Interactive Computer System for the Analysis of Health Care Data." *Medical Care* 14, no. 7 (1976): 603–15.

Murtaugh, C. M.; Cooney, L. M.; DerSimonian, R. R.; Smits, H. L.; and Fetter, R. B. "Nursing Home Reimbursement and the Allocation of Rehabilitation Therapy Resources." *Health Services Research* 23, no. 4 (1988): 468–93.

Owens, R., and Averill, R. F. "The Role of Utilization Management Under PPS." *Healthcare Financial Management* 38, no. 10 (1984): 60–62, 64, 66.

Palmer, G., and Freeman, J. L. "Comparisons of Hospital Bed Utilization in Australia and the United States Using DRGs." *Quality Review Bulletin* 13 (1987): 256–61.

Ryan, J. F.; Fetter, R. B.; and Smits, H. L. "Case Mix of Public Patients in Skilled Nursing Facilities in Connecticut." *Medical Care* 25, no. 1 (1987): 46–51.

Schneider, K. C.; Lichtenstein, J.; Fetter, R. B.; Freeman, J. L.; and Newbold, R. *The New ICD-9-CM Ambulatory Visit Groups Classification Scheme—Definitions Manual*. New Haven, CT: Health Systems Management Group, School of Organization and Management, Yale University, July 1986.

Schneider, K. C.; Lichtenstein, J. L.; Freeman, J. L.; Newbold, R. C.; Fetter, R. B.; Gottlieb, L.; Leaf, P. J.; and Portlock, C. S. "Ambulatory Visit Groups: An Outpatient Classification System." *Journal of Ambulatory Care Management* 11, no. 3 (1988): 1–12.

Smits, H. L.; Fetter, R. B.; and McMahon, L. F. "Variation in Resource Use within DRGs: The Severity Issue." *Health Care Financing Review* annual supplement (November 1984): 71–77.

Sparrow, D. A., and Averill, R. F. "Provision 223: TEFRA's Two-Part Strategy Will Reduce Medicare's Financial Liability to Hospitals." *Healthcare Financial Management* 37, no. 4 (1983): 72–84.

Thompson, J. D. "DRG Prepayment: Its Purpose and Performance." *Bulletin of the New York Academy of Medicine* 64, no. 1 (1988): 25–51.

———. "DRGs and the Length of Stay in the Acute Hospital." *Aging Population: Changing Practice* (May and June 1986): 125–33.

———. "DRGs Broaden Hospitals' Accountability, Responsibility." *Hospital Progress* 62, no. 8 (1981): 46–49.

———. "The Measurement of Nursing Intensity." *Health Care Financing Review* annual supplement (November 1984): 47–55.

———. "One Application of the Diagnosis Related Group Planning Model." In *Topics in Health Care Financing*, 51–65. Rockville, MD: Aspen Systems Publications, 1982.

———. "Prediction of Nurse Resource Use in Treatment of Diagnosis Related Groups." In *Nursing Information Systems*, ed. H. A. Werley and M. R. Grier, 60–78. New York: Springer Publishing Company, 1981.

———. "Prospective Payment and the Volume of Hospital Care." *Health Matrix: The Quarterly Journal of Health Services Management* 3, no. 4 (1985–86): 31–36.

———. "With Cat-Like Tread, the DRGs Are Coming." *Journal of Management in Medicine* 2, no. 3 (1987–88): 193–207.

Thompson, J.D.; Averill, R. F.; and Fetter, R. B. "Planning, Budgeting, and Controlling—One Look at the Future: Case Mix Cost Accounting." *Health Services Research* 14, no. 2 (1979): 111–25.

Thompson, J. D., and Diers, D. "DRGs and Nursing Intensity." *Nursing and Health Care* (October 1985): 435–39.

———. "Management of Nursing Intensity." *Nursing Clinics of North America* 23, no. 3 (1988): 473–92.

Thompson, J. D.; Fetter, R. B.; and Mross, C. D. "Case Mix and Resource Use." *Inquiry* 12, no. 4 (1975): 300–312.

Thompson, J. D.; Fetter, R. B.; and Shin, Y. "One Strategy for Controlling Costs in University Teaching Hospitals." *Journal of Medical Education* 53 (1978): 167–75.

Thompson, J. D., and Grazier, K. L. "Incorporating DRGs into Medical and Management Education." *Journal of Health Administration Education* 2, no. 3 (1984): 261–69.

2

Development

Richard F. Averill

The evolution of the DRGs and their use as the basic unit of payment in a hospital reimbursement system represent a recognition of the fundamental role that a hospital's case mix plays in determining its costs. In the past, such hospital characteristics as teaching status and bed size have been used to attempt to explain substantial cost differences among hospitals. However, these characteristics failed to account adequately for the cost impact of a hospital's case mix. Individual hospitals have often attempted to justify higher cost by contending that they treated a more "complex" mix of patients, the usual contention being that the patients treated were "sicker." Although there has been a consensus in the hospital industry that a more complex case mix results in higher costs, the concept of case-mix complexity has historically lacked a precise definition. The development of the DRGs provided the first operational means of defining and measuring a hospital's case-mix complexity.

CASE-MIX COMPLEXITY

The concept of case-mix complexity initially appears very straightforward. However, clinicians, administrators, and regulators often attach different meanings to the concept depending on their backgrounds and purposes. The term *case-mix complexity* refers to a set of interrelated but

Adapted from *Diagnosis-Related Groups: Definitions Manual*, Fourth Revision (New Haven, CT: Health Systems International, 1987), with permission.

This chapter describes the work of "The New ICD-9-CM Diagnosis Related Groups Classification Scheme," Health Care Financing Administration (HCFA) grants and contracts report, contracts nos. 95P 97499/1-01 and 95P 97499/1-02, between the Health Care Financing Administration and Yale University: Robert B. Fetter, principal investigator; Gail Lasdon, Julian Pettengill, and James Vertrees, project officers; HCFA publication no. 03167. Washington, D.C.: U.S. Department of Health and Human Services, September 1984.

distinct patient attributes, including severity of illness, prognosis, treatment difficulty, need for intervention, and resource intensity. Each of these concepts has a very precise meaning that describes a particular aspect of a hospital's case mix.

— *Severity of illness* refers to the relative levels of loss of function and mortality that may be experienced by patients with a particular disease.

— *Prognosis* refers to the probable outcome of an illness, including the likelihood of improvement or deterioration in the severity of the illness, the likelihood for recurrence, and the probable life span.

— *Treatment difficulty* refers to the patient management problems that a particular illness presents to the health care provider. Such management problems are associated with illnesses without a clear pattern of symptoms, illnesses requiring sophisticated and technically difficult procedures, and illnesses requiring close monitoring and supervision.

— *Need for intervention* relates to the severity of illness that lack of immediate or continuing care would produce.

— *Resource intensity* refers to the relative volume and types of diagnostic, therapeutic, and bed services used in the management of a particular illness.

When clinicians use the notion of case-mix complexity, they mean that the patients treated have a greater severity of illness, present greater treatment difficulty, have poorer prognoses, and have a greater need for intervention. Thus, from a clinical perspective, case-mix complexity refers to the condition of the patients treated and the treatment difficulty associated with providing care. On the other hand, administrators and regulators usually use the concept of case-mix complexity to indicate that the patients treated require more resources and therefore more costly care. Thus, from an administrative or regulatory perspective, case-mix complexity refers to the resource intensity demands that patients place on an institution. While the two interpretations of case-mix complexity are often closely related, they can be very different for certain kinds of patients. For example, while terminal cancer patients are severely ill and have a poor prognosis, they require few hospital resources beyond basic nursing care.

In the past, there has been some confusion regarding the use and interpretation of the DRGs because the aspect of case-mix complexity measured by the DRGs has not been clearly understood. The purpose of the DRGs is to relate a hospital's case mix to the resource demands and associated costs experienced by the hospital. Therefore, a hospital's having a more complex case mix from a DRG perspective means that the hospital treats patients who require more hospital resources but not necessarily that the hospital treats patients having a greater severity of illness, a greater treatment difficulty, a poorer prognosis, or a greater need for intervention.

PATIENT CLASSIFICATION

Given that the purpose of the DRGs is to relate a hospital's case mix to its resource intensity, it was necessary to develop an operational means of determining the types of patients treated and relating each patient type to the resources they consumed. While each patient is unique, groups of patients have demographic, diagnostic, and therapeutic attributes in common that determine their level of resource intensity. By developing clinically similar groups of patients with similar resource intensity, patients can be aggregated into meaningful patient classes. Moreover, if these patient classes covered the entire range of patients seen in an inpatient setting, then collectively they would constitute a patient classification scheme that would provide a means of establishing and measuring hospital case-mix complexity. The DRGs were developed as a patient classification scheme consisting of classes of patients who were similar clinically and in their consumption of hospital resources.

During the process of developing the DRG patient classification scheme, several alternative approaches to constructing the patient classes were investigated. Initially, a normative approach was used in which clinicians defined the DRGs using the patient characteristics that they felt were important for determining resource intensity. Their definitions tended to include an extensive set of specifications, requiring information that might not always be collected through a hospital's medical information system. If the entire range of patients were classified in this manner, the classification would ultimately lead to thousands of DRGs, most of which described patients seen infrequently in a typical hospital. It became evident, therefore, that DRG definition would be facilitated if data from acute care hospitals could be examined to determine the general characteristics and relative frequency of different patient types. In addition, statistical algorithms applied to these data would be useful to suggest ways of forming DRGs that were similar in resource intensity. However, it was also discovered that statistical algorithms applied to historical data in the absence of clinical input would not yield a satisfactory set of DRGs. The DRGs resulting from such a statistical approach, while similar in resource intensity, would often contain patients with a diverse set of characteristics that could not be interpreted from a clinical perspective.

The development of the DRG patient classification scheme thus required that physician judgment, statistical analysis, and verification with historical data be merged into a single process. It was necessary to be able not only to examine large amounts of historical data with statistical algorithms available for suggesting alternative ways of forming DRGs but also to do so in such a way that physicians could review the results at each step to insure that the DRGs formed were clinically coherent.

Basic Characteristics of the DRG Patient Classification Scheme

Given the limitations of previous patient classification schemes and the experience of attempting to develop DRGs with physician panels and statistical analysis, it was concluded that in order for the DRG patient classification scheme to be practical and meaningful it should have the following characteristics:

1. The patient characteristics used in the definition of the DRGs should be limited to information routinely collected on hospital abstract systems.
2. There should be a manageable number of DRGs that encompass all patients seen on an inpatient basis.
3. Each DRG should contain patients with a similar pattern of resource intensity.
4. Each DRG should contain patients who are similar from a clinical perspective (in other words, each class should be clinically coherent).

1. *Patient characteristics.* Restricting the patient characteristics used in the definition of the DRGs to those readily available insured that the DRGs could be extensively applied. Currently, the patient information routinely collected includes age, sex, principal diagnosis, secondary diagnoses, and the surgical procedures performed. Creating DRGs based on information that is collected in only a few settings or on information that is difficult to collect or measure would have resulted in a patient classification scheme that could not be applied uniformly across hospitals. That is not to say that information beyond that currently collected might not be useful for defining the DRGs. As additional information becomes routinely available it must be evaluated to determine if it might result in improvements in the ability to classify patients.

2. *Number of DRGs.* Limiting the number of DRGs to manageable numbers (that is, hundreds of patient classes rather than thousands) insures that, for most of the DRGs, a typical hospital will have enough experience

to allow meaningful comparative analysis to be performed. If there were only a few patients in each DRG, it would be difficult to detect patterns in case-mix complexity and cost performance and to communicate the results to the physician staff.

3. *Resource intensity.* The resource intensity of the patients in each DRG must be similar in order to establish a relationship between the case mix of a hospital and the resources it consumes. Similar resource intensity means that the resources used are relatively consistent across the patients in each DRG. However, some variation in resource intensity will remain among the patients in each DRG. In other words, the definition of the DRG will not be so specific that every patient is identical, but the level of variation will be known and predictable. Thus, while the precise resource intensity of a particular patient cannot be predicted by knowing to which DRG the patient belongs, the average pattern of resource intensity of a group of patients in a DRG can be accurately predicted.

4. *Clinical coherence.* Since one of the major applications of the DRGs is in communicating with the physician community, the patients in each DRG must be similar from a clinical perspective. In other words, the definition of each DRG must be clinically coherent. The concept of clinical coherence requires that the patient characteristics included in the definition of each DRG relate to a common organ system or etiology and that, typically, a specific medical specialty should provide care to the patients in the DRG. For example, patients who are admitted for a dilatation and curettage or a tonsillectomy happen to be similar in terms of most measures of resource intensity, such as length of stay, preoperative stay, operating room time, and use of ancillary services. However, different organ systems and different medical specialties are involved. Thus, the requirement that the DRGs be clinically coherent precludes the possibility of these types of patients being in the same DRG.

A common organ system or etiology and a common clinical specialty are necessary but not sufficient conditions for a DRG to be clinically coherent. In addition, all available patient characteristics that medically would be expected to consistently affect resource intensity should be included in the definition of the DRG. Furthermore, a DRG should not be based on patient characteristics that medically would not be expected to consistently affect resource intensity. For example, patients with appendicitis may or may not have peritonitis. Although these patients are the same from an organ-system, etiology, and medical-specialist perspective, the DRG definitions must form separate patient classes, since peritonitis would increase the resource intensity of appendicitis patients.

The definition of clinical coherence is, of course, dependent on the purpose of the formation of the DRG classification. For the DRGs, the definition of clinical coherence relates to the medical rationale for differences in resource intensity. If, on the other hand, the purpose of the DRGs related to mortality, the patient characteristics that were clinically coherent and, therefore, included in the DRG definitions might be different. Finally, it should be noted that the requirement that the DRGs be clinically coherent caused more patient classes to be formed than would be necessary for explaining resource intensity alone.

Formation of the DRGs

The process of forming the DRGs was begun by dividing all possible principal diagnoses into 23 mutually exclusive principal diagnosis areas, referred to as "major diagnostic categories" (MDCs) (Table 2-1).

Table 2-1: Major Diagnostic Categories

1. Diseases and disorders of the nervous system
2. Diseases and disorders of the eye
3. Diseases and disorders of the ear, nose, and throat
4. Diseases and disorders of the respiratory system
5. Diseases and disorders of the circulatory system
6. Diseases and disorders of the digestive system
7. Diseases and disorders of the hepatobiliiary system and pancreas
8. Diseases and disorders of the musculoskeletal system and connective tissue
9. Diseases and disorders of the skin, subcutaneous tissue, and breast
10. Endocrine, nutritional, and metabolic diseases and disorders
11. Diseases and disorders of the kidney and urinary tract
12. Diseases and disorders of the male reproductive system
13. Diseases and disorders of the female reproductive system
14. Pregnancy, childbirth, and the puerperium
15. Newborns and other neonates with conditions originating in the perinatal period
16. Diseases and disorders of blood and blood forming organs and immunological disorders
17. Myeloproliferative diseases and disorders, and poorly differentiated neoplasms
18. Infectious and parasitic diseases (systemic or unspecified sites)
19. Mental diseases and disorders
20. Alcohol/drug use and alcohol/drug-induced organic mental disorders
21. Injuries, poisonings, and toxic effects of drugs
22. Burns
23. Factors influencing health status and other contacts with health services

Source: Robert B. Fetter, "The New ICD-9-CM Diagnosis-Related Groups Classification Scheme."

The MDCs were formed by physician panels as the first step toward insuring that the DRGs would be clinically coherent. The diagnoses in each MDC correspond to a single organ system or etiology and in general are associated with a particular medical specialty. Thus, in order to maintain the requirement of clinical coherence, no final DRG could contain patients in different MDCs. In general, each MDC was constructed to correspond to a major organ system (for example, respiratory system, circulatory system, digestive system) rather than etiology (such as malignancies or infectious diseases). This approach was used since clinical care is generally organized in accordance with the organ system affected, and not the etiology. Thus, diseases involving both a particular organ system and a particular etiology (for example, malignant neoplasm of the kidney) were assigned to the MDC corresponding to the organ system involved. However, not all diseases or disorders could be assigned to an organ-system-based MDC and a number of residual MDCs were created (such as systemic infectious diseases, myeloproliferative diseases, and poorly differentiated neoplasms). For example, the infectious diseases food poisoning and *Shigella dysenteriae* infection are assigned to the digestive system MDC, and pulmonary tuberculosis is assigned to the respiratory system MDC. On the other hand, infectious diseases that usually involve the entire body, such as miliary tuberculosis and septicemia, are assigned to the systemic infectious disease MDC.

Once the MDCs were defined, each MDC was evaluated to identify those additional patient characteristics that would have a consistent effect on the consumption of hospital resources. Since the presence of a surgical procedure that required the use of the operating room would have a significant effect on the type of hospital resources (for example, operating room, recovery room, anesthesia) used by a patient, most MDCs were initially divided into medical and surgical groups. The medical-surgical distinction is also useful in further defining the clinical specialty involved.

Patients were considered surgical if they had a procedure performed that would require the use of the operating room. Since the patient data generally available do not precisely indicate whether a patient was taken to the operating room, surgical patients were identified on the basis of the procedures that were performed. Physician panels classified every possible procedure code according to whether the procedure would in most hospitals be performed in the operating room. Thus, closed-heart valvotomies, cerebral meninges biopsies, and total cholecystectomies would be expected to require the operating room while thoracentesis, bronchoscopy, and skin sutures would not. If a patient had any procedure that was expected to require the operating room, that patient would be classified as surgical. Once each MDC was divided into medical and surgical categories, then, in general, the surgical patients were further defined according to the precise surgical procedure performed while the medical patients were further defined according to the precise principal diagnosis for which they were admitted to the hospital. The general structure of a typical MDC is shown by the tree diagram in Figure 2-1. In general, specific groups of surgical procedures were defined to distinguish surgical patients by the extent of the surgical procedure performed. For example, the procedure classes defined for the endocrine, nutritional, and metabolic MDC are amputations, adrenal and pituitary procedures, skin grafts and wound debridements, procedures for obesity, parathyroid procedures, thyroid procedures, thyroglossal procedures, and other procedures relating to endocrine, nutritional, or metabolic diseases.

Since patients can have multiple procedures related to their principal diagnosis during a particular hospital stay, and patients may not be assigned to more than one surgical class, the surgical classes in each MDC were defined in a hierarchical order. Patients with multiple procedures would be assigned to the surgical class highest in the hierarchy. For example, if a patient received both a dilatation and curettage and a hysterectomy, the patient would be assigned to the hysterectomy surgical class (Table 2-2). It should be noted that as a result of the surgical hierarchy the ordering of the surgical procedures on the patient abstract has no influence on the assignment of the surgical class and DRG.

In general, specific groups of principal diagnoses were defined for medical patients. Usually the medical classes in each MDC would include a class for neoplasms, symptoms, and specific conditions relating to the organ system involved. For example, the medical classes for the respiratory system MDC are pulmonary embolism, infections, neoplasms, chest trauma, pleural effusion, pulmonary edema and respiratory failure, chronic obstructive pulmonary disease, simple pneumonia, interstitial lung disease, pneumothorax, bronchitis and asthma, respiratory symptoms, and other respiratory diagnoses.

In each MDC there are usually two classes, one medical and one surgical, referred to as "other medical diseases" and "other surgical procedures" respectively. These "other" classes include diagnoses or procedures that are infrequently encountered or not well defined clinically. For example, the "other" medical class for the respiratory system MDC contains the diagnoses "psychogenic respiratory disease" and "respiratory anomalies not otherwise specified," while the "other" surgical class for the female reproductive MDC contains the surgical procedures "liver biopsy" and "exploratory laparotomy." The "other" surgical category contains surgical procedures that, while infrequent, could still reasonably be expected to be performed for a patient in the particular MDC. There are, however, also patients who receive surgical procedures that are completely unrelated to the MDC to which the patient was assigned. An

Figure 2-1: Typical DRG Structure for a Major Diagnostic Category

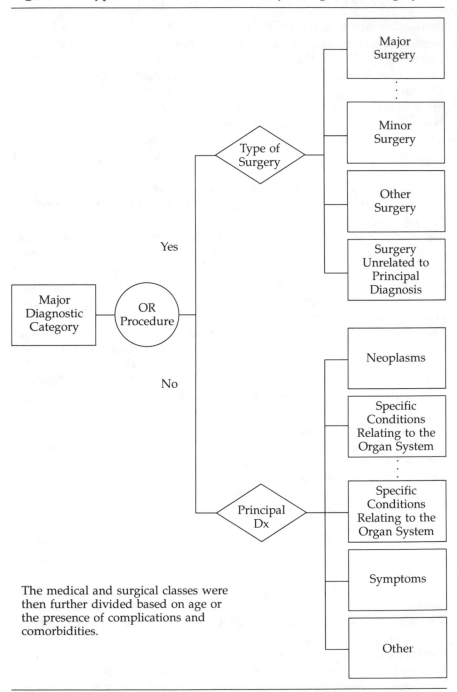

The medical and surgical classes were then further divided based on age or the presence of complications and comorbidities.

Source: *DRG Definitions Manual,* Fourth Revision (New Haven, CT: Health Systems International, Inc., 1987).

Table 2-2: Surgical Classes in MDC 13, Diseases and Disorders of the Female Reproductive System, Listed in Hierarchical Order from Highest to Lowest Rank

---

Pelvic evisceration, radical hysterectomy and radical vulvectomy

Uterus and adnexal procedures

Reconstructive procedures

Vagina, cervix, and vulva procedures

Laparoscopy and incisional tubal interruption

D & C, conization, and radioactive implant

Endoscopic tubal interruption

Other femal reproductive system O.R. procedures

Source: Robert B. Fetter, "The New ICD-9-CM Diagnosis-Related Groups Classification Scheme."

example of such a patient would be one with a principal diagnosis of pneumonia whose only surgical procedure was a transurethral prostatectomy. Such patients are assigned to a surgical class referred to as "unrelated operating room procedures." These patients are ultimately never assigned to a well-defined DRG.

Defining the surgical and medical classes in an MDC required that each surgical or medical class be based on some organizing principle. Examples of organizing principles would be anatomy, surgical approach, diagnostic approach, pathology, etiology, or treatment process. In order for a diagnosis or surgical procedure to be assigned to a particular class, it would be required to correspond to the particular organizing principle for that class. For example, in the urinary system MDC a surgical group was formed for all patients with a procedure on the urethra (that is, the organizing principle was based on anatomy). This surgical group was then further divided according to whether the procedure performed was transurethral (that is, the organizing principle was based on surgical approach).

Once the medical and surgical classes for an MDC were formed, each class of patients was evaluated to determine if complications, comorbidities, or the patient's age would consistently affect the consumption of hospital resources. Physician panels classified each diagnosis code according to whether the diagnosis, when present as a secondary condition, would be considered a substantial complication or comorbidity. A substantial complication or comorbidity was defined as a condition that, in combination with a specific principal diagnosis, would cause an increase in length of stay by at least one day in at least 75 percent of the patients.

For example, sarcoidosis, chronic airway obstruction, and pneumococcal pneumonia are considered substantial complications or comorbidities, while simple goiter and benign hypertension are not. Each medical and surgical class within an MDC was tested to determine if the presence of any substantial comorbidities or complications would consistently affect the consumption of hospital resources. For example, the presence of complications or comorbidities was not significant for patients receiving a carpal tunnel release but was very significant for patients with arrhythmia and conduction disorders.

The same basic list of complications and comorbidities are used across most DRGs. However, depending on the principal diagnosis of the patient, some diagnoses in the basic list of complications and comorbidities may be excluded if they are closely related to the principal diagnosis. For example, urinary retention is a complication or comorbidity for a patient admitted for congestive heart failure but not for a patient admitted for benign prostatic hypertrophy. In addition, in some cases such as newborns or acute myocardial infarction patients, special complications and comorbidity definitions were used in defining the DRGs.

The patient's age was sometimes used in the definition of the DRGs. Pediatric patients (age 17 years or less) were often assigned to separate DRGs. For example, pediatric asthma patients were assigned to a specific DRG.

The final variable used in the definition of the DRGs was the patient discharge status. Separate DRGs were formed for burn patients and newborns if the patients were transferred to another acute care facility. In addition, separate DRGs were formed for patients with alcoholism or drug abuse who left against medical advice, for acute myocardial infarction patients who died, and for newborns who died.

The actual process of forming the DRGs was highly reiterative, involving a combination of statistical results from test data with clinical judgment. At any point during the definition of the DRGs there would often be several patient characteristics that appeared important for understanding the impact on hospital resources. The selection of the patient characteristics to be used and the order in which they would be used was a complex task with many factors examined and weighed simultaneously. The end result of the fourth revision of the DRGs was the creation of 471 patient classes or DRGs that encompass all patients treated in an inpatient setting. In the fourth revision of the Medicare DRGs they are numbered 1–437, 439–467, and 471–475. DRG number 438 is not used in the second, third, or fourth revision. A complete list of the DRGs in the fourth revision is contained in Appendix 2-A.

Since all patients cannot be assigned to a DRG, there are three additional patient classes referred to as classes 468, 469, and 470. If a patient's medical record abstract contains invalid information or if the clinical information on the abstract contains certain types of inconsistencies, the patient may not be assigned to one of the 469 DRGs. These three additional patient classes have been defined to identify the situations in which a patient will not be assigned to one of the 471 DRGs.

Patients are assigned to patient class 468 when all the operating room procedures performed are unrelated to the major diagnostic category of the patient's principal diagnosis. Thus, a patient with a principal diagnosis of congestive heart failure whose only procedure is a cholecystectomy will be assigned to patient class 468, since the cholecystectomy is unrelated to diseases of the circulatory system. Patient abstracts assigned to patient class 468 are often the result of medical record coding errors, such as the coding of the wrong principal diagnosis. However, patients with completely accurate medical record information can also be assigned to patient class 468. Typically, these are patients who are admitted for a particular diagnosis, develop a complication unrelated to the principal diagnosis, and have an operating room procedure performed for the complication. For example, a patient admitted for pneumonia who has benign prostatic hypertrophy and becomes obstructed and receives a transurethral prostatectomy for the benign prostatic hypertrophy would be assigned to patient class 468. Thus, this patient is in class 468 not because of a medical record error but because a pneumonia patient who received a transurethral prostatectomy is clearly atypical both clinically and from a resource perspective and cannot be appropriately associated with a DRG.

Patients are assigned to patient class 469 when a principal diagnosis is given a code that, although it is a valid code according to the *International Classification of Diseases, Ninth Revision, Clinical Modification* (ICD-9-CM), is not precise enough to allow the patient to be assigned to a DRG. For example, ICD-9-CM code 64690 is an unspecified complication of pregnancy with the episode of care unspecified. Thus, this diagnosis code does not indicate the type of complication nor whether the episode of care was antepartum, postpartum, or for delivery. Since the DRG definitions assign patients to different sets of DRGs depending on whether the episode of care was antepartum, postpartum, or for delivery, a patient with a principal diagnosis of 64690 cannot be assigned to a DRG and will be assigned to patient class 469.

It should be noted that patients with a principal diagnosis that is not typically considered a reason to be hospitalized are not assigned to patient class 469. For example, ICD-9-CM code V503, ear piercing, is assigned to DRG 467 and not patient class 469.

Patients are assigned to patient class 470 if certain types of medical record errors that may affect DRG assignment are present. Patients with an invalid or nonexistent ICD-9-CM code as principal diagnosis will be assigned to patient class 470. Patients will also be assigned to patient class 470 if their age, sex, or discharge status is both invalid and necessary for DRG assignment. For example, if a patient has a nonnumeric age or has an age coded greater than 124 years and has a principal diagnosis of asthma with no operating room procedures, the DRG assignment will be to patient class 470 since medical patients with asthma will be assigned to different DRGs depending on their age. On the other hand, if the same patient had a principal diagnosis of hypertension, the DRG assignment would not be to patient class 470 since age is not used in the determination of the DRG for hypertensive patients.

REVISIONS OF THE DRGs

In 1979 hospitals in the United States began coding all diagnostic and surgical procedure information by ICD-9-CM. Since this system represented a significant improvement over previous coding systems, the development of an ICD-9-CM version of the DRGs was initiated between 1980 and 1982. This work was funded by the Health Care Financing Administration through a grant to Yale University.

During the period between January 1982 and the passage of the Prospective Payment System legislation in April 1983, the DRGs as defined by the Yale project were utilized in a great variety of applications, including professional standards review organizations and individual hospitals, and as the basis of the hospital prospective payment system in New Jersey. The initial year of application of the DRGs uncovered a number of technical errors and omissions. The Health Care Financing Administration awarded a contract to Health Systems International, a Connecticut-based consulting firm, to evaluate and correct problems with the DRG definitions annually. In June 1983 the revised DRG definitions were released for use in the Medicare Prospective Payment System. The use of the DRGs as the basis of payment for all Medicare hospital admissions placed the DRG structure under intense scrutiny. During the initial year of the Prospective Payment System numerous questions and issues were raised by hospitals regarding the assignment of specific types of patients to particular DRGs.

In September 1985 the software and documentation for the second revision of the DRGs were released. These modifications were effective for Medicare discharges occurring on or after May 1, 1986. Modifications for the third revision of the DRGs were released in September 1986, effective for Medicare discharges occurring on or after October 1, 1986. Modifications for the fourth revision of the DRGs were released in September 1987, effective for Medicare discharges occurring on or after October 1, 1987.

SUMMARY

The DRGs, as they are now defined, form a manageable, clinically coherent set of patient classes that relate a hospital's case mix to the resource demands and associated costs experienced by the hospital. DRGs are defined on the basis of the principal diagnosis, secondary diagnoses, surgical procedures, age, sex, and discharge status of the patients treated. Through DRGs, hospitals can gain an understanding of the patients being treated, the costs incurred, and, within reasonable limits, the services expected to be required. The classification of patients into DRGs is a constantly evolving process. As coding schemes change, as more comprehensive data are collected, or as medical technology or practice changes, the DRG definitions will be reviewed and revised.

Appendix 2-A: Diagnosis-Related Groups, Fourth Revision

DRG	MDC	Type*	Definition
001	01	P	CRANIOTOMY AGE >17 EXCEPT FOR TRAUMA
002	01	P	CRANIOTOMY FOR TRAUMA AGE >17
003	01	P	CRANIOTOMY AGE 0–17
004	01	P	SPINAL PROCEDURES
005	01	P	EXTRACRANIAL VASCULAR PROCEDURES
006	01	P	CARPAL TUNNEL RELEASE
007	01	P	PERIPH & CRANIAL NERVE & OTHER NERV SYST PROC W CC
008	01	P	PERIPH & CRANIAL NERVE & OTHER NERV SYST PROC W/O CC
009	01	M	SPINAL DISORDERS & INJURIES
010	01	M	NERVOUS SYSTEM NEOPLASMS W CC
011	01	M	NERVOUS SYSTEM NEOPLASMS W/O CC
012	01	M	DEGENERATIVE NERVOUS SYSTEM DISORDERS
013	01	M	MULTIPLE SCLEROSIS & CEREBELLAR ATAXIA
014	01	M	SPECIFIC CEREBROVASCULAR DISORDERS EXCEPT TIA

Continued

* DRG = Diagnosis Related Group; MDC = Major Diagnostic Category; M = Medical DRG; P = Procedure (or Surgical) DRG; CC = Comorbidity or Complication; W = With; W/O = Without.

Reprinted from *Diagnosis-Related Groups: Definitions Manual*, Fourth Revision (New Haven, CT: Health Systems International, 1987), with permission.

Appendix 2-A: Continued

DRG	MDC	Type*	Definition
015	01	M	TRANSIENT ISCHEMIC ATTACK & PRECEREBRAL OCCLUSIONS
016	01	M	NONSPECIFIC CEREBROVASCULAR DISORDERS W CC
017	01	M	NONSPECIFIC CEREBROVASCULAR DISORDERS W/O CC
018	01	M	CRANIAL & PERIPHERAL NERVE DISORDERS W CC
019	01	M	CRANIAL & PERIPHERAL NERVE DISORDERS W/O CC
020	01	M	NERVOUS SYSTEM INFECTION EXCEPT VIRAL MENINGITIS
021	01	M	VIRAL MENINGITIS
022	01	M	HYPERTENSIVE ENCEPHALOPATHY
023	01	M	NONTRAUMATIC STUPOR & COMA
024	01	M	SEIZURE & HEADACHE AGE >17 W CC
025	01	M	SEIZURE & HEADACHE AGE >17 W/O CC
026	01	M	SEIZURE & HEADACHE AGE 0–17
027	01	M	TRAUMATIC STUPOR & COMA, COMA >1 HR
028	01	M	TRAUMATIC STUPOR & COMA, COMA <1 HR AGE >17 W CC
029	01	M	TRAUMATIC STUPOR & COMA, COMA <1 HR AGE >17 W/O CC
030	01	M	TRAUMATIC STUPOR & COMA, COMA <1 HR AGE 0–17
031	01	M	CONCUSSION AGE >17 W CC
032	01	M	CONCUSSION AGE >17 W/O CC
033	01	M	CONCUSSION AGE 0–17
034	01	M	OTHER DISORDERS OF NERVOUS SYSTEM W CC
035	01	M	OTHER DISORDERS OF NERVOUS SYSTEM W/O CC
036	02	P	RETINAL PROCEDURES
037	02	P	ORBITAL PROCEDURES
038	02	P	PRIMARY IRIS PROCEDURES
039	02	P	LENS PROCEDURES WITH OR WITHOUT VITRECTOMY
040	02	P	EXTRAOCULAR PROCEDURES EXCEPT ORBIT AGE >17
041	02	P	EXTRAOCULAR PROCEDURES EXCEPT ORBIT AGE 0–17
042	02	P	INTRAOCULAR PROCEDURES EXCEPT RETINA, IRIS & LENS
043	02	M	HYPHEMA
044	02	M	ACUTE MAJOR EYE INFECTIONS
045	02	M	NEUROLOGICAL EYE DISORDERS
046	02	M	OTHER DISORDERS OF THE EYE AGE >17 W CC
047	02	M	OTHER DISORDERS OF THE EYE AGE >17 W/O CC
048	02	M	OTHER DISORDERS OF THE EYE AGE 0–17
049	03	P	MAJOR HEAD & NECK PROCEDURES
050	03	P	SIALOADENECTOMY

Continued

Appendix 2-A: Continued

DRG	MDC	Type*	Definition
051	03	P	SALIVARY GLAND PROCEDURES EXCEPT SIALOADENECTOMY
052	03	P	CLEFT LIP & PALATE REPAIR
053	03	P	SINUS & MASTOID PROCEDURES AGE >17
054	03	P	SINUS & MASTOID PROCEDURES AGE 0–17
055	03	P	MISCELLANEOUS EAR, NOSE & THROAT PROCEDURES
056	03	P	RHINOPLASTY
057	03	P	T&A PROC, EXCEPT TONSILLECTOMY &/OR ADENOIDECTOMY ONLY, AGE >17
058	03	P	T&A PROC, EXCEPT TONSILLECTOMY &/OR ADENOIDECTOMY ONLY, AGE 0–17
059	03	P	TONSILLECTOMY &/OR ADENOIDECTOMY ONLY, AGE >17
060	03	P	TONSILLECTOMY &/OR ADENOIDECTOMY ONLY, AGE 0–17
061	03	P	MYRINGOTOMY W TUBE INSERTION AGE >17
062	03	P	MYRINGOTOMY W TUBE INSERTION AGE 0–17
063	03	P	OTHER EAR, NOSE & THROAT O.R. PROCEDURES
064	03	M	EAR, NOSE & THROAT MALIGNANCY
065	03	M	DYSEQUILIBRIUM
066	03	M	EPISTAXIS
067	03	M	EPIGLOTTITIS
068	03	M	OTITIS MEDIA & URI AGE >17 W CC
069	03	M	OTITIS MEDIA & URI AGE >17 W/O CC
070	03	M	OTITIS MEDIA & URI AGE 0–17
071	03	M	LARYNGOTRACHEITIS
072	03	M	NASAL TRAUMA & DEFORMITY
073	03	M	OTHER EAR, NOSE & THROAT DIAGNOSES AGE >17
074	03	M	OTHER EAR, NOSE & THROAT DIAGNOSES AGE 0–17
075	04	P	MAJOR CHEST PROCEDURES
076	04	P	OTHER RESP SYSTEM O.R. PROCEDURES W CC
077	04	P	OTHER RESP SYSTEM O.R. PROCEDURES W/O CC
078	04	M	PULMONARY EMBOLISM
079	04	M	RESPIRATORY INFECTIONS & INFLAMMATIONS AGE >17 W CC
080	04	M	RESPIRATORY INFECTIONS & INFLAMMATIONS AGE >17 W/O CC
081	04	M	RESPIRATORY INFECTIONS & INFLAMMATIONS AGE 0–17
082	04	M	RESPIRATORY NEOPLASMS
083	04	M	MAJOR CHEST TRAUMA W CC
084	04	M	MAJOR CHEST TRAUMA W/O CC
085	04	M	PLEURAL EFFUSION W CC
086	04	M	PLEURAL EFFUSION W/O CC

Continued

Appendix 2-A: Continued

DRG	MDC	Type*	Definition
087	04	M	PULMONARY EDEMA & RESPIRATORY FAILURE
088	04	M	CHRONIC OBSTRUCTIVE PULMONARY DISEASE
089	04	M	SIMPLE PNEUMONIA & PLEURISY AGE >17 W CC
090	04	M	SIMPLE PNEUMONIA & PLEURISY AGE >17 W/O CC
091	04	M	SIMPLE PNEUMONIA & PLEURISY AGE 0–17
092	04	M	INTERSTITIAL LUNG DISEASE W CC
093	04	M	INTERSTITIAL LUNG DISEASE W/O CC
094	04	M	PNEUMOTHORAX W CC
095	04	M	PNEUMOTHORAX W/O CC
096	04	M	BRONCHITIS & ASTHMA AGE >17 W CC
097	04	M	BRONCHITIS & ASTHMA AGE >17 W/O CC
098	04	M	BRONCHITIS & ASTHMA AGE 0–17
099	04	M	RESPIRATORY SIGNS & SYMPTOMS W CC
100	04	M	RESPIRATORY SIGNS & SYMPTOMS W/O CC
101	04	M	OTHER RESPIRATORY SYSTEM DIAGNOSES W CC
102	04	M	OTHER RESPIRATORY SYSTEM DIAGNOSES W/O CC
103	05	P	HEART TRANSPLANT
104	05	P	CARDIAC VALVE PROCEDURE W PUMP & W CARDIAC CATH
105	05	P	CARDIAC VALVE PROCEDURE W PUMP & W/O CARDIAC CATH
106	05	P	CORONARY BYPASS W CARDIAC CATH
107	05	P	CORONARY BYPASS W/O CARDIAC CATH
108	05	P	OTHER CARDIOTHORACIC OR VASCULAR PROCEDURES, W PUMP
109	05	P	OTHER CARDIOTHORACIC PROCEDURES W/O PUMP
110	05	P	MAJOR RECONSTRUCTIVE VASCULAR PROC W/O PUMP W CC
111	05	P	MAJOR RECONSTRUCTIVE VASCULAR PROC W/O PUMP W/O CC
112	05	P	VASCULAR PROCEDURES EXCEPT MAJOR RECONSTRUCTION W/O PUMP
113	05	P	AMPUTATION FOR CIRC SYSTEM DISORDERS EXCEPT UPPER LIMB & TOE
114	05	P	UPPER LIMB & TOE AMPUTATION FOR CIRC SYSTEM DISORDERS
115	05	P	PERM CARDIAC PACEMAKER IMPLANT W AMI, HEART FAILURE OR SHOCK
116	05	P	PERM CARDIAC PACEMAKER IMPLANT W/O AMI, HEART FAILURE OR SHOCK
117	05	P	CARDIAC PACEMAKER REVISION EXCEPT DEVICE REPLACEMENT
118	05	P	CARDIAC PACEMAKER DEVICE REPLACEMENT
119	05	P	VEIN LIGATION & STRIPPING
120	05	P	OTHER CIRCULATORY SYSTEM O.R. PROCEDURES

Continued

Appendix 2-A: Continued

DRG	MDC	Type*	Definition
121	05	M	CIRCULATORY DISORDERS W AMI & C.V. COMP DISCH ALIVE
122	05	M	CIRCULATORY DISORDERS W AMI W/O C.V. COMP DISCH ALIVE
123	05	M	CIRCULATORY DISORDERS W AMI, EXPIRED
124	05	M	CIRCULATORY DISORDERS EXCEPT AMI, W CARD CATH & COMPLEX DIAG
125	05	M	CIRCULATORY DISORDERS EXCEPT AMI, W CARD CATH W/O COMPLEX DIAG
126	05	M	ACUTE & SUBACUTE ENDOCARDITIS
127	05	M	HEART FAILURE & SHOCK
128	05	M	DEEP VEIN THROMBOPHLEBITIS
129	05	M	CARDIAC ARREST, UNEXPLAINED
130	05	M	PERIPHERAL VASCULAR DISORDERS W CC
131	05	M	PERIPHERAL VASCULAR DISORDERS W/O CC
132	05	M	ATHEROSCLEROSIS W CC
133	05	M	ATHEROSCLEROSIS W/O CC
134	05	M	HYPERTENSION
135	05	M	CARDIAC CONGENITAL & VALVULAR DISORDERS AGE >17 W CC
136	05	M	CARDIAC CONGENITAL & VALVULAR DISORDERS AGE >17 W/O CC
137	05	M	CARDIAC CONGENITAL & VALVULAR DISORDERS AGE 0–17
138	05	M	CARDIAC ARRHYTHMIA & CONDUCTION DISORDERS W CC
139	05	M	CARDIAC ARRHYTHMIA & CONDUCTION DISORDERS W/O CC
140	05	M	ANGINA PECTORIS
141	05	M	SYNCOPE & COLLAPSE W CC
142	05	M	SYNCOPE & COLLAPSE W/O CC
143	05	M	CHEST PAIN
144	05	M	OTHER CIRCULATORY SYSTEM DIAGNOSES W CC
145	05	M	OTHER CIRCULATORY SYSTEM DIAGNOSES W/O CC
146	06	P	RECTAL RESECTION W CC
147	06	P	RECTAL RESECTION W/O CC
148	06	P	MAJOR SMALL & LARGE BOWEL PROCEDURES W CC
149	06	P	MAJOR SMALL & LARGE BOWEL PROCEDURES W/O CC
150	06	P	PERITONEAL ADHESIOLYSIS W CC
151	06	P	PERITONEAL ADHESIOLYSIS W/O CC
152	06	P	MINOR SMALL & LARGE BOWEL PROCEDURES W CC
153	06	P	MINOR SMALL & LARGE BOWEL PROCEDURES W/O CC
154	06	P	STOMACH, ESOPHAGEAL & DUODENAL PROCEDURES AGE >17 W CC

Continued

Appendix 2-A: Continued

DRG	MDC	Type*	Definition
155	06	P	STOMACH, ESOPHAGEAL & DUODENAL PROCEDURES AGE >17 W/O CC
156	06	P	STOMACH, ESOPHAGEAL & DUODENAL PROCEDURES AGE 0–17
157	06	P	ANAL & STOMAL PROCEDURES W CC
158	06	P	ANAL & STOMAL PROCEDURES W/O CC
159	06	P	HERNIA PROCEDURES EXCEPT INGUINAL & FEMORAL AGE >17 W CC
160	06	P	HERNIA PROCEDURES EXCEPT INGUINAL & FEMORAL AGE >17 W/O CC
161	06	P	INGUINAL & FEMORAL HERNIA PROCEDURES AGE >17 W CC
162	06	P	INGUINAL & FEMORAL HERNIA PROCEDURES AGE >17 W/O CC
163	06	P	HERNIA PROCEDURES AGE 0–17
164	06	P	APPENDECTOMY W COMPLICATED PRINCIPAL DIAG W CC
165	06	P	APPENDECTOMY W COMPLICATED PRINCIPAL DIAG W/O CC
166	06	P	APPENDECTOMY W/O COMPLICATED PRINCIPAL DIAG W CC
167	06	P	APPENDECTOMY W/O COMPLICATED PRINCIPAL DIAG W/O CC
168	06	P	MOUTH PROCEDURES W CC
169	06	P	MOUTH PROCEDURES W/O CC
170	06	P	OTHER DIGESTIVE SYSTEM O.R. PROCEDURES W CC
171	06	P	OTHER DIGESTIVE SYSTEM O.R. PROCEDURES W/O CC
172	06	M	DIGESTIVE MALIGNANCY W CC
173	06	M	DIGESTIVE MALIGNANCY W/O CC
174	06	M	G.I. HEMORRHAGE W CC
175	06	M	G.I. HEMORRHAGE W/O CC
176	06	M	COMPLICATED PEPTIC ULCER
177	06	M	UNCOMPLICATED PEPTIC ULCER W CC
178	06	M	UNCOMPLICATED PEPTIC ULCER W/O CC
179	06	M	INFLAMMATORY BOWEL DISEASE
180	06	M	G.I. OBSTRUCTION W CC
181	06	M	G.I. OBSTRUCTION W/O CC
182	06	M	ESOPHAGITIS, GASTROENT & MISC DIGEST DISORDERS AGE >17 W CC
183	06	M	ESOPHAGITIS, GASTROENT & MISC DIGEST DISORDERS AGE >17 W/O CC
184	06	M	ESOPHAGITIS, GASTROENT & MISC DIGEST DISORDERS AGE 0–17
185	06	M	DENTAL & ORAL DIS EXCEPT EXTRACTIONS & RESTORATIONS, AGE >17

Continued

Appendix 2-A: Continued

DRG	MDC	Type*	Definition
186	06	M	DENTAL & ORAL DIS EXCEPT EXTRACTIONS & RESTORATIONS, AGE 0–17
187	06	M	DENTAL EXTRACTIONS & RESTORATIONS
188	06	M	OTHER DIGESTIVE SYSTEM DIAGNOSES AGE >17 W CC
189	06	M	OTHER DIGESTIVE SYSTEM DIAGNOSES AGE >17 W/O CC
190	06	M	OTHER DIGESTIVE SYSTEM DIAGNOSES AGE 0–17
191	07	P	MAJOR PANCREAS, LIVER & SHUNT PROCEDURES
192	07	P	MINOR PANCREAS, LIVER & SHUNT PROCEDURES
193	07	P	BILIARY TRACT PROC EXCEPT TOT CHOLECYSTECTOMY W CC
194	07	P	BILIARY TRACT PROC EXCEPT TOT CHOLECYSTECTOMY W/O CC
195	07	P	TOTAL CHOLECYSTECTOMY W C.D.E. W CC
196	07	P	TOTAL CHOLECYSTECTOMY W C.D.E. W/O CC
197	07	P	TOTAL CHOLECYSTECTOMY W/O C.D.E. W CC
198	07	P	TOTAL CHOLECYSTECTOMY W/O C.D.E. W/O CC
199	07	P	HEPATOBILIARY DIAGNOSTIC PROCEDURE FOR MALIGNANCY
200	07	P	HEPATOBILIARY DIAGNOSTIC PROCEDURE FOR NON-MALIGNANCY
201	07	P	OTHER HEPATOBILIARY OR PANCREAS O.R. PROCEDURES
202	07	M	CIRRHOSIS & ALCOHOLIC HEPATITIS
203	07	M	MALIGNANCY OF HEPATOBILIARY SYSTEM OR PANCREAS
204	07	M	DISORDERS OF PANCREAS EXCEPT MALIGNANCY
205	07	M	DISORDERS OF LIVER EXCEPT MALIG, CIRR, ALC HEPA W CC
206	07	M	DISORDERS OF LIVER EXCEPT MALIG, CIRR, ALC HEPA W/O CC
207	07	M	DISORDERS OF THE BILIARY TRACT W CC
208	07	M	DISORDERS OF THE BILIARY TRACT W/O CC
209	08	P	MAJOR JOINT & LIMB REATTACHMENT PROCEDURES
210	08	P	HIP & FEMUR PROCEDURES EXCEPT MAJOR JOINT AGE >17 W CC
211	08	P	HIP & FEMUR PROCEDURES EXCEPT MAJOR JOINT AGE >17 W/O CC
212	08	P	HIP & FEMUR PROCEDURES EXCEPT MAJOR JOINT AGE 0–17
213	08	P	AMPUTATION FOR MUSCULOSKELETAL SYSTEM & CONN TISSUE DISORDERS
214	08	P	BACK & NECK PROCEDURES W CC
215	08	P	BACK & NECK PROCEDURES W/O CC

Continued

Appendix 2-A: Continued

DRG	MDC	Type*	Definition
216	08	P	BIOPSIES OF MUSCULOSKELETAL SYSTEM & CONNECTIVE TISSUE
217	08	P	WND DEBRID & SKN GRFT EXCEPT HAND, FOR MUSCSKELET & CONN TISS DIS
218	08	P	LOWER EXTREM & HUMER PROC EXCEPT HIP, FOOT, FEMUR AGE >17 W CC
219	08	P	LOWER EXTREM & HUMER PROC EXCEPT HIP, FOOT, FEMUR AGE >17 W/O CC
220	08	P	LOWER EXTREM & HUMER PROC EXCEPT HIP, FOOT, FEMUR AGE 0–17
221	08	P	KNEE PROCEDURES W CC
222	08	P	KNEE PROCEDURES W/O CC
223	08	P	MAJOR SHOULDER/ELBOW PROC, OR OTHER UPPER EXTREMITY PROC W CC
224	08	P	SHOULDER, ELBOW OR FOREARM PROC, EXC MAJOR JOINT PROC, W/O CC
225	08	P	FOOT PROCEDURES
226	08	P	SOFT TISSUE PROCEDURES W CC
227	08	P	SOFT TISSUE PROCEDURES W/O CC
228	08	P	MAJOR THUMB OR JOINT PROC, OR OTH HAND OR WRIST PROC W CC
229	08	P	HAND OR WRIST PROC, EXCEPT MAJOR JOINT PROC, W/O CC
230	08	P	LOCAL EXCISION & REMOVAL OF INT FIX DEVICES OF HIP & FEMUR
231	08	P	LOCAL EXCISION & REMOVAL OF INT FIX DEVICES EXCEPT HIP & FEMUR
232	08	P	ARTHROSCOPY
233	08	P	OTHER MUSCULOSKELET SYS & CONN TISS O.R. PROC W CC
234	08	P	OTHER MUSCULOSKELET SYS & CONN TISS O.R. PROC W/O CC
235	08	M	FRACTURES OF FEMUR
236	08	M	FRACTURES OF HIP & PELVIS
237	08	M	SPRAINS, STRAINS, & DISLOCATIONS OF HIP, PELVIS & THIGH
238	08	M	OSTEOMYELITIS
239	08	M	PATHOLOGICAL FRACTURES & MUSCULOSKELETAL & CONN TISS MALIGNANCY
240	08	M	CONNECTIVE TISSUE DISORDERS W CC
241	08	M	CONNECTIVE TISSUE DISORDERS W/O CC
242	08	M	SEPTIC ARTHRITIS
243	08	M	MEDICAL BACK PROBLEMS
244	08	M	BONE DISEASES & SPECIFIC ARTHROPATHIES W CC
245	08	M	BONE DISEASES & SPECIFIC ARTHROPATHIES W/O CC

Continued

Appendix 2-A: Continued

DRG	MDC	Type*	Definition
246	08	M	NON-SPECIFIC ARTHROPATHIES
247	08	M	SIGNS & SYMPTOMS OF MUSCULOSKELETAL SYSTEM & CONN TISSUE
248	08	M	TENDONITIS, MYOSITIS & BURSITIS
249	08	M	AFTERCARE, MUSCULOSKELETAL SYSTEM & CONNECTIVE TISSUE
250	08	M	FX, SPRN, STRN & DISL OF FOREARM, HAND, FOOT AGE >17 W CC
251	08	M	FX, SPRN, STRN & DISL OF FOREARM, HAND, FOOT AGE >17 W/O CC
252	08	M	FX, SPRN, STRN & DISL OF FOREARM, HAND, FOOT AGE 0–17
253	08	M	FX, SPRN, STRN & DISL OF UPARM, LOWLEG EX FOOT AGE >17 W CC
254	08	M	FX, SPRN, STRN & DISL OF UPARM, LOWLEG EX FOOT AGE >17 W/O CC
255	08	M	FX, SPRN, STRN & DISL OF UPARM, LOWLEG EX FOOT AGE 0–17
256	08	M	OTHER MUSCULOSKELETAL SYSTEM & CONNECTIVE TISSUE DIAGNOSES
257	09	P	TOTAL MASTECTOMY FOR MALIGNANCY W CC
258	09	P	TOTAL MASTECTOMY FOR MALIGNANCY W/O CC
259	09	P	SUBTOTAL MASTECTOMY FOR MALIGNANCY W CC
260	09	P	SUBTOTAL MASTECTOMY FOR MALIGNANCY W/O CC
261	09	P	BREAST PROC FOR NON-MALIGNANCY EXCEPT BIOPSY & LOCAL EXCISION
262	09	P	BREAST BIOPSY & LOCAL EXCISION FOR NON-MALIGNANCY
263	09	P	SKIN GRAFT &/OR DEBRID FOR SKN ULCER OR CELLULITIS W CC
264	09	P	SKIN GRAFT &/OR DEBRID FOR SKN ULCER OR CELLULITIS W/O CC
265	09	P	SKIN GRAFT &/OR DEBRID EXCEPT FOR SKIN ULCER OR CELLULITIS W CC
266	09	P	SKIN GRAFT &/OR DEBRID EXCEPT FOR SKIN ULCER OR CELLULITIS W/O CC
267	09	P	PERIANAL & PILONIDAL PROCEDURES
268	09	P	SKIN, SUBCUTANEOUS TISSUE & BREAST PLASTIC PROCEDURES
269	09		OTHER SKIN, SUBCUT TISS & BREAST PROC W CC
270	09		OTHER SKIN, SUBCUT TISS & BREAST PROC W/O CC
271	09	M	SKIN ULCERS
272	09	M	MAJOR SKIN DISORDERS W CC
273	09	M	MAJOR SKIN DISORDERS W/O CC

Continued

Appendix 2-A: Continued

DRG	MDC	Type*	Definition
274	09	M	MALIGNANT BREAST DISORDERS W CC
275	09	M	MALIGNANT BREAST DISORDERS W/O CC
276	09	M	NON-MALIGANT BREAST DISORDERS
277	09	M	CELLULITIS AGE >17 W CC
278	09	M	CELLULITIS AGE >17 W/O CC
279	09	M	CELLULITIS AGE 0–17
280	09	M	TRAUMA TO THE SKIN, SUBCUT TISS & BREAST AGE >17 W CC
281	09	M	TRAUMA TO THE SKIN, SUBCUT TISS & BREAST AGE >17 W/O CC
282	09	M	TRAUMA TO THE SKIN, SUBCUT TISS & BREAST AGE 0–17
283	09	M	MINOR SKIN DISORDERS W CC
284	09	M	MINOR SKIN DISORDERS W/O CC
285	10	P	AMPUTAT OF LOWER LIMB FOR ENDOCRINE, NUTRIT, & METABOL DISORDERS
286	10	P	ADRENAL & PITUITARY PROCEDURES
287	10	P	SKIN GRAFTS & WOUND DEBRID FOR ENDOC, NUTRIT & METAB DISORDERS
288	10	P	O.R. PROCEDURES FOR OBESITY
289	10	P	PARATHYROID PROCEDURES
290	10	P	THYROID PROCEDURES
291	10	P	THYROGLOSSAL PROCEDURES
292	10	P	OTHER ENDOCRINE, NUTRIT & METAB O.R. PROC W CC
293	10	P	OTHER ENDOCRINE, NUTRIT & METAB O.R. PROC W/O CC
294	10	M	DIABETES AGE >35
295	10	M	DIABETES AGE 0–35
296	10	M	NUTRITIONAL & MISC METABOLIC DISORDERS AGE >17 W CC
297	10	M	NUTRITIONAL & MISC METABOLIC DISORDERS AGE >17 W/O CC
298	10	M	NUTRITIONAL & MISC METABOLIC DISORDERS AGE 0–17
299	10	M	INBORN ERRORS OF METABOLISM
300	10	M	ENDOCRINE DISORDERS W CC
301	10	M	ENDOCRINE DISORDERS W/O CC
302	11	P	KIDNEY TRANSPLANT
303	11	P	KIDNEY, URETER & MAJOR BLADDER PROCEDURES FOR NEOPLASM
304	11	P	KIDNEY, URETER & MAJOR BLADDER PROC FOR NON-NEOPL W CC
305	11	P	KIDNEY, URETER & MAJOR BLADDER PROC FOR NON-NEOPL W/O CC

Continued

Appendix 2-A: Continued

DRG	MDC	Type*	Definition
306	11	P	PROSTATECTOMY W CC
307	11	P	PROSTATECTOMY W/O CC
308	11	P	MINOR BLADDER PROCEDURES W CC
309	11	P	MINOR BLADDER PROCEDURES W/O CC
310	11	P	TRANSURETHRAL PROCEDURES W CC
311	11	P	TRANSURETHRAL PROCEDURES W/O CC
312	11	P	URETHRAL PROCEDURES, AGE >17 W CC
313	11	P	URETHRAL PROCEDURES, AGE >17 W/O CC
314	11	P	URETHRAL PROCEDURES, AGE 0–17
315	11	P	OTHER KIDNEY & URINARY TRACT O.R. PROCEDURES
316	11	M	RENAL FAILURE
317	11	M	ADMIT FOR RENAL DIALYSIS
318	11	M	KIDNEY & URINARY TRACT NEOPLASMS W CC
319	11	M	KIDNEY & URINARY TRACT NEOPLASMS W/O CC
320	11	M	KIDNEY & URINARY TRACT INFECTIONS AGE >17 W CC
321	11	M	KIDNEY & URINARY TRACT INFECTIONS AGE >17 W/O CC
322	11	M	KIDNEY & URINARY TRACT INFECTIONS AGE 0–17
323	11	M	URINARY STONES W CC, &/OR ESW LITHOTRIPSY
324	11	M	URINARY STONES W/O CC
325	11	M	KIDNEY & URINARY TRACT SIGNS & SYMPTOMS AGE >17 W CC
326	11	M	KIDNEY & URINARY TRACT SIGNS & SYMPTOMS AGE >17 W/O CC
327	11	M	KIDNEY & URINARY TRACT SIGNS & SYMPTOMS AGE 0–17
328	11	M	URETHRAL STRICTURE AGE >17 W CC
329	11	M	URETHRAL STRICTURE AGE >17 W/O CC
330	11	M	URETHRAL STRICTURE AGE 0–17
331	11	M	OTHER KIDNEY & URINARY TRACT DIAGNOSES AGE >17 W CC
332	11	M	OTHER KIDNEY & URINARY TRACT DIAGNOSES AGE >17 W/O CC
333	11	M	OTHER KIDNEY & URINARY TRACT DIAGNOSES AGE 0–17
334	12	P	MAJOR MALE PELVIC PROCEDURES W CC
335	12	P	MAJOR MALE PELVIC PROCEDURES W/O CC
336	12	P	TRANSURETHRAL PROSTATECTOMY W CC
337	12	P	TRANSURETHRAL PROSTATECTOMY W/O CC
338	12	P	TESTES PROCEDURES, FOR MALIGNANCY
339	12	P	TESTES PROCEDURES, NON-MALIGNANCY AGE >17
340	12	P	TESTES PROCEDURES, NON-MALIGNANCY AGE 0–17
341	12	P	PENIS PROCEDURES

Continued

Appendix 2-A: Continued

DRG	MDC	Type*	Definition
342	12	P	CIRCUMCISION AGE >17
343	12	P	CIRCUMCISION AGE 0–17
344	12	P	OTHER MALE REPRODUCTIVE SYSTEM O.R. PROCEDURES FOR MALIGNANCY
345	12	P	OTHER MALE REPRODUCTIVE SYSTEM O.R. PROC EXCEPT FOR MALIGNANCY
346	12	M	MALIGNANCY, MALE REPRODUCTIVE SYSTEM W CC
347	12	M	MALIGNANCY, MALE REPRODUCTIVE SYSTEM W/O CC
348	12	M	BENIGN PROSTATIC HYPERTROPHY W CC
349	12	M	BENIGN PROSTATIC HYPERTROPHY W/O CC
350	12	M	INFLAMMATION OF THE MALE REPRODUCTIVE SYSTEM
351	12	M	STERILIZATION, MALE
352	12	M	OTHER MALE REPRODUCTIVE SYSTEM DIAGNOSES
353	13	P	PELVIC EVISCERATION, RADICAL HYSTERECTOMY & RADICAL VULVECTOMY
354	13	P	UTERINE, ADNEXA PROC FOR NON-OVARIAN/ADNEXAL MALIG W CC
355	13	P	UTERINE, ADNEXA PROC FOR NON-OVARIAN/ADNEXAL MALIG W/O CC
356	13	P	FEMALE REPRODUCTIVE SYSTEM RECONSTRUCTIVE PROCEDURES
357	13	P	UTERINE & ADNEXA PROC FOR OVARIAN OR ADNEXAL MALIGNANCY
358	13	P	UTERINE & ADNEXA PROC FOR NON-MALIGNANCY W CC
359	13	P	UTERINE & ADNEXA PROC FOR NON-MALIGNANCY W/O CC
360	13	P	VAGINA, CERVIX & VULVA PROCEDURES
361	13	P	LAPAROSCOPY & INCISIONAL TUBAL INTERRUPTION
362	13	P	ENDOSCOPIC TUBAL INTERRUPTION
363	13	P	D&C, CONIZATION & RADIO-IMPLANT, FOR MALIGNANCY
364	13	P	D&C, CONIZATION EXCEPT FOR MALIGNANCY
365	13	P	OTHER FEMALE REPRODUCTIVE SYSTEM O.R. PROCEDURES
366	13	M	MALIGNANCY, FEMALE REPRODUCTIVE SYSTEM W CC
367	13	M	MALIGNANCY, FEMALE REPRODUCTIVE SYSTEM W/O CC
368	13	M	INFECTIONS, FEMALE REPRODUCTIVE SYSTEM
369	13	M	MENSTRUAL & OTHER FEMALE REPRODUCTIVE SYSTEM DISORDERS
370	14	P	CESAREAN SECTION W CC

Continued

Appendix 2-A: Continued

DRG	MDC	Type*	Definition
371	14	P	CESAREAN SECTION W/O CC
372	14	M	VAGINAL DELIVERY W COMPLICATING DIAGNOSES
373	14	M	VAGINAL DELIVERY W/O COMPLICATING DIAGNOSES
374	14	P	VAGINAL DELIVERY W STERILIZATION &/OR D&C
375	14	P	VAGINAL DELIVERY W O.R. PROC EXCEPT STERIL &/OR D&C
376	14	M	POSTPARTUM & POST ABORTION DIAGNOSES W/O O.R. PROCEDURE
377	14	P	POSTPARTUM & POST ABORTION DIAGNOSES W O.R. PROCEDURE
378	14	M	ECTOPIC PREGNANCY
379	14	M	THREATENED ABORTION
380	14	M	ABORTION W/O D&C
381	14	P	ABORTION W D&C, ASPIRATION CURETTAGE OR HYSTEROTOMY
382	14	M	FALSE LABOR
383	14	M	OTHER ANTEPARTUM DIAGNOSES W MEDICAL COMPLICATIONS
384	14	M	OTHER ANTEPARTUM DIAGNOSES W/O MEDICAL COMPLICATIONS
385	15		NEONATES, DIED OR TRANSFERRED TO ANOTHER ACUTE CARE FACILITY
386	15		EXTREME IMMATURITY OR RESPIRATORY DISTRESS SYNDROME, NEONATE
387	15		PREMATURITY W MAJOR PROBLEMS
388	15		PREMATURITY W/O MAJOR PROBLEMS
389	15		FULL TERM NEONATE W MAJOR PROBLEMS
390	15		NEONATE W OTHER SIGNIFICANT PROBLEMS
391	15		NORMAL NEWBORN
392	16	P	SPLENECTOMY AGE >17
393	16	P	SPLENECTOMY AGE 0–17
394	16	P	OTHER O.R. PROCEDURES OF THE BLOOD AND BLOOD FORMING ORGANS
395	16	M	RED BLOOD CELL DISORDERS AGE >17
396	16	M	RED BLOOD CELL DISORDERS AGE 0–17
397	16	M	COAGULATION DISORDERS
398	16	M	RETICULOENDOTHELIAL & IMMUNITY DISORDERS W CC
399	16	M	RETICULOENDOTHELIAL & IMMUNITY DISORDERS W/O CC
400	17	P	LYMPHOMA & LEUKEMIA W MAJOR O.R. PROCEDURE
401	17	P	LYMPHOMA & NON-ACUTE LEUKEMIA W OTHER O.R. PROC W CC

Continued

Appendix 2-A: Continued

DRG	MDC	Type*	Definition
402	17	P	LYMPHOMA & NON-ACUTE LEUKEMIA W OTHER O.R. PROC W/O CC
403	17	M	LYMPHOMA & NON-ACUTE LEUKEMIA W CC
404	17	M	LYMPHOMA & NON-ACUTE LEUKEMIA W/O CC
405	17		ACUTE LEUKEMIA W/O MAJOR O.R. PROCEDURE AGE 0–17
406	17	P	MYELOPROLIF DISORD OR POORLY DIFF NEOPL W MAJ O.R. PROC W CC
407	17	P	MYELOPROLIF DISORD OR POORLY DIFF NEOPL W MAJ O.R. PROC W/O CC
408	17	P	MYELOPROLIF DISORD OR POORLY DIFF NEOPL W OTHER O.R. PROC
409	17	M	RADIOTHERAPY
410	17	M	CHEMOTHERAPY
411	17	M	HISTORY OF MALIGNANCY W/O ENDOSCOPY
412	17	M	HISTORY OF MALIGNANCY W ENDOSCOPY
413	17	M	OTHER MYELOPROLIF DIS OR POORLY DIFF NEOPL DIAG W CC
414	17	M	OTHER MYELOPROLIF DIS OR POORLY DIFF NEOPL DIAG W/O CC
415	18	P	O.R. PROCEDURE FOR INFECTIOUS & PARASITIC DISEASES
416	18	M	SEPTICEMIA AGE >17
417	18	M	SEPTICEMIA AGE 0–17
418	18	M	POSTOPERATIVE & POST-TRAUMATIC INFECTIONS
419	18	M	FEVER OF UNKNOWN ORIGIN AGE >17 W CC
420	18	M	FEVER OF UNKNOWN ORIGIN AGE >17 W/O CC
421	18	M	VIRAL ILLNESS AGE >17
422	18	M	VIRAL ILLNESS & FEVER OF UNKNOWN ORIGIN AGE 0–17
423	18	M	OTHER INFECTIOUS & PARASITIC DISEASES DIAGNOSES
424	19	P	O.R. PROCEDURE W PRINCIPAL DIAGNOSES OF MENTAL ILLNESS
425	19	M	ACUTE ADJUST REACT & DISTURBANCES OF PSYCHOSOCIAL DYSFUNCTION
426	19	M	DEPRESSIVE NEUROSES
427	19	M	NEUROSES EXCEPT DEPRESSIVE
428	19	M	DISORDERS OF PERSONALITY & IMPULSE CONTROL
429	19	M	ORGANIC DISTURBANCES & MENTAL RETARDATION
430	19	M	PSYCHOSES
431	19	M	CHILDHOOD MENTAL DISORDERS
432	19	M	OTHER MENTAL DISORDER DIAGNOSES
433	20		ALCOHOL/DRUG ABUSE OR DEPENDENCE, LEFT AMA

Continued

Appendix 2-A: Continued

DRG	MDC	Type*	Definition
434	20		ALC/DRUG ABUSE OR DEPEND, DETOX OR OTH SYMPT TREAT W CC
435	20		ALC/DRUG ABUSE OR DEPEND, DETOX OR OTH SYMPT TREAT W/O CC
436	20		ALC/DRUG DEPENDENCE W REHABILITATION THERAPY
437	20		ALC/DRUG DEPENDENCE, COMBINED REHAB & DETOX THERAPY
438	20		NO LONGER VALID
439	21	P	SKIN GRAFTS FOR INJURIES
440	21	P	WOUND DEBRIDEMENTS FOR INJURIES
441	21	P	HAND PROCEDURES FOR INJURIES
442	21	P	OTHER O.R. PROCEDURES FOR INJURIES W CC
443	21	P	OTHER O.R. PROCEDURES FOR INJURIES W/O CC
444	21	M	MULTIPLE TRAUMA AGE >17 W CC
445	21	M	MULTIPLE TRAUMA AGE >17 W/O CC
446	21	M	MULTIPLE TRAUMA AGE 0–17
447	21	M	ALLERGIC REACTIONS AGE >17
448	21	M	ALLERGIC REACTIONS AGE 0–17
449	21	M	POISONING & TOXIC EFFECTS OF DRUGS AGE >17 W CC
450	21	M	POISONING & TOXIC EFFECTS OF DRUGS AGE >17 W/O CC
451	21	M	POISONING & TOXIC EFFECTS OF DRUGS AGE 0–17
452	21	M	COMPLICATIONS OF TREATMENT W CC
453	21	M	COMPLICATIONS OF TREATMENT W/O CC
454	21	M	OTHER INJURY, POISONING & TOXIC EFFECT DIAG W CC
455	21	M	OTHER INJURY, POISONING & TOXIC EFFECT DIAG W/O CC
456	22		BURNS, TRANSFERRED TO ANOTHER ACUTE CARE FACILITY
457	22	M	EXTENSIVE BURNS W/O O.R. PROCEDURE
458	22	P	NON-EXTENSIVE BURNS W SKIN GRAFT
459	22	P	NON-EXTENSIVE BURNS W WOUND DEBRIDEMENT OR OTHER O.R. PROC
460	22	M	NON-EXTENSIVE BURNS W/O O.R. PROCEDURE
461	23	P	O.R. PROC W DIAGNOSES OF OTHER CONTACT W HEALTH SERVICES
462	23	M	REHABILITATION
463	23	M	SIGNS & SYMPTOMS W CC
464	23	M	SIGNS & SYMPTOMS W/O CC
465	23	M	AFTERCARE W HISTORY OF MALIGNANCY AS SECONDARY DIAGNOSIS
466	23	M	AFTERCARE W/O HISTORY OF MALIGNANCY AS SECONDARY DIAGNOSIS

Continued

Appendix 2-A: Continued

DRG	MDC	Type*	Definition
467	23	M	OTHER FACTORS INFLUENCING HEALTH STATUS
468	**		UNRELATED OPERATING ROOM PROCEDURES
469	**		PRINCIPAL DIAGNOSIS INVALID AS DISCHARGE DIAGNOSIS
470	**		UNGROUPABLE
471	08	P	BILATERAL OR MULTIPLE MAJOR JOINT PROCS OF LOWER EXTREMITY
472	22	P	EXTENSIVE BURNS W O.R. PROCEDURE
473	17		ACUTE LEUKEMIA W/O MAJOR O.R. PROCEDURE AGE >17
474	04		RESPIRATORY SYSTEM DIAGNOSIS WITH TRACHEOSTOMY
475	04	M	RESPIRATORY SYSTEM DIAGNOSIS WITH VENTILATOR SUPPORT

3

Refinement

Jean L. Freeman, Robert B. Fetter, Hayoung Park, Karen C. Schneider, Jeffrey L. Lichtenstein, William A. Bauman, Charles C. Duncan, John S. Hughes, Daniel H. Freeman, Jr., and George R. Palmer

The diagnosis-related groups (DRGs) have evolved over the past 20 years from a series of revisions designed to accommodate updates in diagnostic and procedure coding, changes in medical practice patterns, and advances in medical technology. Selected groups have also been redefined on the basis of findings from studies evaluating the system's clinical coherence and predictive validity. Before the introduction of Medicare's Prospective Payment System (PPS) in 1983, these modifications represented major changes in both the structure and content of the groups and were largely implemented under research projects conducted by the Health Systems Management Group at Yale University. Since 1983 the system has been reviewed and revised yearly for the Medicare program by the Health Care Financing Administration. States with all-payer systems have also introduced revisions, particularly to the pediatric groups.

While these enhancements have considerably improved the system's ability to measure more precisely the complexity of a hospital's case mix, there is still concern that the DRGs do not adequately account for one factor potentially associated with complexity—the severity of a patient's illness. This has been a particularly important issue since the implementation of DRGs for payment purposes. If patients with greater severity cost more to treat and DRGs do not adequately differentiate

This chapter describes the work of "DRG Refinement with Diagnostic Specific Comorbidities and Complications: A Synthesis of Current Approaches to Patient Classification," (final report of cooperative agreements nos. 15-C-98930/1-01 and 17-C-98930/1-0251 between the Health Care Financing Administration (HFCA) and Yale University: Robert B. Fetter, principal investigator; Jean L. Freeman, co-principal investigator; Harry L. Savitt, project officer; January 1989.

them, then hospitals having a higher proportion of such cases may be faced with rates under PPS that are too low to cover the costs of providing services. There is also some concern that hospitals may refuse to treat patients they perceive as very ill and more costly to treat. Hence, it is often argued that not adjusting for severity of illness may lead to payment inequities and limited access to care for selected groups of patients.

A number of patient classification schemes, representing alternatives or refinements to the DRGs, have attempted to address this issue. They include disease staging; the Severity of Illness Index; the Computerized Severity of Illness Index; "patient management categories"; the Medical Illness Severity Grouping System (MEDISGRPs); Acute Physiology and Chronic Health Evaluation (APACHE); and the Body Systems Approach of the Commission on Professional and Hospital Activities (CPHA). Each of these classification schemes has its own particular strengths and weaknesses. In fact, each is based on a different concept of severity, such as "risk of death" for disease staging and "total burden of illness" for the Severity of Illness Index.

While severity of illness may not be defined or measured consistently across systems, there is general agreement that patients with two or more diagnoses tend to be "sicker" than patients with a single, relatively minor condition. Moreover, the level and type of services required to treat some diseases or perform some procedures is likely to depend on the presence of other diagnoses. For example, patients with elective surgery and major complications on average require more nursing care, laboratory tests, units of blood, medications, and routine services than patients with no major complications or comorbidities.

A study conducted at Yale University with funding from the Health Care Financing Administration refined the DRGs using diagnosis and procedure-specific comorbidities and complications to define the more complex types of patients with higher levels of resource utilization. The refinement approach therefore incorporates important contributions from previous DRG development studies and research projects related to the development of alternative patient classification schemes. This chapter provides a brief overview of these schemes and describes the goals, methods, and findings of the DRG refinement study.

OVERVIEW OF SEVERITY CLASSIFICATION SYSTEMS

Disease Staging

Disease staging defines increasing levels of disease severity in terms of biological progression and complications (such as infection, obstruction, or hemorrhage).[1] Under this system, diseases are first assigned to one of

420 "staged disease categories" and then divided into four stages of increasing severity, which describe the extent of complications and systemic involvement: (1) conditions with no complications, (2) problems limited to an organ or system, (3) multiple site involvement, (4) death. Physicians initially developed criteria for each stage based on objective clinical findings (clinical disease staging). The stages were then operationally defined by combinations of diagnostic codes from the *International Classification of Diseases, Ninth Revision, Clinical Modification*, or ICD-9-CM (coded disease staging). Since stages are disease-specific, they are not comparable across diseases. That is, a stage 2 for one condition (for example, cancer) may not necessarily represent the same level of severity as a stage 2 for another condition (for example, diabetes).

Although the stages were not specifically constructed to differentiate patients with respect to utilization patterns, there is some evidence that patients with a more severe stage use more resources than those with a less severe stage.[2,3] There is also evidence that a redefinition of selected DRGs based on disease staging results in groups with "greater clinical validity" and "greater homogeneity in resource consumption."[4]

A patient level severity scale (Q-Scale) based on disease staging has recently been developed that incorporates the stages of each patient's diseases into a single measure.[5] The measure is expressed as a percentage of the average severity of some population (for example, Medicare beneficiaries). Q-Scale values may be used to adjust for severity both within and across DRGs. For example, a patient's Q-Scale of 150 within a given DRG indicates that this patient's severity level is 50 percent higher than the population's average severity for that DRG.

"Patient Management Categories"

"Patient management categories" (PMCs) differentiate patients according to the diagnostic and therapeutic services required for their care. That is, patients "requiring a different diagnostic and treatment strategy for effective care" are classified into different PMCs.[6] The system initially partitions patients into 47 disease modules or disease groups. Each group is then divided into PMCs on the basis of selected elements of the Uniform Hospital Discharge Data Set (UHDDS), particularly diagnoses and procedures. Like disease staging, the categories were initially described by clinicians and then operationally defined in terms of specific combinations of diagnostic and procedure codes. Physician panels also specified a set of services required to treat a typical patient within each PMC. In addition, a "normative cost weight" was developed for each PMC.

Three contributions from the PMC research regarding the association between additional diagnoses and hospital resource use have important implications for DRG refinement. First, the physicians constructing the PMCs recognized that "several interrelated diagnoses may, in fact, represent only one manifestation...of a single disease process."[7] Hence, the presence of additional diagnoses may not indicate a comorbid condition requiring a different set or increased quantity of hospital services to treat. Second, a hierarchy of PMCs was developed for each disease group, ranging from categories representing the more severely ill or difficult-to-treat patients to the least complicated types of cases. Third, analyses of hospital cost data aggregated by PMC revealed that more severely ill patients were "not necessarily the most costly to manage."[8]

CPHA's Body Systems Approach

The Body Systems Approach of the Commission on Professional and Hospital Activities (CPHA) defines increasing levels of disease severity according to the number of body systems affected.[9] The method involves assigning each diagnosis (principal and additional) on a patient's discharge abstract to a "major diagnostic category" (MDC), which is based on the DRG definition of those categories. The number of distinct MDCs represented is then the patient's severity score. Developers of the system have found that "average length of stay increases as the number of body systems affected increases."[10]

Severity of Illness Index

Horn's Severity of Illness Index (SII) is a four-level severity score assigned to a patient based on the values of seven variables "related to patient burden of illness."[11] These seven variables are:

— Stage of the principal diagnosis
— Concurrent interacting conditions
— Rate of response to therapy
— Impairment remaining after therapy
— Complications of the principal diagnosis
— Dependency on hospital staff
— Extent of non-operating-room procedures

Assignment of a severity score by this method involves two steps. First, a specially trained abstractor reviews the record and scores each of the above variables into one of four levels of increasing severity. The rater then assigns an overall score, ranging from 1 to 4, "by implicitly integrating the values of these seven variables."[12]

Analyses indicate that three of the variables (stage, complications, and interacting conditions) account for 68 to 75 percent of the variation in the overall severity index.[13] Stage of the principal diagnosis is defined as "the peak extent of organ involvement as manifested in peak symptoms and disability during hospitalization."[14] While it is conceptually very similar to disease staging, the clinical and coded definitions are *not* the same. Complications of the principal diagnosis include additional diagnoses that are "direct consequences of the principal diagnosis disease process," adverse effects of the patient's therapy, and hospital-acquired diseases, such as nosocomial infections.[15] Additional diagnoses, other than complications, that affect the course of hospitalization are considered interactions.

Computerized Severity Index (CSI)

The CSI is an outgrowth or "second generation" version of Horn's manual Severity of Illness Index.[16] It measures severity in terms of the patient's total burden of illness, expressed as the extent and interaction of diseases. Under this system, severity criteria sets have been developed for over 700 diagnostic categories based on aggregations of the ICD-9-CM codes. These criteria sets define four levels of severity within each group as a function of signs and symptoms, laboratory tests, and radiological findings. For example, the criteria for determining the severity of pneumonia are based in part on pulse rate, temperature, white blood cell count, and pleural discomfort. A patient is assigned a severity score from 1 to 4 for each diagnosis. An overall severity score is derived from a weighted combination of the severity levels corresponding to each diagnosis (principal and additional). The CSI system and MEDISGRPs (described below) are similar in that each is based on a broad set of clinical findings. The major difference is that CSI scores are disease-specific and the MEDISGRPs score is not.

Medical Illness Severity Grouping System (MEDISGRPs)

The Medical Illness Severity Grouping System (MEDISGRPs) utilizes objective clinical findings to classify patients into one of five groups based on severity at admission, where severity is defined in terms of "potential for organ failure."[17] Subsequent evaluations may be performed during the course of the patient's hospital stay to monitor response to therapy.

Assignment of an admission severity score is a three-step process. First, a patient's chart is reviewed and key clinical findings (KCFs) are recorded. KCFs are "objective indicators of an abnormal situation" and include results from laboratories and radiology and pathology tests as well as findings from the physical examination. In the second step each KCF is assigned to a severity class or level based on the likelihood of organ failure. Criteria for this assignment have been developed by Medi-Qual Systems, Inc., but the information is not publicly available.

Finally, an overall severity score from 0 to 4 is assigned to a patient on the basis of the level of severity for each KCF (see Table 3-1). Brewster et al.[18] provide a general description of patients within each severity score. It should be noted that the MEDISGRPs severity score is not disease-specific and a patient's most severe KCF may not be related to the principal reason for admission.

Subsequent reviews evaluate acute or subacute morbidity arising during the course of a hospital stay.[19] For these reviews, the MEDISGRPs algorithm assigns patients to one of three levels: no significant morbidity, minor morbidity, or major morbidity.

Acute Physiology and Chronic Health Evaluation (APACHE II)

APACHE II is a severity-of-illness classification system based on 12 physiologic measures: vital signs (heart rate, mean blood pressure, respiratory rate, temperature, and Glasgow Coma Score), findings obtained from venous blood tests (hematocrit and white blood cell count, serum potassium, serum sodium, and serum creatinine), and results of arterial blood gas tests (serum pH and PaO_2).[20] Values for these tests are categorized into five levels of increasing abnormality. Corresponding weights are then attached to each level ranging from 0 (normal) to 4 (highly abnormal). These 12 measurements are obtained on patients within 24

Table 3-1: MEDISGRPs Admission Severity Scores

Score	Meaning
0	No significant findings
1	Minimal findings, indicating a low potential for organ failure
2	Either acute findings connoting a short time course with an unclear potential for organ failure, or severe findings with high potential for organ failure
3	Both acute and severe findings indicating a high potential for imminent organ failure
4	Critical findings indicating the presence of organ failure

Source: A. C. Brewster, B. G. Karlin, L. A. Hyde, C. M. Jacobs, R. C. Bradbury, and Y. M. Chae, "MEDISGRPs: A Clinically Based Approach to Classifying Hospital Patients at Admission," *Inquiry* 22 (1985): 377–87.

hours of admission. Weights corresponding to the categories containing each patient's test results are then totaled across all 12 measurements. The sum of these weights, plus weights assigned for age and chronic health status, yields the patient's total APACHE II severity score.

The system was designed principally to describe groups of intensive care unit patients and to evaluate their care. It has been found that APACHE II scores are strongly associated with hospital mortality.

Summary

Developers of these severity classification techniques have proposed ways in which their systems might be used to replace or refine DRGs for payment, management, and quality control purposes. These methods of patient classification, however, are actually derived from different definitions of severity. Disease staging, for example, defines severity in terms of risk of death. The Severity of Illness Index attempts to measure severity in terms of total burden of illness. For MEDISGRPs, severity is defined in terms of potential for organ failure. Finally, CPHA's Body Systems Approach defines increasing levels of disease severity by the number of body systems affected.

In spite of these conceptual differences in definition of severity, the operational definitions of these systems—how they place patients into severity categories—are remarkably similar in one important respect. Most have considered additional diagnoses—diagnoses other than the principal—as extremely important factors in their models of resource use. In particular, disease staging operationally defines severity levels (stages) with combinations of ICD-9-CM codes that describe the extent of complications and systemic involvement. Likewise, "patient management categories" were initially described by clinicians and then operationally defined in terms of specific combinations of diagnosis and procedure codes. Finally, two of the variables used to construct the Severity of Illness Index—concurrent interacting conditions and complications of the principal diagnosis—assess the impact of additional diagnoses.

DRGs currently incorporate information on patients' additional diagnoses at the fourth or final level of the classification scheme. The general structure of the system is illustrated in Figure 1-4 (page 15). First, all patients are initially assigned to one of 23 "major diagnostic categories" (MDCs) on the basis of their principal diagnosis code. Second, within each MDC patients are categorized as surgical or medical based on the presence or absence, respectively, of an operating room procedure. Third, medical patients are categorized into subgroups based on principal diagnosis and surgical patients into subgroups based on operating room procedures. These subgroups of medical and surgical patients are usually referred to as adjacent DRGs or ADRGs. Examples of medical ADRGs from the respiratory system are pulmonary embolism, pleural effusion, simple pneumonia and pleurisy, and bronchitis and asthma. Examples of surgical ADRGs from the nervous system are craniotomy, spinal procedures, and carpal tunnel release. Finally, each of the surgical and nonsurgical ADRGs may be divided further on the basis of other variables, including whether or not the patient had a substantial comorbidity or complication.

A substantial comorbidity or complication is defined by a list of diagnosis codes that a panel of physicians felt would increase the length of stay by at least one day for 75 percent of the patients. This list covers a broad spectrum of disease conditions from major acute illnesses, such as heart attack and stroke, to relatively minor acute illnesses and chronic conditions, such as otitis media and chronic obstructive pulmonary disease.

In summary, while there are diverse ways of defining severity, research into alternative measures of patient classification has provided considerable evidence that DRG definitions could be improved by differentiating patients with respect to specific comorbidities and complications. In particular, a hierarchy of additional diagnoses, which may be specific to particular diagnostic and procedure categories, is supported by other models of the disease process and its treatment in the hospital setting.

OBJECTIVES OF DRG REFINEMENT

The principal objective of DRG refinement was to replace the list of substantial comorbidities and complications (CCs) with sets of CCs that represent different levels of resource use. The ultimate goal was to build a model whose structure is illustrated in Figure 3-1. Under this model there are classes of additional diagnoses, each associated with a different level or type of hospital services for a given ADRG. Based on previous research, it was expected that this gradient would differ depending on the diagnostic or procedure category. That is, certain additional diagnoses would have a strong influence on resource use in one ADRG but not in another.

DEVELOPMENT OF CC CLASSES

The construction of ADRG-specific categories of CCs was a multistage process that involved both statistical analyses of hospital discharge data

Figure 3-1: Proposed Structure of DRG Classification with Refinement

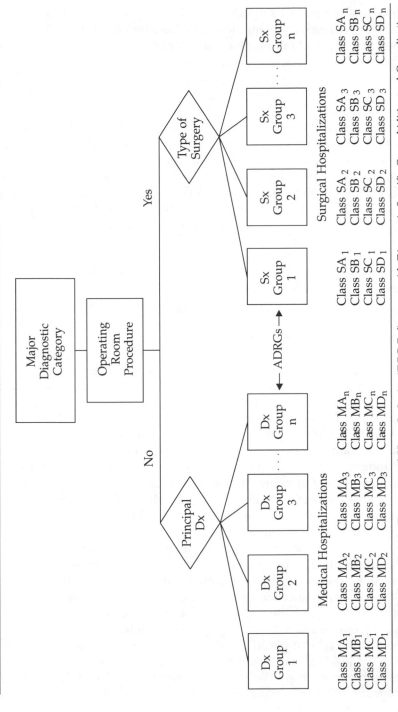

Source: Robert B. Fetter, Jean L. Freeman, and Harry L. Savitt, "DRG Refinement with Diagnostic Specific Comorbidities and Complications: A Synthesis of Current Approaches to Patient Classification."

and clinical review of the findings. Methods pertaining to the four principal stages of model development are described in detail in the study's final report. A brief summary of each stage is presented in this chapter.

Stage 1

In the first step of stage 1, the impact of comorbidities and complications (CCs) on hospital charges and length of stay was examined for patients in ADRGs from MDC 4, diseases and disorders of the respiratory system. Mean charges and lengths of stay were calculated for all individual additional diagnoses from the DRG CC list that appeared for any patient within an ADRG. These individual CC diagnoses were then aggregated into groups based on their clinical similarity and the similarity of their impact on resource use.

These groups of CCs very closely resembled the original medical DRGs, except that diagnoses not on the CC list had been eliminated. Therefore, for subsequent analyses, the CC diagnoses were assembled into "CADRGs" (which are in effect "CC groups") based on the ADRG that the CC would be assigned as a principal diagnosis.[21] For example, the ADRG and CADRG for the diagnostic category "hypertension" are given in Table 3-2. On the left are listed all the principal diagnosis codes that define this group and on the right are all the codes from the CC list that fall into this category as additional diagnoses. Note that only the subset of malignant hypertension codes are part of the CC list. This initial grouping of CC codes into categories was performed for two reasons. First, some preliminary analyses suggested these categories were clinically reasonable, with some exceptions that were edited. Moreover, aggregating the 2,958 CC codes into 136 CADRGs greatly facilitated the implementation and interpretation of the subsequent data analyses.

Once the CADRGs were formed, members of the study's physician panel identified those additional diagnoses (CADRGs) that they expected to be associated with increased resource utilization for each ADRG. Toward this end, some general guidelines were developed from the literature to identify the potentially significant CADRGs. These guidelines are based on the expectation that the presence of additional diagnoses will affect resource use if those diagnoses influence either the hospital course of treatment or the patient's response to therapy. On the basis of previous research, these diagnoses may be broadly classified into three groups: (1) complications of the principal diagnosis that require a prolonged hospital stay and more specialized services to treat, (2) other disease processes (comorbidities) that require additional diagnostic and therapeutic services during the hospitalization, and (3) conditions that

Table 3-2: Diagnosis Codes in the ADRG and CADRG for Hypertension

ADRG		CADRG	
4010	MALIGNANT HYPERTENSION	4010	MALIGNANT HYPERTENSION
4011	BENIGN HYPERTENSION		
4019	HYPERTENSION NOS		
40200	MAL HYPERTEN HRT DIS NOS	40200	MAL HYPERTEN HRT DIS NOS
40210	BEN HYPERTEN HRT DIS NOS		
40290	HYPERTENSIVE HRT DIS NOS		
4040	MAL HYPERT HRT/ RENAL DIS	4040	MAL HYPERTEN HRT/ RENAL DIS
4041	BEN HYPERT HRT/ RENAL DIS		
4049	HYPERT HRT/RENAL DIS NOS		
40501	MAL RENOVASC HYPERTENS	40501	MAL RENOVASC HYPERTENS
40509	MAL SECOND HYPERT NEC	40509	MAL SECOND HYPERTEN NEC
40511	BENIGN RENOVASC HYPERTEN		
40519	BENIGN SECOND HYPERT NEC		
40591	RENOVASC HYPERTENSION		
40599	SECOND HYPERTENSION NEC		

Source: "DRG Refinement with Diagnostic Specific Comorbidities and Complications."

arise as a result of the hospital stay or as a direct result of the services provided.

Complications of the principal diagnosis include additional diagnoses that are direct consequences of or in some sense caused by the principal disease process. For example, gastrointestinal bleeding is a possible complication of diverticular disease. Comorbidities represent diseases and disorders that are actively managed or may affect the active management of the conditions (procedures) in the ADRG. Hence, comorbidity CADRGs should either require additional acute care services to treat beyond that normally provided to patients in the ADRG or prolong the patient's response to therapy. Finally, complications of treatment include adverse effects of the patient's therapy and hospital-acquired diseases. Such CADRGs would include potential complications of surgery (for example, pulmonary embolism) and complications that may arise as a result of the hospital stay (for example, aspiration pneumonia and decubitus ulcer).

Stage 2

After the physicians generated their initial hypotheses regarding the effect of these CADRGs on resource use within an ADRG, discharge data for adult patients in Maryland and California hospitals were screened with a forward selection procedure that identified the statistically significant associations. Under the forward selection process, variables were added (but not deleted) one at a time to the regression model according to the values of their partial F statistics. That is, at each step the variable selected to enter the model had the largest significant F statistic among the variables that were not included in the model at the $p < .10$ level. This interactive process continued until no more variables met the inclusion criteria ($p < .10$).

Descriptive statistics were also generated in this stage to identify any anomalies or outliers in the data. Of particular interest were sets of observations about which the model did not predict well. Two variables, temporary tracheostomy and early death (death within two days of admission), were found to be strongly associated with unusually long and short lengths of stay, respectively. The effect of these variables on resource use was the focus of special substudies conducted by members of the physician panel.[22] In terms of the analysis, discharges of patients with these characteristics were isolated as special subgroups ("early death" and "temporary tracheostomy") and the regression executed on the remaining observations in the data base.

Stage 3

Classes were then assigned to those additional diagnoses in the third stage that were either selected by the regression model or hypothesized as significant by the physicians. The algorithm for assigning classes to the medical and surgical hospitalizations in each data base was based on both length of stay and charges, and on absolute as well as percentage increases (see Table 3-3). That is, both increases in length of stay and charges for patients in each CADRG were examined relative to the group of baseline patients with no substantial comorbidities and complications in terms of both days and charges as well as percentage increases. With respect to Maryland data, for example, class B CADRGs for the medical hospitalizations are those where the difference was greater than one week or $3,000 or the increase in charges or days was over 150 percent. Lower bounds for the classes B, C, and D were essentially the same for medical

Table 3-3: Criteria Used for Class Assignment of CADRGs

DL = (mean LOS for patients with the CADRG) − (mean LOS for baseline patients)

DC = (mean charge for patients with the CADRG) − (mean charge for baseline patients)

RL = DL/(mean LOS for baseline patients)

RC = DC/(mean charge for baseline patients)

Medical Hospitalizations

Maryland

Class B if DL > 7 or DC > 3,000 or RL > 1.5 or RC > 1.5
         C if 1 < DL ≤ 7 or 400 < DC ≤ 3,000 or .2 < RL ≤ 1.5 or .2 < RC ≤ 1.5
         D if DL ≤ 1 or DC ≤ 400 or RL ≤ .2 or RC ≤ .2

California

Class B if DL > 7 or DC > 4,500 or RL > 1.5 or RC > 1.5
         C if 1 < DL ≤ 7 or 600 < DC ≤ 4,500 or .2 < RL ≤ 1.5 or .2 < RC ≤ 1.5
         D if DL ≤ 1 or DC ≤ 600 or RL ≤ .2 or RC ≤ .2

Surgical Hospitalizations

Maryland

Class A if DL > 14 or DC > 9,000 or RL > 3 or RC > 3
         B if 7 < DL ≤ 14 or 4,500 < DC ≤ 9,000 or 1.5 < RL ≤ 3 or 1.5 < RC ≤ 3
         C if 1 < DL ≤ 7 or 600 < DC ≤ 4,500 or .2 < RL ≤ 1.5 or .2 < RC ≤ 1.5
         D if DL ≤ 1 or DC ≤ 600 or RL ≤ .2 or RC ≤ .2

California

Class A if DL > 14 or DC > 15,000 or RL > 3 or RC > 3
         B if 7 < DL ≤ 14 or 7,500 < DC ≤ 15,000 or 1.5 < RL ≤ 3 or 1.5 < RC < 3
         C if 1 < DL ≤ 7 or 1,000 < DC ≤ 7,500 or .2 < RL ≤ 1.5 or .2 < RC ≤ 1.5
         D if DL ≤ 1 or DC ≤ 1,000 or RL ≤ .2 or RC ≤ .2

Source: "DRG Refinement with Diagnostic Specific Comorbidities and Complications."

and surgical hospitalizations, but differed across the two data bases.[23] Class boundaries were based on (1) a review of the distribution of patients with respect to these differences, (2) whether or not the contents of the classes were reasonable from a clinical perspective, and (3) the original definition of a CC (hence the one-day threshold for class D). The algorithm is hierarchical, so that CADRGs meeting the criteria for multiple classes were assigned the highest class.

It was found in preliminary analyses that additional diagnoses had a much stronger effect for surgical cases than for medical hospitalizations. The stronger association between additional diagnoses and resource use for surgical cases was attributed to the patients' having two serious conditions—surgery and a major illness. When the trauma of surgery is added to the trauma of a severe medical condition, the patient becomes more severely ill than when there is the same medical condition and no surgery. In particular, surgical patients with some CCs were provided over three times the services that patients with no CCs received. These additional diagnoses for surgical patients were considered "catastrophic" in their effect on resource use. A fourth class (class A) was therefore created for these extreme cases.

Stage 4

Findings from both the California and Maryland data bases were then examined and reviewed by the physician panel for clinical interpretability. Of particular interest was whether a given CADRG, or additional diagnosis category, had the same effect (was assigned the same class) across all the different types of medical and surgical hospitalizations. In other words, the physicians looked for the presence of interactions—instances where, for example, the additional diagnosis was a class B for one principal diagnosis category and class C for another.

To facilitate this review, a number of tables were constructed to summarize the results. One of these summaries presented the percentage distribution of medical and surgical discharges in the two data bases by class for each additional diagnosis category or CADRG. Table 3-4 provides information from this table for a few high-volume CADRGs. It presents, for selected CADRGs, the percent of medical discharges with the CADRG that were assigned class B, C, and D. The percent is based on Maryland and California discharges combined. These selected CADRGs represent the two trends found in reviewing the table, either (1) a large proportion of the discharges in one category, indicating a consistent effect across different types of medical hospitalizations; or (2) an equal distribution of discharges across two or three classes, indicating the presence of interactions or differential resource use by ADRG.

It was this latter set of CADRGs that required the most review. In particular, the physicians reviewed the class assignment for these CADRGs by individual ADRGs. They identified those ADRGs where the different pattern of resource use could be interpreted in light of some underlying model of the disease or treatment process.

In constructing the final model it was decided to assign each CADRG first to a class (M_B, M_C, M_D for medical hospitalizations; S_A, S_B, S_C, S_D for

Table 3-4: Percent Distribution of Discharges in Maryland and California Data Bases by Class within Selected High-Frequency CADRGs

	Class		
Medical Discharges	*B*	*C*	*D*
Other disorders of the eye	5.6	90.5	3.9
Respiratory infections and inflammations	97.8	1.9	0.2
Cardiac arrest, unexplained	95.8	4.1	0.1
Specific cerebrovascular disorders exc TIA	63.8	35.3	0.9
Pneumothorax	51.2	46.8	2.0
Gastrointestinal hemorrhage	44.1	54.0	1.9

Source: "DRG Refinement with Diagnostic Specific Comorbidities and Complications."

surgical hospitalizations) based on how the majority of discharges in the combined Maryland and California data bases were assigned. Then, ADRG exceptions were made under the following conditions:

— Both data bases provided strong evidence of an interaction.

— The physician panel agreed on a plausible explanation for the differential resource use.

— The ADRG contained a high volume of patients relative to other ADRGs.

For example, the CADRG for pneumothorax was part of class M_B for all ADRGs except those with related diagnoses—lung cancer, major chest trauma, pleural effusion, pulmonary symptoms, and other pulmonary disorders. For those ADRG exceptions, pneumothorax was part of class M_C. This not only makes sense medically but is borne out by the data.

FINAL DRG REFINEMENT MODEL

The analyses and clinical review conducted in the four stages resulted in the DRG refinement model illustrated in Figure 3-2. Under this model, patients are initially assigned to one of 23 major diagnostic categories (MDCs) based on their principal diagnosis code. These MDCs are identical to the ones defined under the fifth revision of the DRGs.

Within each MDC, except MDC 3 (diseases and disorders of the ear, nose, and throat), patients with a temporary tracheostomy are isolated as an initial group and are not considered further in the classification process. The remaining patients are then categorized as surgical or medical based on the presence or absence, respectively, of an operating room

Figure 3-2: Structure of Refined DRG Classification with Medical and Surgical Classes of Additional Diagnoses*

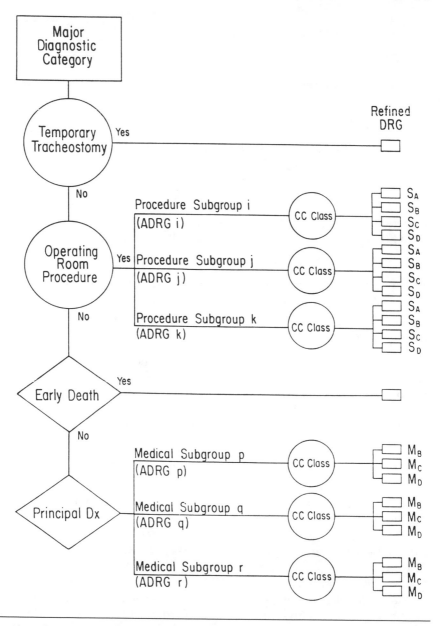

*Some exceptions to the system-wide definition of classes are made for specific ADRGs.
Source: "DRG Refinement with Diagnostic Specific Comorbidities and Complications."

procedure. In MDC 3 the initial tracheostomy group contains only medical patients with a temporary tracheostomy, since the procedure is often part of the normal course of treatment for surgical patients.

Medical patients who died within two days of admission form a separate DRG referred to as "early death." All other medical patients (that is, those *not* classified as "early death" or temporary tracheostomy) are placed in subgroups based on their principal diagnosis. Likewise, the remaining surgical patients (that is, those *not* classified as "temporary tracheostomy") are placed in subgroups according to the operating room procedures performed on them. These medical and surgical subgroups are referred to as adjacent DRGs or ADRGs. The remaining medical patients (that is, those *not* classified as "early death" or "temporary tracheostomy") are placed in subgroups based on their principal diagnosis and the remaining surgical patients (that is, those *not* classified as "temporary tracheostomy") in subgroups by operating room procedures.

Finally, patients in each of the medical and surgical ADRGs are divided into final groups (DRGs) based on classes of additional diagnoses developed in stages 1 through 4 of the study. The classes for medical hospitalizations represent subsets of additional diagnoses on the fifth revision's comorbidities and complications (CC) list that have a major (M_B), moderate (M_C), and minor/no (M_D) effect on resource use. Likewise, for surgical hospitalizations the classes represent those with a catastrophic (S_A), major (S_B), moderate (S_C), and minor/no (S_D) effect. For completeness, M_D and S_D contain both (1) additional diagnoses on the CC list that were neither expected by the physician panel to increase resource use nor found to be associated with charges or length of stay in the utilization analyses and (2) all additional diagnoses not on the CC list.

For the most part, the composition of the medical classes is the same for the medical ADRGs and the composition of the surgical classes is the same for surgical ADRGs. That is, there are standard or generic sets of diagnosis codes that define the classes for all medical (M_B, M_C, M_D) and surgical (S_A, S_B, S_C, S_D) hospitalizations. Examples of diagnoses in the generic classes are given in Table 3-5.

There are some exceptions, however, to the generic definitions of the classes for specific ADRGs. As was discussed above, exceptions were made in constructing the model when the data indicated an additional diagnosis had a differential effect on resource use depending on the patient's principal diagnosis (medical ADRG) or major operating room procedure (surgical ADRG). In general, the exceptions are of two types. First, exceptions exist when the additional diagnosis commonly occurs as part of the disease process and does not require additional services to treat. For example, pleural effusion is a member of the generic class B

Table 3-5: Examples of Diagnoses in Medical and Surgical Classes

Medical Classes	Surgical Classes
	A Catastrophic 0388 OTHER SPECIFIED SEPTICEMIAS 436 CEREBROVASCULAR ACCIDENT 4100 ACUTE MYOCARDIAL INFARCTION OF ANTEROLATERAL WALL
B Major 0388 OTHER SPECIFIED SEPTICEMIAS 436 CEREBROVASCULAR ACCIDENT 4100 ACUTE MYOCARDIAL INFARCTION OF ANTEROLATERAL WALL	*B Major* 4372 HYPERTENSIVE ENCEPHALOPATHY 5609 UNSPECIFIED INTESTINAL OBSTRUCTION 6826 CELLULITIS OF LEG, EXCEPT FOOT
C Moderate 1629 MALIGNANT NEOPLASM OF BRONCHUS AND LUNG, UNSPECIFIED 4919 UNSPECIFIED CHRONIC BRONCHITIS 5715 CIRRHOSIS OF LIVER WITHOUT MENTION OF ALCOHOL 5609 UNSPECIFIED INTESTINAL OBSTRUCTION 4372 HYPERTENSIVE ENCEPHALOPATHY 6826 CELLULITIS OF LEG, EXCEPT FOOT	*C Moderate* 1629 MALIGNANT NEOPLASM OF BRONCHUS AND LUNG, UNSPECIFIED 4919 UNSPECIFIED CHRONIC BRONCHITIS 5715 CIRRHOSIS OF LIVER WITHOUT MENTION OF ALCOHOL
D Minor 4011 BENIGN HYPERTENSION 4660 ACUTE BRONCHITIS 7242 LUMBAGO	*D Minor* 4011 BENIGN HYPERTENSION 4660 ACUTE BRONCHITIS 7242 LUMBAGO

Source: "DRG Refinement with Diagnostic Specific Comorbidities and Complications."

for most medical ADRGs. However, for the ADRG corresponding to pulmonary embolism it is a member of class C. Second, exceptions exist when the additional diagnosis complicates in some way the treatment of the principal diagnosis or surgical procedure. For example, additional

Table 3-6: Matrix Representation of DRG Refinement with Estimated Mean Charges for Medicare Patients, 1986

Medical Hospitalizations

Diagnostic Category	Class		
	M_B	M_C	M_D
Spinal disorders and injuries	$10,855	$5,386	$4,507
Specific cerebrovascular disorders except TIA	$10,639	$5,776	$4,348
Simple pneumonia and pleurisy	$ 8,238	$5,026	$3,721
Heart failure and shock	$ 8,142	$4,521	$3,447
Esophagitis, gastroenteritis, and miscellaneous digestive diseases	$ 6,663	$3,042	$2,292
Medical back problems	$ 6,517	$3,706	$2,892
Diabetes, age >35	$ 8,080	$3,660	$2,656
Other factors influencing health status	$ 4,676	$2,482	$1,630

Source: "DRG Refinement with Diagnostic Specific Comorbidities and Complications."

diagnoses indicating spinal disorders are members of the generic class C for most medical hospitalizations. However, for the ADRGs corresponding to medical back problems and rehabilitation they are part of class B.

With the refinement model, a hospital's product lines can therefore be represented as a matrix of disease and procedure categories by classes. Table 3-6 is a portion of that matrix for the medical hospitalizations. The rows are the principal diagnosis subcategories (ADRGs) from spinal disorders and injuries to other factors influencing health status. Listed are selected high frequency groups particularly for the Medicare population. The cells then contain information about the production process, in this case the mean charges for Medicare patients in 1986. Note the gradient in charges across classes. M_D is the baseline class containing patients with no or minor CCs. Average charges increase about $1,000 from D to C and about $3,000 to $4,000 from C to B.

CONCLUSION

In several ways, the DRGs refined in this manner represent a substantial improvement over the current version of the groups. First of all, the underlying rationale for this approach is based on previous DRG development studies and the work of others involved in alternative case-mix classification systems. As was noted above, specific combinations of principal and additional diagnoses have been used to define different levels of severity and complexity of treatment in disease staging, "patient management categories," and the Severity of Illness Index, as well as in CPHA's Body Systems Approach. Hence, the refinements are an extension of an already well-established base of research.

Second, by identifying patients with very serious conditions (such as septicemia or stroke) in the class structure, the clinical coherence of the scheme has been considerably enhanced. Moreover, the refined scheme may decrease incentives to "dump" or undertreat what are perceived to be the more costly types of patients.

Third, these refinements do not represent a radical departure from the current structure of the DRGs. The basic components of the classes, the CADRGs, are consistent with disease definitions at a higher level of the scheme. Moreover, implementation of the refined DRGs still requires only information that commonly appears on a hospital discharge abstract. In fact, the inherent matrix representation of the refined model makes the scheme conceptually and operationally much simpler than the old system. This matrix structure, with some modifications, will be evaluated for neonates in future research projects.

Finally, although the severity issue motivated this set of refinements, it is important to emphasize that the aim of the study was not a refinement based on severity as defined in terms of risk of death or organ failure. Rather, the goal was consistent with the original objective of DRGs: to identify groups of patients with similar resource profiles. This was accomplished by defining more precisely a hospital's product lines in terms of patient characteristics—comorbidities and complications—with different levels of resource use. In this light, the classes should be considered an adjustment for case complexity regardless of what made the case more complex.

ACKNOWLEDGMENTS

We would like to thank Jane Gau, Li-Qian Liu, Hsiao-Hsing Lo, Martin Mador, and Chunwei Wang for computer programming, and Thomas McGuire for technical assistance.

REFERENCES

1. M. D. Gonella, M. C. Hornbrook, and D. Z. Louis, "Staging of Disease: A Case-Mix Measurement," *Journal of the American Medical Association* 251, no. 5 (1984): 637–44.
2. J. E. Conklin, J. E. Lieberman, C. A. Barnes, and D. Z. Louis, "Disease Staging: Implications for Hospital Reimbursement and Management," *Health Care Financing Review*, supplement (1984): 13–22.
3. M. L. Garg, D. Z. Louis, W. A. Giliebe, C. S. Spirka, J. K. Skipper, and R. R. Parekh, "Evaluating Inpatient Costs: The Staging Mechanism," *Medical Care* 16, no. 3 (1978): 191–201.
4. Conklin et al., "Disease Staging," 20.
5. J. G. Christoffersson, J. E. Conklin, and J. Gonella, "The Impact of Severity of Illness on Hospital Costs," *DRG Monitor* 6, no. 1 (1988): 1–8.
6. W. W. Young, "Incorporating Severity of Illness and Comorbidity in Case-Mix Measurement," *Health Care Financing Review*, supplement (1984): 23–31.
7. Young, "Incorporating Severity," 24.
8. Young, "Incorporating Severity," 26.
9. S. Mendenhall, "DRGs Must Be Changed to Take Patient's Illness Severity into Account," *Modern Healthcare* 14, no. 15 (1984): 86–88.
10. Mendenhall, "DRGs Must Be Changed," 88.
11. S. D. Horn, P. D. Sharkey, and D. A. Bertram, "Measuring Severity of Illness: Homogeneous Case Mix Groups," *Medical Care* 21, no. 1 (1983): 14–30.
12. Ibid., 15.
13. S. D. Horn, "Measuring Severity: How Sick Is Sick? How Well Is Well?" *Healthcare Financial Management* (October 1986): 21–32.
14. Horn, "Measuring Severity of Illness," 26.
15. Ibid., 28.
16. Ibid.
17. A. C. Brewster, B. G. Karlin, L. A. Hyde, C. M. Jacobs, R. C. Bradbury, and Y. M. Chae, "MEDISGRPs: A Clinically Based Approach to Classifying Hospital Patients at Admission," *Inquiry* 22 (1985): 377–87.
18. Ibid.
19. L. I. Iezzoni, M. A. Moskowitz, and S. Asu, *The Ability of MEDISGRPs and Its Clinical Variables to Predict Cost and In-Hospital Death* (report to the Health Care Financing Administration under agreement no. 18-C-98526/1-04, July 1988).

20. D. P. Wagner and E. A. Draper, "Acute Physiology and Chronic Health Evaluation (APACHE II) and Medicare Reimbursement," *Health Care Financing Review* supplement (1984): 91–105.

21. The CC list appears in the *DRG Definitions Manual*, fifth revision (New Haven, CT: Health Systems International, 1987), 565–666.

22. J. S. Hughes, J. Lichtenstein, L. Magno, and R. B. Fetter, "Improving DRGs: Use of Procedure Codes for Assisted Respiration to Adjust for Complexity of Illness," *Medical Care*, in press.

23. Lower (and upper) bounds for charges were based on estimated charges per patient day, which differed in medical and surgical discharges.

Part II

Use of DRGs for Managing Hospital Resources

4

The Product-Line Management Model

Robert B. Fetter and Jean L. Freeman

The development of the DRG classification scheme was motivated largely by the desire to apply industrial management methods to hospital management. DRGs have allowed administrators to view the use and cost of hospital services in terms of "product lines." In the context of these product lines, various aspects of production and operations management commonly employed by manufacturing firms—quality control, cost accounting, and product selection and design—can be applied to hospitals for the purpose of increasing efficiency and quality of care.

This chapter describes the organizational structure required for the implementation of the product-line approach. The first section contrasts the traditional approach to hospital management, which focused on the functioning of a hospital's departments, with the product-line approach, which focuses on the set of services provided to each patient.

The next section explains the emphasis of product-line (or "matrix") management on both efficiency and effectiveness. Department managers are chiefly responsible for the efficient production of intermediate products, and physicians are responsible for the effective utilization of these products in treating patients. Unlike traditional hospital management structures, the product-line approach explicitly integrates physicians into the hospital's organizational structure.

The matrix model was originally applied to management in industry. It was, for example, incorporated in the space program to merge the work of managers and engineers. Because matrix management focuses on the final product, it is also referred to as product-line management. The identification of final "products" in hospitals allows the matrix model to

Portions of this chapter are adapted from Robert B. Fetter and Jean L. Freeman, "Diagnosis Related Groups: Product Line Management within Hospitals." *Academy of Management Review* 11, no. 1 (1986): 41–54, with the permission of the *Academy of Management Review*.

be applied to the hospital setting. The performance of both physicians and department managers can be monitored by analyzing resource use in the production of a hospital's products, that is, the care of patients in the various DRGs.

TRADITIONAL HOSPITAL MANAGEMENT

Traditionally, hospitals have been organized around operating departments, such as laboratory, radiology, and laundry. Department managers were responsible for expenditures in their departments; physicians were not formally integrated into this system.

The hospital chart in Figure 4-1 illustrates the position of the physician in a typical hospital. Physicians are loosely linked to the chain of command, as indicated by the dotted line. In the United States, very few physicians are hospital employees. Most serve as independent entrepreneurs using the hospital and its facilities on behalf of their patients. The various operating departments report to the associate directors and the associate directors report to the chief executive officer (CEO). There are two distinct types of operating departments—direct patient care departments (such as intensive care and operating room) and indirect patient care or overhead departments (such as linen service and housekeeping).

This structure implies that by managing the departments that produce various direct and indirect services employed in the diagnosis and treatment of illness, one is managing the institution. But the final product of a hospital is not clean linen, nutritional meals, or appropriate medications. Rather, the product of the hospital is the bundle of services, ordered by the physician and delivered to the patient in recognition of his or her needs. The hospital's products are its treated patients. If the services a hospital provides are not those that a patient needs, the hospital is not successful, even though it may produce and render services efficiently.

EFFICIENCY VERSUS EFFECTIVENESS

Both physicians and management influence hospital costs. If department managers do not produce services efficiently or if physicians order unnecessary services, then patient treatment costs may be excessive. Because of the unique contribution of each group, it is necessary to define their individual and collective responsibilities explicitly.

Management is chiefly responsible for the production of what we will call "intermediate products." Intermediate products are the goods and services provided by the various operating departments. They are referred to as intermediate products because they are used in the process

Figure 4-1: Typical Hospital Organization Chart

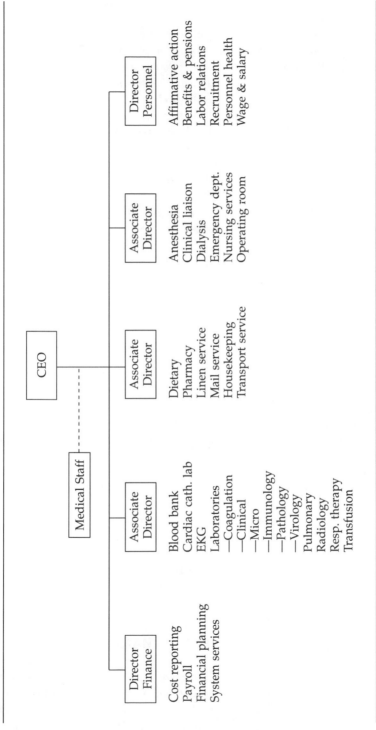

Source: Robert B. Fetter and Jean L. Freeman, "Product Line Management within Hospitals."

of treating a patient—a patient whose treatment, or bundle of services, is the final "product" of a hospital. It is in the production of these intermediate products that one can talk of the *efficiency* of production.

Efficiency refers to the production of a service at the lowest marginal cost (given a certain level of quality). Management is responsible for producing a service, such as a laboratory test, at the lowest cost and at a certain quality level. If a hospital is inefficient in the production of these intermediate products, the total cost of its ultimate product—treated patients—will be higher than necessary. Management alone is responsible and accountable for the production efficiency of these intermediate products.

While efficiency is a measure of the relative inputs required to produce a given output, effectiveness is a measure of success in producing a desired outcome. *Effectiveness* refers to the degree of success at achieving a desired outcome relative to the process employed. Using additional labor and materials in the production of a "standard" x-ray would constitute a lowered efficiency of production. Ordering more x-rays than are necessary to complete a given diagnosis would constitute a less effective use of resources.

Effectiveness is found in the utilization of the intermediate products that are necessary to diagnose and treat patients. Physicians utilize these intermediate products in "producing" different types of patient care and are thus responsible for the *effectiveness* with which they employ these resources. The definition of the effective use of the intermediate products will vary from DRG to DRG and from hospital to hospital, but, whatever the standard, it is clearly the responsibility of the physician to decide which services are needed.

It is clear that an organizational structure must monitor the efficiency of the production of intermediate products as well as the effective utilization of those products. Otherwise, the structure will capture only half the story. The appropriate structure will explicitly integrate the physician into the organization's management; this structure will manage patient care from both an efficiency and an effectiveness orientation. The following section will examine the evolution of the matrix structure in manufacturing and explore its uses in hospital management and financing.

MATRIX MANAGEMENT IN MANUFACTURING

The concept of matrix management evolved in the early 1960s. It was originally implemented by the aerospace industry in the effort to put a man on the moon. The matrix structure met the need of the space program to merge the work of managers and engineers in the process of manufacturing complex and unique products. Matrix management is useful in situations where groups of highly trained professionals with distinct sets of skills are joined in the production of a complex product.

Matrix management is a dual-authority management structure that places emphasis on technical progress as well as product development. The matrix consists of product designers (engineers) across the top and managers of individual support services, the intermediate products, along the side. The engineers, or program managers, are responsible for product development and the managers oversee the support services necessary to produce the product. At the intersection of these two axes one can assign responsibility to the manager of the support department or the product manager or both.

In Table 4-1 each product (guidance system, fuselage, landing mechanism) required the work of several intermediate product centers. The engineer who designed the product determined the type and amount of work required of each of the intermediate product centers in the production of the product. The designer of the guidance system, for example, used services from the Electronic Shop, Computer Design, and Material Engineering support centers. Both the product designer and the managers of the participating support centers would be held responsible for the guidance system, depending on whether the issue was one of efficiency or effectiveness as defined above.

There are both advantages and disadvantages to the matrix model. The environment must be conducive to matrix management for the benefits to outweigh the drawbacks. While matrix management encourages teamwork and joint responsibility, it discourages unity of command and breaks down the chain of authority found in a hierarchical organizational structure. Although matrix management creates managers conversant

Table 4-1: Matrix Management Model in the Aerospace Industry, Final Products (Engineers)

	Guidance System	Fuselage	Landing Mechanism
Foundry		X	
Electronic shop	X		X
Computer design	X	X	X
Material engineer	X	X	X

Source: Robert B. Fetter and Jean L. Freeman, "Diagnosis Related Groups: Product Line Management within Hospitals."

with both technical and marketing personnel, it also creates conflicts among managers whose authority and responsibilities overlap and whose priorities seem at times inconsistent.

The matrix model fits the hospital setting, where we find, as we did in the aerospace industry, highly trained professionals with distinct sets of skills (that is, physicians, technicians, managers of services) joined in the production of a complex and unique product (the treatment of a patient). Yet matrix management has been avoided in hospitals for several reasons. Hospitals have lacked a product definition, and because the matrix structure focuses on the final product, a clearly defined product is essential to matrix management. In addition, hospitals have lacked an incentive for cost containment. The revenue-optimizing orientation of the hospital made management-physician cooperation unnecessary; it was to the benefit of the hospital to focus on revenue rather than cost.

DRGs have provided a set of product definitions that are explicit, and, with the advent of the Prospective Payment System, the same across all hospitals. Prospective payment has also changed the revenue-maximizing orientation of the hospital to one of cost control. The emergence of product definitions and the shift in focus to cost containment is giving hospital managers the ability, and the incentive, to adopt a matrix management structure.

PRODUCT-LINE MANAGEMENT IN HOSPITALS

The use of matrix management in a hospital setting was first proposed by Duncan Neuhauser in the early 1970s.[1] Neuhauser defined a matrix organization as both a hierarchical chain of command (vertical coordination through departmentalization) and a lateral chain of command (horizontal coordination across departments). The simultaneous horizontal and vertical chains of command create dual lines of responsibility and authority.

In the aerospace industry matrix products were defined on the horizontal axis and support services along the vertical axis. Products and support services must also be defined for the clinical matrix, or product-line, model. Support services for the matrix structure will correspond generally to the traditional operating departments. Types of patients or DRGs will constitute our "final product." Since it would be difficult for a hospital to use all 467 DRGs and have 467 final product definitions and corresponding management modes, the DRGs may be aggregated into clusters that conform to clinical practices. Each group of DRGs is called a "clinical management service." Table 4-2 shows a DRG clustering for gynecology clinical management service.

Table 4-2: Grouping DRGs into a Clinical Management Service

Gynecology Management Service
DRG
353 PELVIC EVISCERATION, RADICAL HYSTERECTOMY & VULVECTOMY
354 NON-RADICAL HYSTERECTOMY, AGE ≥ 70 AND/OR CC
355 NON-RADICAL HYSTERECTOMY, AGE ≤ 70 W/O CC
356 FEMALE REPRODUCTIVE SYSTEM RECONSTRUCTIVE PROCEDURES
357 UTERUS & ADNEXA PROC FOR MALIGNANCY
358 UTERUS & ADNEXA PROC FOR NON-MALIGNANCY EXCEPT TUBAL INT
359 TUBAL INTERRUPTION FOR NON-MALIGNANCY
360 VAGINA, CERVIX & VULVA PROCEDURES
361 LAPAROSCOPY & ENDOSCOPY (FEMALE) EXCEPT TUBAL INTER
362 LAPAROSCOPIC, TUBAL INTERRUPTION
363 D&C, CONIZATION & RADIO-IMPLANT FOR MALIGNANCY
364 D&C, CONIZATION EXCEPT FOR MALIGNANCY
365 OTHER FEMALE REPRODUCTIVE SYSTEM O.R. PROCEDURES
366 MALIGNANCY, FEMALE REPROD SYSTEM AGE ≥ 70 &/OR CC
367 MALIGNANCY, FEMALE REPROD SYSTEM AGE ≤ 70 W/O CC
368 INFECTIONS, FEMALE REPROD SYSTEM
369 MENSTRUAL & OTHER FEMALE REPRODUCTIVE SYSTEM DISORDERS

Source: Robert B. Fetter and Jean L. Freeman, "Diagnosis Related Groups: Product Line Management within Hospitals."

Once the clinical management services and the clinical support services have been defined, the clinical matrix, or product-line, structure can be set up. Table 4-3 applies the manufacturing matrix structure to the hospital setting. Across the top are the final products (clinical management services or DRGs) and along the side are intermediate products (clinical support services). Like the engineer in the previous example, the physician puts together the bundle of services that he or she feels are necessary for the final product—the treatment of a particular patient. And like the support service managers in industry, the clinical support service managers in a hospital produce and deliver requested services. At the intersection of a clinical management service and an intermediate product center (marked with an X in Table 4-3), the dual effects on patient care can be assessed.

In this matrix structure each product (a DRG in a clinical management service) requires services from several intermediate product centers. The physician determines the type and intensity of the service required in the production of the product. For example, the pediatrician will use services from the laboratory, radiology, and dietary clinical support services.

Table 4-3: Product-Line Management Model

	Final Products (Physicians) Clinical Management Services		
Intermediate Products (Clinical Support Service Manager)	*Cardiology*	*Pediatrics*	*General Surgery*
Laboratory	X	X	X
Radiology	X	X	X
Dietary	X	X	X
Physical therapy	X		X

Source: Robert B. Fetter and Jean L. Freeman, "Diagnosis Related Groups: Product Line Management within Hospitals."

In choosing the bundle of services necessary to treat the patient, the physician in charge leads the patient care team composed of personnel (for example, nurse, radiologist, pathologist, technician, therapist, dietician, social worker) who deliver support services from their respective departments (such as nursing, radiology, pathology, operating room, physical therapy, dietary, social services). The teams are formed around each patient for the duration of his or her stay. Thus, as patients are admitted and discharged, patient-centered teams with different compositions will be forming, dissolving, and re-forming.

Physician groups defined by a clinical management service are responsible for determining the mix of the hospital's resources necessary to diagnose and treat each type of patient in their service. The exact nature of the group of physicians will vary among hospitals as a function of the hospital's degree of specialization and the size of its medical staff. There are logical groupings of physicians responsible for the care of specific types of patients. Such physician groups as cardiologists, pediatricians, and general surgeons can be linked to specific subsets of DRGs for which they are primarily responsible (Figure 4-2). They are accountable for any significant variance from the standard of either a physician group, the industry, or the community in the use of resources for their defined groups of patients.

This matrix approach to organization, involving groups of physicians responsible for defined groups of patients and managers responsible for clinical support services, allows the organization to assign specific organizational authority and responsibility.

Figure 4-2: Product-Line Management Organizational Chart

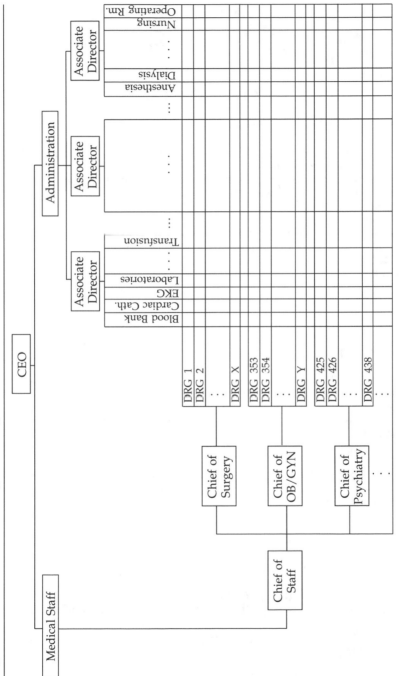

Source: Robert B. Fetter and Jean L. Freeman, "Product-Line Management within Hospitals."

REFERENCE

1. D. Neuhauser, "The Hospital as a Matrix Organization," *Hospital Administration* 17 (1972): 8–25.

SELECTED BIBLIOGRAPHY

Berry, R. E. "Product Heterogeneity and Hospital Cost Analysis." *Inquiry* 7 (1970): 67–75.

———. "Cost and Efficiency in the Production of Hospital Services." *Milbank Memorial Fund Quarterly* 52 (1974): 291–313.

Chase, R. B., and Aquilano, N. J. *Production and Operations Management.* Homewood, IL: Richard D. Irwin, 1977.

Feldstein, M. S. "Hospital Cost Variation and Case-Mix Differences." *Medical Care* 3 (1965): 95–103.

Fetter, R. B. *The New ICD-9-CM Diagnosis-Related Groups Classification Scheme.* Health Care Financing Administration publication no. 03167. Washington, D.C.: U.S. Government Printing Office, 1983.

Fetter, R. B.; Shin, Y.; Freeman, J.; Averill, R. F.; and Thompson, J. D. "Case Mix Definition by Diagnosis-Related Groups." *Medical Care* 18, supplement (1980).

Harris, J. E. "The Internal Organization of Hospitals: Some Economic Implications." *Bell Journal of Economics* 8 (1977): 467–82.

Lave, J. R. "A Review of the Methods Used to Study Hospital Costs." *Inquiry* 3 (1966): 57–81.

Lave, J. R. and Lave, L. B. "Estimated Cost Function for Pennsylvania Hospitals." *Inquiry* 7 (1970): 3–14.

———. "Hospital Cost Functions." *American Economic Review* 60 (1970): 379–95.

———. "The Extent of Role Differentiation among Hospitals." *Health Services Research* 6 (1971): 15–38.

Lee, M. L., and Wallace, R. L. "Problems in Estimating Multiproduct Cost Functions: An Application to Hospitals." *Western Economic Journal* 11 (1973): 350–63.

Levitt, T. "Production-Line Approach to Service." *Harvard Business Review* 50, no. 5 (1972): 41–52.

National Center for Health Statistics. *Health, United States, 1982.* Department of Health and Human Services publication no. (PHS) 83-1232 (Public Health Service). Washington, D.C.: U.S. Government Printing Office, 1983.

Neuhauser, D. "The Hospital As a Matrix Organization." *Hospital Administration* 17, no. 4 (1972): 8–25.

Ruchlin, H. S., and Levenson, I. "Measuring Hospital Productivity." *Health Services Research* 9 (1974): 308–23.

Sonquist, J. A., and Morgan, J. N. *The Detection of Interaction Effects.* Ann Arbor, MI: Institute for Social Research, The University of Michigan, 1964.

Thompson, J. D.; Averill, R. F.; and Fetter, R. B. "Planning, Budgeting and Controlling—One Look at the Future: Case-Mix Cost Accounting." *Health Services Research* 14 (1979): 111–25.

Young, D. W., and Saltman, R. B. "Prospective Reimbursement and the Hospital Power Equilibrium: A Matrix-Based Management Control System." *Inquiry* 20 (1983): 20–33.

5

Cost Accounting and Budgeting

Ian R. Chandler, Robert B. Fetter, and Robert C. Newbold

The products of a hospital are patient treatment processes. The costs incurred in patient treatment include general hospital overheads (such as administration) as well as the direct costs for tests, procedures, and nursing care. The accurate assignment of responsibility for costs requires an accounting system that distinguishes costs associated with the production of a unit of service (for example, a chest x-ray) from costs associated with the quantity of services (for example, number of chest x-rays) that are ordered. Clinical departments (such as radiology) must be held accountable for the efficiency with which they perform tests and procedures, while individual physicians must be held accountable for the number and types of tests and procedures that they order.

This chapter discusses the structure of a cost-accounting system that assigns costs to patient care processes. It discusses the use of such a system for preparing budgets and for analyzing differences in hospital or department costs from one reporting period to the next.

HOSPITAL ACCOUNTING SYSTEMS

The financial structure of a traditional hospital, like its organizational structure, is centered on the operating departments. The hospital's financial position can be determined by examining the costs and revenues derived from all the operating departments within the hospital. Hospitals typically maintain two distinct accounting systems. The first determines the hospital's financial and cash position at any time or across any time

This chapter describes the work of a project to develop a Clinical Care Program Management System between United Health Services (UHS) and Yale University, April 15, 1983 through June 30, 1984, supported in part by the Hartford Foundation: Robert B. Fetter, principal investigator; Karen Schneider, project director; Norman Goodman, UHS project director.

period and is used, both inside and outside the hospital, as a general indicator of the hospital's financial condition. The balance sheet, income statement, and fund flow statements are products of this system.

The second system is a managerial accounting system that provides information for internal management purposes. It provides financial information to help department heads run their departments. Each head of a department is assumed to be responsible for the financial integrity of that department. Traditional accounting methods in hospitals do not allocate costs to individual patients.

Case-mix accounting is an extension of traditional managerial accounting systems that allocates costs from clinical departments to patients. Department accounts provide information concerning most measures of productivity, such as minutes of direct labor per meal, or direct materials cost per radiological examination. Costs are allocated to patients by adding up the number of each type of radiological procedure or laboratory test, or the number of nursing care hours used to treat each patient. Just as the clinical department heads are responsible for the costs of producing laboratory tests or radiological exams, so individual physicians are responsible for the ways in which these intermediate products are combined to treat patients.

For example, suppose that a certain patient required 14 hours of general nursing care, two hours of intensive care nursing, 45 minutes of operating room time, and ten meals. If the labor and materials costs of one hour of general nursing, one hour of intensive care nursing, one minute of operating room time, and one meal are known, then these costs can be allocated to that patient. If costs are aggregated over all patients in a DRG, they can be used to monitor and evaluate the cost performance of physicians, and to develop budget projections based on change in case mix. Cost data can also be used to manage efficient production of services, and to set prices for services and types of cases.

Different costs will serve different purposes. Direct marginal costs are perhaps the best measure for comparing the performance of different physicians, while both total and marginal costs can be used for pricing. Costs that are localized to specific departments can be used for evaluating the cost effectiveness of those departments in performing tests or procedures. Collection of detailed information is essential, because it has a direct bearing on the quality of the reports that can be generated.

For example, nursing costs can be recorded by the day, by the hour, or by the minute; surgical services can be accounted for by time spent in the operating room, by type of procedure, or by both. There are trade-offs between data accuracy and the time and expense involved in collecting data. For example, under ordinary circumstances the lump sum of laundry costs consumed by the laboratory will probably give sufficient detail.

However, if there is a sudden rise in laundry costs for the laboratory, it may be necessary to break them down into costs for lab coats, linen, and other laundry.

The managerial accounting system must give hospital management great flexibility in structuring accounts and data collection. Collecting complete data on all the activities of the hospital is usually not necessary. Rather, it is important to have a broad overview of what is going on with the ability to perform detailed cost investigations when they are warranted. The cost-accounting structure described in the next section offers this kind of flexibility.

Structure of Accounts

The cost-accounting system presented here has three levels of detail. The first examines costs for the hospital as a whole, and the distribution of costs among the various cost centers of the hospital. The second considers individual cost centers, and the distribution of costs for any given cost center over the tests or procedures performed by that cost center. The third level of detail examines the mix of tests, procedures, and nursing care used to treat individual patients, and assigns responsibility for the mix of tests and procedures to the physicians involved. Tables 5-1 through 5-6 and Appendices 5-A and 5-B give an outline of this structure.

Allocation of Overheads to Direct Cost Centers

Table 5-2 shows the allocation statistics used to allocate costs from the overhead cost centers to the direct cost centers. These statistics will function as relative value units for carrying out cost allocations. For example, costs for laundry are allocated on the basis of the number of pounds of laundry processed for that cost center during the reporting period. Thus, when laundry costs are allocated to the medicine 1 and radiology cost centers, it will be in the ratio of 5,897:258. Hence, if laundry expenses came to $10,000 for the reporting period, and if medicine 1 and radiology were the *only* cost centers in the hospital, then laundry expenses would be allocated as follows:

$$\$10,000 \ \times \ \frac{5,897}{5,897 + 258} \ = \ \$9580.83 \text{ (Allocated to medicine 1)}$$

$$\$10,000 \ \times \ \frac{258}{5,897 + 258} \ = \ \$419.17 \text{ (Allocated to radiology)}$$

In general, the statistics used to allocate overhead costs to direct cost centers may allocate some of these costs back to the overhead cost centers themselves. A mathematical technique for dealing with this problem is

Table 5-1: Cost Elements for the Hospital as a Whole

Overhead Cost Centers	*Physicians*
Administration	Dr. A
Maintenance	Dr. B
Housekeeping	Dr. C
Building and grounds	Dr. D
Data processing	Dr. E
Laundry	Dr. F
Cafeteria	Dr. G
Libraries	Dr. H
Photocopying	Dr. I
Accounting	Dr. J
Communication	Dr. K
Staff residence	Dr. L
.	.
.	.
.	.

Direct Cost Centers	
Medicine 1	
Medicine 2	
Surgery 1	*Laboratory Product Line*
Surgery 2	Blood glucose level
Orthopedics	Blood sodium level
Pediatrics	Blood potassium level
Gynecology	Blood bicarbonate level
Psychiatry	RBC iron level
Laboratory ⟶	Complete blood count
Pharmacy	PTT
Blood bank	Platelet count
Radiology	Reticulocyte count
Physical therapy	Urine glucose level
Occupational therapy	
.	.
.	.
.	.
.	

described in Appendix 5-C. Through use of this technique, it is possible to ensure that all overhead costs will be allocated appropriately to the direct cost centers.

Detailed Costs for Direct Cost Centers

Table 5-3 shows an explosion of laboratory costs into detailed cost centers. These include both fixed and variable labor and materials as well as allocated overheads. Explicit separation of fixed and variable costs is very

Table 5-2: Allocation of Overheads to Direct Cost Centers

Overhead Cost Centers	*Direct (Clinical) Cost Centers*			
	Medicine 1	$\cdots$	*Radiology*	$\cdots$
Administration (total expense)	$103,492	$\cdots$	$188,300	$\cdots$
Maintenance (floor space)	10,292 sq. ft.	$\cdots$	12,846 sq. ft.	$\cdots$
Housekeeping (no. of beds)	29 beds	$\cdots$	3 beds	$\cdots$
Building (floor space)	10,292 sq. ft.	$\cdots$	9,846 sq. ft.	$\cdots$
Data processing (no. of terminals)	5 terminals	$\cdots$	17 terminals	$\cdots$
Laundry (lbs. laundry)	5,897 lbs.		258 lbs.	
Cafeteria (no. of employees)	17 employees		23 employees	
. . .	. . .		. . .	

important for marginal pricing decisions and budgeting. Overheads must be considered separately since they are not costs for which the laboratory director is directly responsible. However, they need to be considered in calculating the overall cost of laboratory services. Such a breakdown of costs can also be done for the clinical wards, such as medicine or surgery. In these cases, they would include salaries for both nurses and physicians, and materials costs for the wards. They might also include costs for operating room, recovery room, and anesthesiology as allocated overheads, although these last items could also be treated as direct cost centers in their own right.

Costing of Tests and Procedures

Implicit in this formulation of hospital cost accounting is the notion that every clinical cost center will have some sort of "intermediate product line." For a laboratory or radiology cost center, this is straightforward conceptually, since the intermediate product line consists of the tests or procedures performed by the department. The same is true for departments such as surgery or obstetrics, where the product line consists of surgical procedures or normal births, and also hours of preoperative or

Table 5-3: Detailed Costs for Direct Cost Centers

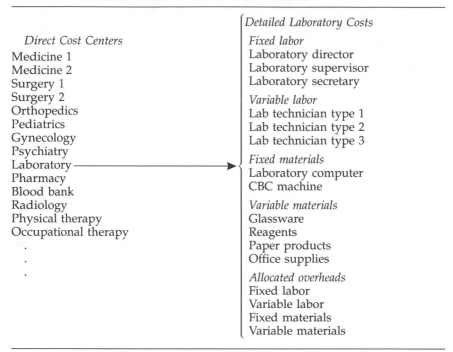

Direct Cost Centers	*Detailed Laboratory Costs*
	Fixed labor
Medicine 1	Laboratory director
Medicine 2	Laboratory supervisor
Surgery 1	Laboratory secretary
Surgery 2	*Variable labor*
Orthopedics	Lab technician type 1
Pediatrics	Lab technician type 2
Gynecology	Lab technician type 3
Psychiatry	*Fixed materials*
Laboratory	Laboratory computer
Pharmacy	CBC machine
Blood bank	
Radiology	*Variable materials*
Physical therapy	Glassware
Occupational therapy	Reagents
.	Paper products
.	Office supplies
.	*Allocated overheads*
	Fixed labor
	Variable labor
	Fixed materials
	Variable materials

postoperative nursing care. With departments such as psychiatry or medicine, things are a bit more problematical. Here, the patient is often being treated for chronic illness, and may be in the hospital for a period of observation. The work that internists or psychiatrists do on the patient is often not easy to quantify in terms of "procedures." In this case, perhaps the best measure to use for allocating costs is just the number of consults or number of minutes or hours spent by physicians with the patients, as well as number of hours or days of nursing care.

The laboratory department has been chosen for an example of the costing of an intermediate product line because it is fairly intuitive. Table 5-4 shows the allocation of laboratory costs to tests conducted by the laboratory department. There are five broad categories of costs that must be distributed over all the tests performed by the laboratory. These include fixed and variable labor and materials costs, as well as allocated overheads (also in the form of fixed and variable labor and materials).

Statistics for variable labor costs can be found by recording the amount of time spent by each of the different types of technicians on each

Table 5-4: Costing of Tests and Procedures; Example: Laboratory

Detailed Costs	Laboratory Tests			
	CBC	PTT	Sodium	· · ·
Fixed labor				
Laboratory director	$0.27	$0.57	$0.06	· · ·
Laboratory supervisor	0.30	0.63	0.07	· · ·
Laboratory secretary	0.18	0.19	0.03	· · ·
Variable labor				
Lab technician type 1	0.27	1.67	0.00	· · ·
Lab technician type 2	0.35	1.90	0.00	· · ·
Lab technician type 3	0.00	0.00	0.35	· · ·
Laboratory aides	0.15	0.15	0.15	· · ·
Fixed materials				
Laboratory computer	0.16	0.16	0.06	· · ·
CBC machine	1.02	0.05	0.00	· · ·
Variable materials				
Glassware	0.02	0.02	0.01	· · ·
Reagents	0.12	0.39	0.08	· · ·
Paper products	0.02	0.02	0.02	· · ·
Office supplies	0.05	0.05	0.05	· · ·
Allocated overheads				
Fixed labor	0.02	0.04	0.02	· · ·
Variable labor	0.15	0.31	0.15	· · ·
Fixed materials	0.03	0.06	0.03	· · ·
Variable materials	0.12	0.25	0.12	· · ·
Totals	$3.23	$6.36	$1.20	· · ·

of the different tests. Dividing the amount of time spent on a particular type of test by the number of tests performed will give the time required to perform a single test, and hence the cost of a single test. Statistics for variable materials costs can similarly be determined by recording the amounts of different types of materials (reagents, glassware, etc.) consumed in performing each of the tests.

Statistics for fixed labor are somewhat less intuitive, and can be arrived at by a number of different methods. One is to find the average labor time (without regard to labor category) for all of the variable labor inputs to the tests, and use this average to allocate fixed labor costs. Another is to use total cost for each of the tests (that is, total inputs of all direct labor and materials except fixed labor). Other methods include estimating the time spent by supervisors training technicians to perform certain tests, or by secretaries processing reports on different tests. Whatever method is chosen for allocating fixed labor costs, it must be appropriate for the local circumstances.

Fixed materials costs (equipment) can be arrived at by dividing the replacement cost of a piece of equipment by the estimated number of tests that it will perform. For example, if a particular machine has an expected life of about five years, performs 10,000 tests per year, and has a replacement cost of $25,000, then the cost per test would be:

$$\frac{\$25,000}{5 \times 10,000} = \$0.50 \text{ per test}$$

Allocated overheads for fixed and variable labor and materials can likewise be mapped into tests in a manner appropriate to local circumstances.

Allocation of Costs to Patients

Once costs have been allocated to tests and procedures (or hours of nursing time, or visits by consultants, etc.) they must be allocated to patients. This is simple conceptually, since it just involves adding up the number of tests or procedures performed on every patient treated by the hospital. In practice, there are important data collection problems, since hospitals may not have this information available for all clinical departments. If this is the case, then the best thing to do is to use detailed information where it exists, and elsewhere to use a set of relative value units obtained from other sources. Various methods for allocating cost from direct cost centers to DRGs are described in Appendix 5-D.

One set of statistics that can be used is derived from a 1985 state of Maryland hospital data base and represents average charges for radiology, laboratory, pharmacy, operating room, therapy, drugs, and supplies per case, and average charges for patient meals per day. These charges are averaged over all of the patients treated in hospitals in Maryland during 1985. A recent study of nursing care carried out at Yale University can be used to estimate the relative amount of nursing care consumed by patients in each of the DRGs on a per-day basis.[1] It should be noted that the Maryland statistics are for DRGs, and therefore do not include outpatients. Thus, either the outpatients must be excluded (the hospital must arrive at an estimate of the fraction of costs that pertain to inpatients for each of the clinical cost centers) or the hospital has to generate its own statistics for mapping costs to outpatients.

If detailed local information does exist, then of course it should be used in preference to the sets of statistics mentioned above (the statistics will probably give costs that are in error by 20 percent or 30 percent or more for some DRGs). Table 5-5 shows the in-hospital statistics for the laboratory cost center for all of the hospital's patients and Table 5-6 shows the same information for Dr. A's patients only. These statistics are simply a record of the numbers of various tests performed for the patients in each of the DRGs. Note that the numbers in Table 5-5 represent the sum of statistics over all of the physicians practicing in the hospital. Physicians can thus be treated as responsibility centers, and can be held accountable for the mix of tests and procedures that they use in treating patients. Alternately, they can be grouped together (for example, all orthopedic surgeons) so that a group of them can be treated collectively as a responsibility center.

Summary of Cost Mapping

The hospital general ledger line items must be grouped into cost centers. There are two broad categories and several subcategories:

— Overhead cost centers

— Direct cost centers

  — Inpatient services (for example, medicine, surgery)

  — Ancillary services (for example, radiology, pharmacy)

Table 5-5: Allocation of Costs to Patients (All Patients)

Cost Center: LABORATORY
Physician: ALL PHYSICIANS

(Table shows number of tests performed for all patients in the hospital.)

Number of Patients in Each DRG:	2	3	2		1,493
	DRG 1	DRG 2	DRG 3	· · ·	Totals
Test Name					
Blood glucose	57	83	60	· · ·	20,439
Blood sodium	28	45	48	· · ·	17,495
Blood potassium	12	18	12	· · ·	5,570
Blood bicarbonate	31	43	17	· · ·	21,379
Blood iron	6	4	0	· · ·	6,379
CBC	12	19	9	· · ·	9,801
PTT	2	0	0	· · ·	873
Platelet	13	22	19	· · ·	3,805
Reticulocytes	3	0	0	· · ·	661
Urine glucose	12	31	18	· · ·	10,328

Table 5-6: Allocation of Costs to Patients (One Physician)

Cost Center: LABORATORY
Physician: DR. A
(Table shows number of tests performed for patients of Dr. A only.)

Number of Patients for Dr. A	2	1	0		63
	DRG 1	*DRG 2*	*DRG 3*	$\cdots$	*Totals*
Test Name					
Blood glucose	57	12	0	$\cdots$	341
Blood sodium	28	14	0	$\cdots$	568
Blood potassium	12	9	0	$\cdots$	86
Blood bicarbonate	31	12	0	$\cdots$	919
CBC	12	5	0	$\cdots$	405
PTT	2	0	0	$\cdots$	7
Platelet	13	8	0	$\cdots$	155
Reticulocytes	3	0	0	$\cdots$	14
Blood iron	6	2	0	$\cdots$	79
Urine glucose	12	9	0	$\cdots$	222
.	.	.	.		.
.	.	.	.		.
.	.	.	.		.

— Outpatient services (for example, clinics, ambulatory surgery)

— Other (for example, emergency room, volunteer services)

The overheads must be allocated to the direct cost centers as demonstrated in Table 5-2.

For each of the direct (clinical) cost centers, one of two options must be selected:

— The hospital may define a series of sub-cost centers for various categories of labor and supplies, and must also define a product line for that cost center. It must relate the labor and supplies costs to the product line by means of allocation statistics, as demonstrated in Table 5-4. It must also keep a record of which tests and procedures have been performed on patients in each of the DRGs (including a record of the physician ordering the test, if possible), as demonstrated in Tables 5-5 and 5-6.

— Alternately, the hospital may use preexisting outside allocation statistics (such as the Maryland data base statistics or the Yale nursing statistics) to allocate costs to patients. Since the Yale and Maryland data are designed for use with DRGs, and DRGs handle inpatients only, the hospital must also arrive at some estimate of the fractions of costs for the cost centers that are used to treat inpatients.

The hospital must then assign costs to clinical cost centers, procedures, physicians, and DRGs to answer a variety of questions regarding costing, budgeting, and variance analysis. Figure 5-1 is a schematic outline of this process.

CASE-MIX COST ANALYSIS

Detailed DRG costing information is the basis for hospital financial reports on cost, cost projection, cost control, charges for services, and

Figure 5-1: Schematic of Cost Mapping

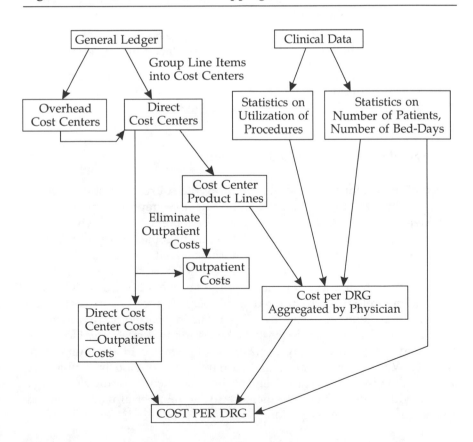

reimbursement policies. Average costs per DRG are useful for purposes of gross cost projections and budgeting, but identifying the sources of waste requires more detailed analysis. Even though a DRG may exhibit little change in average cost from one year to the next, there may still be some patients within that DRG whose costs are quite high relative to the norm. Cost and quality outliers need to be examined to determine whether they are a result of normal statistical fluctuation or systematic waste.

There are several reasons why the consumption of resources in a hospital may change from one reporting period to the next. These include:

— Changes in case mix (the number of each type of patient treated by the hospital)

— Changes in the mix of procedures performed on various types of patients (for example, computerized tomography scans [CT-scans] may now be performed in preference to chest x-rays)

— Changes in the efficiency with which these procedures are performed (that is, the mix of resources used to perform a chest x-ray or a CT-scan)

— Changes in the costs of resources that the hospital must purchase to perform the procedures (inflation of labor and materials costs)

The example in the following section illustrates how a case-mix cost analysis can be used to discover and explain cost variances that occur over time. (Chapter 7 presents a more detailed discussion of cost-variance analysis.)

An Example: Cardiac Pacemaker Implants

Hospital management would like to know the source of cost differences between the 1985 reporting period and the 1986 reporting period. The first step is an examination of the report in Table 5-7, which shows cost variances for each of the hospital's clinical management services (CMS or clinical specialty) over 1985–1986. From this table, it can be seen that there has been a general increase in costs that cannot be accounted for entirely by changes in the number of patients or the number of bed-days. Cardiology and neurology both suffered a 20 percent increase in costs. The number of patients increased by 15 percent in neurology; this increase may account for most of the cost increases for that specialty. However, cardiology experienced only a 5.2 percent increase in the number of patients. When to investigate an increase in costs is obviously a subjective matter, but in this context, a 20 percent increase in costs for the cardiology service with only a 5.2 percent increase in the number of patients would appear to merit an investigation.

Table 5-7: Variance within All Clinical Management Services for One Year

Clinical Management Services Variance, 1985–86

CMS	No. of Patients	Variance		
		Patient	Bed Days	Cost
Cardiology	3,550	+ 5.2%	+10.6%	+20.0%
Gastroenterology	2,000	− 2.2%	− 4.2%	+ 3.5%
General medicine	1,437	− 1.5%	− 5.5%	− 1.1%
Endocrinology	562	+10.6%	− 5.2%	+ 0.2%
Neurology	1,325	+15.0%	+12.3%	+20.0%
Oncology	792	+10.2%	− 1.0%	+17.5%
General surgery	1,578	− 1.2%	− 0.2%	− 2.0%
CT surgery	675	− 1.7%	− 5.2%	+ 1.2%
Urology	794	− 6.6%	−12.5%	− 4.0%
Pediatrics	851	+10.2%	+ 1.2%	+14.3%
Psychiatry	523	−15.0%	−20.0%	− 5.0%

Table 5-8 is a more detailed description of the information in Table 5-7, showing cost variances for each of the DRGs within the cardiology service. Most of these cost variances appear to be significant, and one DRG in particular, DRG 116, shows an extreme cost variance. The 64.5 percent increase in cost for this DRG is combined with a 2.9 percent increase in the number of patients, indicating that little of the cost increase is due to a rise in the number of patients.

Table 5-8: Variance within One Clinical Management Service over One Year

Cardiology Management Service, 1985–86

DRG	No. of Patients	Variance		
		Patient	Bed Days	Cost
.	.	.	.	.
.	.	.	.	.
.	.	.	.	.
115 PERM CARD PACEMKR W	128	+6.7%	+0.5%	+18.9%
116 PERM CARD PACEMKR W/O	71	+2.9%	+2.4%	+64.5%
117 CARD PACEMKR REPLACE	147	+8.9%	+1.8%	+32.9%
118 CARD PACEMKR GEN REP	59	−8.2%	+4.9%	+22.0%
.	.	.	.	.
.	.	.	.	.
.	.	.	.	.

While Table 5-8 documents an increase in costs for the cardiology DRGs, it does not give any clues as to the sources of these cost increases. Perhaps the patients treated in 1986 were more seriously ill, or perhaps there were problems with staff or administrative inefficiency, or perhaps the patients treated in 1985 were just not receiving good-quality care. To determine the sources of cost increases, the data must be analyzed in

Table 5-9: Costs per Final Cost Center for DRG 116

DRG 116, PERMANENT CARDIAC PACEMAKER W/O AMI OR CHF, 1985–86

Final Cost Center	1985 Unit Cost	1986 Unit Cost	Difference	Precent Change
1. DIETARY	$ 70	$ 91	$ 21	30%
2. ADMITTING	25	29	4	16%
3. BILLING	173	263	90	52%
4. HOTEL	146	209	63	43%
5. NURSING	646	788	142	22%
6. HOUSE STAFF	66	86	20	30%
7. MEDICAL RECORDS	18	29	11	61%
8. SOCIAL SERVICES	14	21	6	50%
9. NEWBORN INTEN. CARE	—	—	—	—
10. INTENSIVE CARE	11	260	249	2,163%
11. CORONARY CARE	383	360	−23	−6%
12. OPERATING ROOM	220	258	38	17%
13. RECOVERY ROOM	7	14	7	100%
14. ANESTHESIA	16	202	39	24%
15. DELIVERY ROOM	—	—	—	—
16. DIAGNOSTIC RADIO.	161	263	102	63%
17. RADIOISOTOPES	6	12	7	116%
18. RADIOTHERAPY	—	3	3	—
19. LABORATORY	248	591	343	138%
20. EKG, EEG	48	56	7	17%
21. MED-SURG. SUPPLIES	2,228	3,708	1,480	66%
22. PHYSICAL MEDICINE	12	28	18	134%
23. RESPIRATORY THERAPY	39	139	100	256%
24. IV THERAPY	35	61	26	74%
25. PHARMACY	106	268	162	153%
26. RENAL DIALYSIS	30	50	20	66%
27. RENAL TRANSPLANT	—	—	—	—
28. UROLOGY	—	—	—	—
29. EMERGENCY ROOM	13	18	5	38%
30. CLINICS	3	3	—	—
31. OUTPATIENT	—	—	—	—
32. MISCELLANEOUS	38	41	3	8%
			$2,943	

more detail. Reports such as those shown in Table 5-9 would be produced for each of the DRGs with significant cost increases.

Table 5-10 contains detailed information on DRG 116 costs, after including data on the number of patients and number of bed-days for both years. There were only two additional patients in 1986, but a total cost increase of 64.5 percent. Most of this increase (92.82 percent) is accounted for by increases in per-patient costs, while only 4.03 percent is accounted for by increases in volume (number of patients). There is also a 28.6 percent increase in bed-days per patient. This length of stay increase accounts for about a third of the total cost increase, and it may be worthwhile to ask medical staff to account for this.

These cost increases have a ripple effect throughout the institution. A rise in costs on cardiology floors does not necessarily mean that hospital support services have become less efficient. In Table 5-9, it can be seen that increases in dietary and nursing costs seem largely related to and commensurate with the 28.6 percent length of stay increase. Had these costs stayed the same despite the increased workload, the increase in efficiency would have gone unnoticed if the DRG variances had not been taken into account. However, laboratory, pharmacy, and respiratory therapy showed considerably larger cost increases than can be accounted for by the 28.6 percent length of stay increase. For laboratory, costs

Table 5-10: Variance within a DRG over One Year

DRG 116, PERMANENT CARDIAC PACEMAKER W/O AMI OR CHF, 1985–86

	1985 Volume/ Cost	1986 Volume/ Cost	Difference	Percent Change
Number of patients	69	71	2	2.9%
Total cost	$271,037	$446,079	$175,042	64.5%
Cost per case	$3,928	$6,283	$2,355	60.0%
Cost per day	$431	$535	$104	24.1%
Average LOS (days)	9.1	11.7	2.6	28.6%
Total charges	$269,104	$370,307	$101,203	37.6%
Average charges per case	$3,900	$5,215	$1,315	33.7%
Ratio: cost/charge	1.007	1.205		

		Accounted for by		
	Total	Volume	Unit Cost	Unexplained Interaction
Cost change	$175,041	$7,056	$162,470	$5,515
Percent of total		4.03%	93%	3.15%

increased by 138 percent, from $248 to $591 per case. It is not clear from this statistic whether this is a result of the ordering of more or different laboratory tests, or whether it is due to inefficiency on the part of the laboratory itself.

The dramatic cost changes in intensive care of +2,163 percent suggests that something unusual has happened in this area. Upon investigation, it turns out that this change is a result of the difference in the way patients were treated for pacemaker implants over the two years. The hospital has increased its complement of intensive care beds, and more patients are receiving their postoperative care in the intensive care unit rather than the coronary care unit. For this reason, a more appropriate analysis might be to combine the statistics for the two cost centers.

Further investigation reveals that the alarming increase in medical-surgical supplies costs ($1,480) is due to a change in the cost of the pacemaker itself. The pharmacy cost increase from $106 to $268 could be a result of a change in the type of antibiotics employed, or a decrease in the efficiency of the pharmacy, and would have to be investigated. If a further level of detail is required, costs for laboratory, pharmacy, etc., can be broken down further to check for specific increases in the utilization of different types of labor or materials. In this way, the analysis of cost variances proceeds from a gross level to a fine level, from clinical services to specific tests and procedures.

Other Reports

In addition to examining cost variance, reports can identify the most and least profitable DRGs and departments and the DRGs with the highest charges. Table 5-11 gives a summary of total hospital costs distributed across the 24 major diagnostic categories. It may be instructive to compare this information with costs from previous years, from other hospitals, or from budget estimates. Table 5-12 shows 11 DRGs that together account for 26.7 percent of the hospital's total costs. Efforts at cost containment might well be directed at these DRGs. Table 5-13 compares the hospital's costs with the national averages for some DRGs. This will give some idea of how efficient the hospital is in relation to other hospitals in treating patients in various DRGs.

Case-Mix Budgeting

The costing process can be run in reverse to prepare budgets. First, estimates must be made of the number of patients whom the hospital will treat in each of the DRGs during the coming year. By multiplying these numbers by this year's *variable* costs, an estimate can be made of the DRG

Table 5-11: Patient Cost by Major Diagnostic Category, Hospital B, 1983

MDC No.	Major Diagnostic Category	No. of Patients	All Costs		
			Total	Percent	Per Patient
1.	D/D* NERVOUS SYSTEM	979	$1,286,358	9.9	$1,314.00
2.	D/D EYE	225	236,538	1.8	1,051.30
3.	D/D EAR, NOSE & THROAT	436	423,356	3.3	971.00
4.	D/D RESPIRATORY SYSTEM	670	1,227,122	9.4	1,831.50
5.	D/D CIRCULATORY SYSTEM	899	1,729,681	13.3	1,924.00
6.	D/D DIGESTIVE SYSTEM	1,235	1,735,411	13.4	1,405.20
7.	D/D HEPATOBILIARY SYSTEM & PANCREAS	313	574,855	4.4	1,836.60
8.	D/D MUSCULOSKELETAL SYSTEM ...	729	1,103,891	8.5	1,514.30
9.	D/D SKIN, SUB. TISSUE & BREAST	321	350,089	2.7	1,090.60
10.	ENDOCRINE, NUTRITIONAL & METABOLIC D/D	508	530,892	4.1	1,045.10
11.	D/D KIDNEY & URINARY TRACT	150	215,487	1.7	1,436.60
12.	D/D MALE REPRODUCTIVE SYSTEM	126	176,955	1.4	1,404.40
13.	D/D FEMALE REPRODUCTIVE SYSTEM	117	127,460	1.0	1,089.40
14.	PREGNANCY, CHILDBIRTH & PUERPERIUM	707	660,431	5.1	934.10
15.	NEWBORNS & OTHER NEONATES ...	132	240,920	1.9	1,825.20
16.	D/D BLOOD & BLOOD FORMING ORGANS	77	98,668	0.8	1,281.40
17.	MYELOPROLIFERATIVE DISORDERS	80	74,301	0.6	928.80
18.	INFECTIOUS & PARASITIC DISEASES	103	171,592	1.3	1,665.90
19.	MENTAL DISEASES & DISORDERS	241	406,547	3.1	1,686.90
20.	SUBSTANCE USE & ORGANIC DISORDERS	147	150,808	1.2	1,025.90
21.	INJURIES, POISON. & TOXIC DRUG EFFECTS	455	649,500	5.0	1,427.50
22.	BURNS	17	15,021	0.1	883.60
23.	FACTORS INFLUENCING HEALTH STAT & ...	37	35,811	0.3	967.90
24.	UNASSIGNABLE	393	764,986	5.9	1,946.50

*D/D = Diseases and disorders of the ...

Table 5-12: Percent of Costs by DRG, Hospital B, 1983

DRG No.	Diagnosis Related Group	No. of Patients	Total DRG Costs	Percent Costs	Cum. Percent Costs
468	UNRELATED OR PROC	150	$559,967	4.3	4.3
373	VAGINAL DELIVERY W/O CC	526	454,580	3.5	7.8
14	SPECIFIC CEBER DISORDER EXC TIA	160	437,315	3.4	11.2
121	HEART FAILURE & SHOCK	138	393,221	3.0	14.2
442	OTHER OR PROC FOR INJUR W CC	49	327,627	2.5	16.7
294	DIABETES AGE >36	174	263,033	2.0	18.8
210	HIP & FEMUR PROC EXC MAJ JT W CC	61	252,194	1.9	20.7
184	ESOPH GASTRO MISC DIG DISORD 0–11	181	221,696	1.1	22.4
167	APPENDECTOMY W/O CC	186	200,839	1.5	24.0
89	SIMPLE PNEUMONIA & PLEURISY W	82	194,214	1.5	25.4
429	ORGANIC DISTURB & MENTAL RETARDATION	59	164,658	1.3	26.7

Table 5-13: Costs per DRG, Hospital B against National Average, 1983

		MDC 5, CIRCULATORY SYSTEM			
		Hospital B		U.S. Hospital Average	
DRG		No. of Patients	Cost per Patient	No. of Patients	Cost per Patient
121	CIRCULATORY DISORD W AMI & CV COMPL	47	$3,136	77	$5,518
122	CIRCULATORY DISORD W AMI W/O C.V.	43	$2,314	285	$4,208
123	CIRCULATORY DISORD W AMI, EXPIRED	22	$1,504	259	$2,144
124	CIRC DIS EXC AMI W CARD CATH & COMP DI	3	$1,363	571	$1,410
125	CIRC DIS EXC AMI W CARD CATH W/O COMP	8	$4,186	4	$8,230
126	ACUTE & SUBACUTE ENDOCARDITIS	6	$2,657	418	$3,051
127	HEART FAILURE & SHOCK	138	$1,993	60	$1,939

variable costs for the coming year (not yet accounting for inflation). The cost-mapping algorithm can then be inverted to map these projected variable costs back into the clinical services, back into the overheads, and finally back to the general ledger of the hospital. Then, inflation factors can be estimated for labor and materials for the coming year, and multiplied by both the fixed and variable costs in the general ledger. Finally, these projected general ledger costs can be sent back through the cost-mapping algorithm to produce budgets for the hospital departments and estimated DRG costs for the coming year. A schematic outline of this process is given in Figure 5-2.

Figure 5-2: Schematic Outline of Case-Mix Budgeting

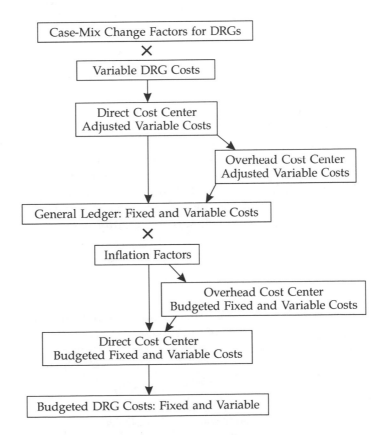

Central to the budgeting process is an initial separation of the general ledger into fixed and variable components. Fixed costs do not vary with patient volume and change only under special circumstances, while variable costs change with patient volume. It is not always clear whether certain costs should be considered fixed or variable. For example, if the laboratory director is unwilling to decrease the number of laboratory technicians even in the face of projected decreases in demand for laboratory services, then the salaries of laboratory technicians can be regarded as fixed.

One problem with formulating budgets for hospitals is that medical technology is changing rapidly. It may therefore be of value to get a certain amount of clinical input into the budgeting process. If certain technologies will come into use during the coming year, estimated costs for these can be factored into the budgeting process at different levels. If radiology is going to buy a new CT scanner, its anticipated cost could be added to the general ledger. If it is known that physicians will use a different mix of antibiotics, then this can be reflected in the matrix relating pharmacy drugs to DRGs.

Budget reports can be prepared at the end of the forecasted period to compare actual with budgeted costs. The sources of cost variation can then be identified. First, the actual inflation factors and the actual case-mix changes must be taken into account. (Also, if necessary, known cost changes, such as a new CT scanner, or changes in medical practice can be taken into account.) Variation that remains between actual and budgeted costs will then consist of variation due to unanticipated changes in physician practice (ordering different mixes of tests and procedures) and changes in the efficiency of clinical departments. Detailed examination of the cost variances for individual departments, and practice changes of individual physicians, will help to identify areas where costs are out of line.

ACKNOWLEDGMENTS

We would like to thank Daniel Gautier and Jean-Marie Rodrigues for demonstrating the work of the French PMSI Project, which further developed this cost-accounting model in several French hospitals.

REFERENCE

1. R. B. Fetter, J. D. Thompson, J. F. Ryan, D. Diers, J. L. Freeman, S. H. Lo, and R. C. Newbold, *Diagnosis Related Groups (DRGs) and Nursing Resources* (final report, grant no. 15-C-98500/1-02, Health Care Financing Administration; New

Haven, CT: Health Systems Management Group, School of Organization and Management, Yale University, November 1987).

SELECTED BIBLIOGRAPHY

Berry, R. E. "Product Heterogeneity and Hospital Cost Analysis." *Inquiry* 7 (1970): 67–75.

Buck, C. R., Jr. "Point of View—Hospitals Produce What They Are Paid For: Costs and Patient Days." *Health Care Management Review* 2 (Fall 1977): 59–65.

Feldstein, M. S. "Hospital Cost Variation and Case-Mix Differences." *Medical Care* 3 (1965): 95–103.

Fetter, R. B. *Development, Testing, and Evaluation of a Prospective Case Payment Reimbursement System*. Final report, Social Security Administration, Health Care Financing Administration contract no. 600–75–0180. New Haven, CT: Health Systems Management Group, School of Organization and Management, Yale University, January 1981.

Fetter, R. B.; Thompson, J. D.; and Mills, R. "A System for Cost and Reimbursement Control in Hospitals." *The Yale Journal of Biology and Medicine* 49, no. 2 (1976): 123–36.

Fetter, R. B.; Mills, L. M.; and Mills, R. E. "A System for Concurrent Patient Care Evaluation." Paper presented at the Operations Research Society of America and Institute of Management Sciences meeting in Las Vegas, November 1975.

Fetter, R. B.; Mills, R.; Riedel, D. C.; and Thompson, J. D. "The Application of Diagnostic Specific Cost Profiles to Cost and Reimbursement Control in Hospitals." *Journal of Medical Systems* 1 (November 1977): 137–49.

Griffith, J. R.; Hancock, W.; and Munson, F. C. (eds.). *Cost Control in Hospitals*. Ann Arbor, MI: Health Administration Press, 1976.

Holder, W. W. "Hospital Budgeting: State of the Art." *Hospital and Health Services Administration* 23, no. 2 (1978): 57.

Lave, J. R., and Lave, L. B. "Hospital Cost Functions." *American Economic Review* 60 (1970): 379–95.

———. "Estimated Cost Functions for Pennsylvania Hospitals." *Inquiry* 7 (1970): 3–14.

Lee, M. L., and Wallace, R. L. "Problems in Estimating Multiproduct Cost Functions: An Application to Hospitals." *Western Economic Journal* 11 (1973): 350–63.

Levitt, T. "Production-Line Approach to Service." *Harvard Business Review* 50 (1972): 41–52.

Neuhauser, D. "The Hospital as a Matrix Organization." *Hospital Administration* 17 (1972): 8–25.

Ruchlin, H. S., and Levenson, I. "Measuring Hospital Productivity." *Health Services Research* 9 (1974): 308–23.

Thompson, J. D.; Averill, R. F.; and Fetter, R. B. "Planning, Budgeting, and Controlling—One Look at the Future: Case-Mix Cost Accounting." *Health Services Research* 14 (1979): 111–25.

Thompson, J. D.; Fetter, R. B.; and Mross, C. D. "Case Mix and Resource Use." *Inquiry* 12, no. 4 (1975): 300–312.

Thompson, J. D.; Fetter, R. B.; and Shin, Y. "One Strategy for Controlling Costs in University Teaching Hospitals." *Journal of Medical Education* 53, no. 3 (1978): 167–75.

Appendix 5-A: Initial and Final Cost Center Allocation Statistics

Cost Center	Initial Cost Center Allocation Statistics	Final Cost Center Allocation Statistics
Overhead General Services		
Depreciation—building and fix	Square feet	
Depreciation—equipment	Equipment values	
Employee health	Gross salary	
Operations and maintenance	Square feet	
Laundry/linen	Pounds of laundry	
Housekeeping	Hours worked	
Dietary—food*	Meals served	
Dietary—other*	Meals served	
Cafeteria	Number of employees	
Maintenance of personnel	Employees housed	
Medical records*	Medical record time	
Social services	Social service time	
Interns and residents	Number of interns and residents	
Supervision of physicians	Time	
Central services	Number of requisitions	
Pharmacy	Number of requisitions	
Nursing administration	Time	
Nonpatient phones	Number of lines	
Data processing	Time	
Purchasing	Cost of purchases	
Audiovisual	Time	
General administration	Total expenses	
Ancillary Services		
OR/recovery rooms		Time
Anesthesia		Charges
Delivery rooms		Charges
Radiology		Standard costs
Laboratory		Standard costs
EKG		RVU
EEG		RVU
Physical therapy		RVU
Occupational therapy		Charges
Speech pathology		Charges
Audiology		Charges
Inhalation therapy		RVU
Blood		RVU
IV therapy		RVU
G.I. laboratory		RVU

Continued

Appendix 5-A: Continued

Cost Center	Initial Cost Center Allocation Statistics	Final Cost Center Allocation Statistics
Cost of mecial supplies		Actual costs
Cost of drugs		Actual costs
Renal dialysis		Charges
CT-scan		Charges
Biomedical		Charges
Direct Inpatient General Services		
Inpatients (acute care)		Non-ICU weighted LOS
Intensive care		ICU/CCU LOS
Neonatal (premature nursery)		LOS in neonatal
Routine nursery		LOS in routine nursery
General nursing service		Non-ICU weighted LOS
Intensive nursing		ICU/CCU LOS
Admitting		One per patient
Cashier, A/R		Total number of charges on bills
Inpatient dietary		Weighted LOS
Inpatient medical records		1 + [LOS/7]
Other Cost Centers		
Miscellaneous		One per patient
Emergency room		Charges
Non-Inpatient Cost Centers		
Clinics service		No
Ambulatory surgery		costs
Family practice		allocated
Drug abuse		to
Skilled nursing facility		patients

*These cost centers have an overhead component as well as a direct care component.
Reprinted from J. L. Freeman, R. B. Fetter, R. C. Newbold, J.-M Rodrigues, and D. Gautier, "Development and Adaptation of a Hospital Cost and Budgeting Model for Cross-National Use," *Journal of Management in Medicine* 1, no. 1 (June 1986): 38–57.

Appendix 5-B: Typical Hospital Chart of Accounts with Overhead and DRG Allocation Statistics

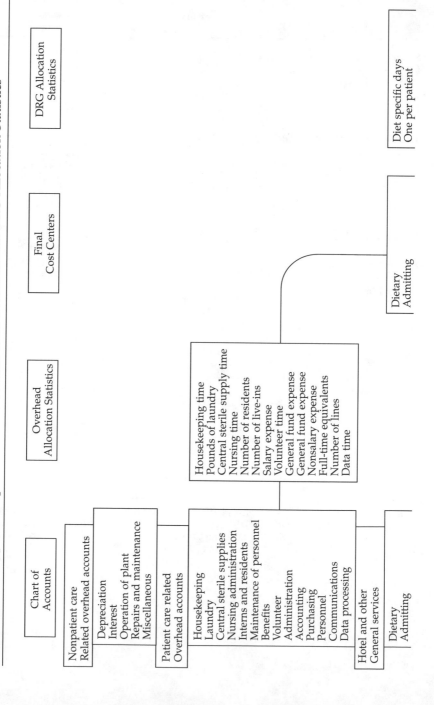

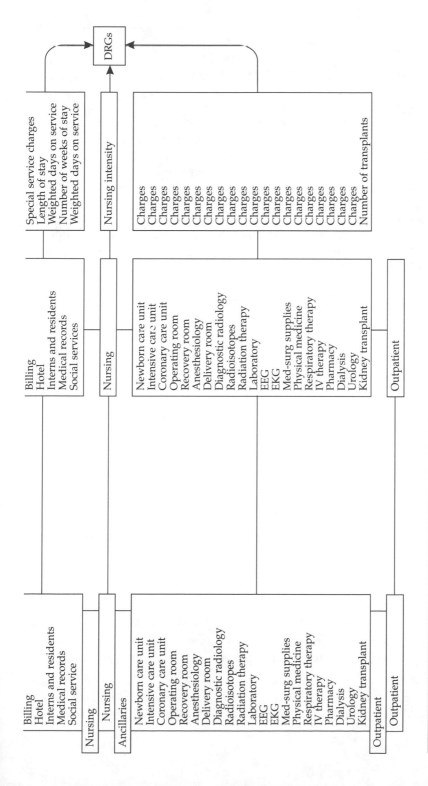

Reprinted from J. D. Thompson, R. F. Averill, and R. B. Fetter, "Planning, Budgeting, and Controlling—One Look at the Future: Case-Mix Cost Accounting," *Health Services Research* 14, no. 2 (Summer 1979): 116, with the permission of the Hospital Research and Educational Trust.

APPENDIX 5-C:
OVERHEAD COST ALLOCATIONS

When costs from an overhead cost center are allocated to direct (clinical) cost centers, some of their costs are typically allocated back to themselves. Thus, some of the costs from the administration cost center are consumed by the administration department itself. Likewise, some of the cafeteria costs are consumed in feeding cafeteria workers. In order to arrive at accurate average DRG costs, it is essential that all overhead costs be included; hence, even those costs initially allocated back to the overhead cost centers must ultimately be assigned to some direct cost center.

The overhead cost allocation technique shown here is called the "reciprocal" method, and approximates the "multiple distribution" method shown below.

Steps in the Multiple-Distribution Process

Step 1: $\hat{C}^{(1)} = C^{(0)}F, C^{(1)} = C^{(0)}G$

Step 2: $\hat{C}^{(2)} = C^{(1)}F + \hat{C}^{(1)} = C^{(0)}GF + C^{(0)}F, C^{(2)} = C^{(1)}G = C^{(0)}G^2$

Step 3: $\hat{C}^{(3)} = C^{(2)}F + \hat{C}^{(2)} = C^{(0)}G^2F + C^{(0)}GF + C^{(0)}F, C^{(3)}$
$$= C^{(0)}G^3$$

$$\cdot \qquad \cdot$$
$$\cdot \qquad \cdot$$
$$\cdot \qquad \cdot$$

Step n: $\hat{C}^{(n)} = C^{(0)}[G^{n-1} + G^{n-2} + ... + G + I]F, C^{(n)} = C^{(n)}G^n$

where

$\hat{C}^{(k)}$ represents the costs allocated from the overhead cost centers to the direct cost centers in iteration k

$C^{(k)}$ represents the costs allocated from the overhead cost centers back into themselves in iteration k

F   represents the fractions of costs in the overhead cost centers to be allocated to the direct cost centers in any given iteration

G   represents the fractions of costs in the overhead cost centers to be allocated back to themselves in any given iteration

Observe that the sum of the elements in any row of the (GF) matrix must equal one. For this reason, the multiple-distribution process allocates more and more costs to the direct-cost centers with each iteration, while correspondingly fewer costs are allocated back to the overheads.

Direct Costs

$$\hat{c}_1 \cdots \hat{c}_k$$

Overhead Costs

$c_1 \cdots c_i$

g_{11}	g_{12}	$\cdots$	g_{1i}	f_{11}	$\cdots$	f_{1k}
g_{21}	g_{22}	$\cdots$	g_{2i}	f_{21}	$\cdots$	f_{2k}
.	.	$\cdots$	.	.	$\cdots$	.
.	.	$\cdots$	.	.	$\cdots$	.
.	.	$\cdots$	.	.	$\cdots$	.
g_{i1}	g_{i2}	$\cdots$	g_{ii}	f_{i1}	$\cdots$	f_{ik}

G   F

It is possible to derive a closed form of the multiple distribution in the limiting case as the number of iterations tends to infinity. From linear algebra, we know that if $(I-G)^{-1}$ is nonsingular, and if $\operatorname{Lim} n \to \infty \sum_{k=0}^{n} G^k$ converges, then $(I - G)^{-1}$ exists, and $(I - G)^{-1} = \operatorname{Lim} n \to \infty \sum_{k=0}^{n} G^k$. Because the multiple-distribution process satisfies the requirements for an absorbing Markov chain,[1] these conditions hold, so a closed form of the multiple distribution is:

$$\hat{C} = C^{(0)}(I - G)^{-1}F.$$

Furthermore, the matrix $P = (I - G)^{-1}F$, sometimes called the "traceback" matrix, is an $i \times k$ matrix that gives the proportion of costs at each overhead cost center being allocated to each direct cost center, something not readily available from the multiple-distribution process. This matrix shows how much each of the overhead cost centers contributes to the costs of each direct cost center.

Reference

1. J. Kemeny and J. Snell, *Finite Markov Chains* (Princeton, NJ: P. Van Nostrand Company, Inc., 1960), 22, 26.

APPENDIX 5-D:
ALLOCATION OF COSTS FROM DIRECT COST
CENTERS TO DRGs

If detailed procedure costing cannot be performed on some clinical cost center because of a lack of readily available data, it is necessary to arrive at an alternative method of cost allocation that can be used in lieu of procedure costs. The most common methods of cost allocation are described below.

Cost-to-Charge Ratio

In this method of allocation, costs are compared with patient service charges. Total costs are calculated for a particular service, and are compared with total patient charges for the same service. A cost-to-charge ratio is calculated, and this becomes the statistic for allocating costs. This is a simple but crude method of allocating costs, since costs are not usually proportional to charges.

For example, suppose that the food service cost center had total costs of $500,000 for a certain year, and that the total charges for meals came to $700,000. The cost-to-charge ratio is then ($500,000/$700,000) = 0.71. Thus, if a patient meal had a charge of $4.25, the costs allocated to that meal would be: $4.25 × 0.71 = $3.02.

Weighted Length of Stay

Length of stay is a convenient measure for allocating costs for services that are used daily, such as patient accommodations or patient meals. The cost of a single unit of service can be estimated for patients in each of the DRGs, and then costs can be allocated to these patients on the basis of the number of weighted bed-days.

Using weighted length of stay to allocate nursing costs is more complicated because nursing intensity varies considerably for different types of patients. There is also variation between institutions, and variation from day to day during a patient's stay. Nevertheless, as has been demonstrated in the 1987 Yale study "Diagnosis Related Groups (DRGs) and Nursing Resources," it is possible to arrive at length-of-stay nursing weights for each of the DRGs.

Actual Cost

For some items, the actual costs are known and can be allocated to patients directly. Perhaps the best example is medications: all that is necessary to arrive at the cost for each patient is to count the number of units consumed by each patient and multiply this number by the number of patients. For example, if the cost of one unit of drug A is $15.00 from the general ledger, and if indirect pharmacy costs (heating, administration, maintenance, etc.) are $8.00 per unit of medication, then the cost of one unit of drug A administered to a patient is $23.00.

Relative Value Units

Relative value units (RVUs) are weighted measures of resource consumption based on the relative amount of time and materials required to produce a particular service. RVUs can be developed by assigning a base weight to the least expensive procedure and calculating the relative weights of the other procedures as follows:

$$\frac{\text{Weight of}}{\text{procedure X}} = \frac{\text{Weight of least expensive}}{\text{procedure (procedure Y)}} \times \frac{\text{Cost of procedure X}}{\text{Cost of procedure Y}}$$

Even though total hospital costs will change, relative value units will remain relatively constant from year to year. Allocating costs to patients is then a simple matter of adding up the numbers of each type of procedure performed, and multiplying by the appropriate RVUs. The fraction of department costs to be allocated to a particular patient can then be found by dividing this number by the total RVUs for the department, and multiplying by total department costs.

For example, if a department had total costs of $500,000, and a particular patient had three tests of type Y performed, and tests of type Y had an RVU of 3.27, and the sum of the products of tests and RVUs for the department was 47,389.25, then the costs allocated to this patient would be:

$$\$500,000 \times \frac{3 \times 3.27}{47,387.25} = \$103.50$$

Standard Cost

In standard costing, unit costs are calculated for all of the materials and labor categories in a department. The number of units of each of these categories that are consumed in performing a particular procedure are then calculated, and the standard cost can be found by summing up the products of unit costs and units consumed. Table 5-D-1 shows the cost per unit and number of units consumed in producing an x-ray study, and also the total standard cost.

Table 5-D-1: Costs, Hospital X, Department of Radiology

	Standard	Unit Cost	Standard Cost
(No.) 1928			
(Name) Abdomen X-Ray Flat and Erect			
Category			
I. Direct labor	$ .31	$5.73	$ 1.78
1. Transport			
2. Supervisory/special	0	22.83	0
3. Regular tech.	.25	14.45	3.61
		Subtotal	$ 5.39
II. Direct material			
1. Films			
A. No. of films			
(Adjusted by E = .03)			
8 × 10	0	.38	$ 0
10 × 12	0	.52	0
11 × 14	0	.75	0
14 × 14	0	.89	0
14 × 17	2.40	1.08	2.59
7 × 17	0	.23	0
9 × 9	0	.42	0
		Subtotal	$ 2.59
2. Supplies ($ amount adjusted by F = .28)	1.28	0	0
III. Departmental overhead expenses			
1. Room equipment/facility cost			
A. General and tomography	0	16.79	$ 0
B. Skull bones	0	60.86	0
C. General	.22	8.66	1.91
D. General	0	11.22	0
E. Fluoroscopy	0	42.73	0
F. Fluoroscopy	0	46.07	0
G. Fluoroscopy	0	59.58	0
H. Mammography	0	42.95	0
I. Special procedures	0	29.43	0
J. I.V.P.	0	28.85	0
K. I.V.P.	.09	34.05	3.06
L. Ultrasound	0	32.93	0
		Subtotal	$ 4.97
2. Darkroom expense — total films	2.40	.07	$ .17
3. General overhead			
A. Total tech. time	.25	24.87	$ 6.22
IV. Allocated overhead			
1. Total tech. time	.25	28.83	$ 7.21
	Standard cost		$26.55

6

Nursing Resources

John D. Thompson and Donna Diers

> The effective management of nursing resources requires a linkage between the costs of services and the patients who receive them....
>
> It is somewhat ironic that nursing intensity measurement would be the last element in the DRG system to be developed. No other hospital service has been examined more frequently than routine nursing care.[1]

Whearsen the DRG-based prospective reimbursement methodology was originally tested in New Jersey in 1980, there was a specific requirement, engineered by the New Jersey State Nurses' Association (NJSNA), for a study of ways to allocate or assign nursing intensity to DRGs.[2] This provision was in part responsible for NJSNA's support for the DRG implementation. The intent of the study was to recognize the perception of nurses that DRGs would imperfectly capture nursing resources since the variables that determine nursing resources were not part of DRG construction. On the assumption that an interpretable model would evolve, DRGs could be "weighted" by a nursing intensity factor that would be reflected in reimbursement rates.

The study produced an instrument, Resource Intensity Measures (RIMs), to measure nursing resource use.[3] The research began with the assumption that nursing resource consumption and DRG assignment were *independent*. Thus DRGs (actually MDCs) were the last, not the first,

Based in part on "Diagnosis Related Groups and Nursing Resources," final project report, grant no. 15-C-98500/1-02 between the Health Care Financing Administration (HCFA) and Yale University: Robert B. Fetter and John D. Thompson, principal investigators; Jeanette F. Ryan, project director; Patricia Willis, project officer; November 1987. The study team was Donna Diers, Jean L. Freeman, Sophie H. Lo, and Robert C. Newbold. The nursing advisory committee was Elizabeth Draper, Phyllis Giovannetti, and Margaret D. Sovie. Linda Lewandowski, Susan Molde, and Joyce Potter were nursing consultants. The statements contained in this chapter are solely those of the authors and do not necessarily reflect the views or policies of the Health Care Financing Administration.

classifying variable and the RIMs measure required that new nursing data be collected. A length of stay (LOS) weight was derived and nursing time was adjusted according to the skill mix of the staff. Time spent by licensed practical nurses (LPNs) and by nurses' aides was scaled down by a wage factor. Intensive care and pediatrics were never included, and an arbitrary trim point of 32 days of stay was assumed.

The RIMs measure included a number of questionable assumptions and arbitrary decision rules that were counterintuitive for nurses and prompted serious debate.[4,5] Although RIMs were never implemented as part of New Jersey's reimbursement methodology, the effort illuminated most of the issues pertinent to studying nursing intensity: the necessity for a per-case measure, the separation of intensive or special care from routine care, the importance of patient classification as the base, the difficulty of attaching all of nursing time to specific patients in order to have a comparable measure across hospitals, the handling of aberrant cases or "outliers," and the complexity of breaking nursing costs out of the rest of hospital costs and charges for analysis.

The present chapter discusses these and additional issues with particular attention to the uses to which measurements of nursing intensity might be put.

DRGs AND NURSING INTENSITY

Like physicians, nurses think of tending to individual patients; daily change in patients' condition is central. The DRG-based per-case methodology runs counter to their experience of their work. In addition, nurses have believed that variables other than the ones used to form DRGs are important in determining daily variation in nursing intensity, a point that assumed political form in the American Nurses' Association testimony to Congress when prospective payment was being considered.[6]

Official American nursing argues that the "medical model" embodied in medical diagnosis (and thus DRGs) does not explain nursing practice, and there is a powerful thrust in the nursing community toward the construction of alternative labeling systems or "nursing diagnoses." The North American Nursing Diagnosis Association (NANDA) has orchestrated the move toward a system of classification of patient conditions. NANDA hopes that nursing diagnosis might one day be parallel to or be included within the International Classification of Diseases (ICD), much as the American Psychiatric Association developed the classification of psychiatric disorders, the Diagnostic and Statistical Manual or DSM III, included for the first time in the ninth revision of ICD codes.

While NANDA has approved a short list of "accepted" nursing diagnoses, there is not uniform agreement on the process of their formation or on their content.[7] Present efforts appear directed toward establishing MDC-like categories, under which more specific patient conditions could be listed.

There are conceptual and technical problems with the notion of using nursing diagnoses within DRGs for nursing intensity measurement. We do not propose to discuss this complex issue in detail here. In theory, it should be possible to put nursing diagnoses into hierarchies much as medical diagnoses are in the DRG system.

Unlike medical diagnoses, which can be assigned with some reliability and which do not change once assigned unless the diagnosis changes, it is in the nature of nursing diagnoses that not only do they change, but also they *should*. A patient's pain or constipation should be relieved, for example, and that nursing diagnosis would then disappear from the list, whereas a patient's appendicitis may be cured with an appendectomy, but the patient still had documented appendicitis. Further, nursing diagnoses occur daily, repeatedly, and in multiple combinations.

For our purposes, the importance of the nursing diagnosis research is that it points up the possibility that patient conditions in addition to diagnosis or surgical procedures may play a part in the allocation of nursing resources. Halloran has shown that nursing diagnosis *in combination* with DRGs explains a greater proportion of the variability in nursing time than DRGs alone.[8,9] To date, however, the nursing diagnosis work has not been applied to per-case (or per-DRG) analysis of nursing intensity and no studies have distinguished intensive or special care from routine care.

SPECIAL CARE

Intensive care services developed from postoperative recovery rooms, which became adjuncts of operating rooms during the nursing shortage of World War II. The recovery room was considered a special part of the operating room and thus fell into the category of ancillary services. Special charges were usually levied; afterwards, when intensive care units (ICUs) began to blossom, the costing convention carried over. Although a special charge is usually assigned for these kinds of services, it is not considered as ancillary service income but as an additional revenue under the classification of "room and board." These services are a substitute, though a more expensive one, for the regular nursing care given to patients in their hospital beds. This peculiar characteristic of separate charges without separate costing has made the management of resources in special care units a very touchy problem.

Intensive care is intensive *nursing* care. The staffing ratio is usually 1:1 or 1:2, and it is estimated that, on average, patients receive 17 hours of nursing care for every day of ICU stay. The relatively stable staffing formula and the fact that a different charge is made for ICU or special care services suggests that the ICU portion of a patient's stay must be treated separately in any model of analysis of nursing intensity.

Today, special care units, for which different room and board charges are assessed, include medical, surgical, pediatric, and neonatal intensive care units; burn units; telemetry and stepdown units; hospice units; and in-hospital birth centers. Charges are higher than regular room rates in all but the last two. As the number and kinds of special care beds have grown, the use of them as reflected by days in special care has grown even more rapidly and is of particular interest in the treatment of selected DRGs. The growth in special care was documented first by Rockwell, then by Draper, and then by Thompson.[10-12] The differential use of special care across hospitals is a new area of inquiry.

There are several ways to account for the relative volume of nursing used in special care units of general hospitals. The first is to track the growth of intensive care days over a period of time in a group of hospitals serving a describable population. Such an examination should include experience prior to, as well as after, the institution of prospective payment. A second approach would be to analyze the pattern of the provision of intensive care for each of the hospitals. Variation in the use of these services across hospitals could be elucidated and a determination made as to whether a given hospital was following the overall trend. Finally, certain characteristics of hospitals that seem to influence the relative number of intensive care days can be examined.

Table 6-1 traces the growth of intensive care days (excluding neonatal ICU days) in the 35 general hospitals in Connecticut from 1973 to 1987. Over the 15-year period, intensive care days increased by 50.44 percent. The growth from 1977 on was at a fairly constant rate and did not change much on the implementation of prospective payment in 1984. The annual rate of growth picked up again in 1987. It appears that prospective payment did not radically influence the pattern of growth of intensive care services in the general hospitals in Connecticut.

The growth across individual hospitals in intensive care days from 1983 to 1987 was also examined. The relative use of intensive care in each hospital was defined as the ratio of intensive care days to routine care days given to adult medical-surgical patients, multiplied by 100. There was an overall increase in intensive care days of 5.33 ratio points between 1983 and 1987. In only four hospitals was there a decrease in the ratio, and these decreases were quite small (Table 6-2). The growth rate in the first

Table 6-1: Intensive Care Days except Neonatal ICU, Connecticut General Hospitals, 1973–1987

Year	Days in Intensive Care Units	Yearly Percent Increase	Percent Increase from 1973
1973	124,852		
1974	128,679	3.14	3.14
1975	136,280	5.91	9.15
1976	157,877	15.85	26.45
1977	157,492	− 0.24	26.14
1978	160,314	1.79	28.40
1979	163,356	1.90	30.84
1980	165,911	1.56	32.89
1981	170,724	2.90	36.74
1982	173,324	1.52	38.82
1983	178,330	2.89	42.83
1984	183,637	2.98	47.08
1985	183,892	0.14	47.29
1986	183,544	− 0.18	47.01
1987	187,828	2.33	50.44

Source: The Connecticut Hospital Association.

three-quarters of the hospitals is erratic since different hospitals added intensive care days at different rates. However, the eight hospitals at the bottom of the list that had relatively more ICU days in 1983 also used more ICU days in 1987.

The major finding of interest, however, is the variation in the ratios, from 2.92 in hospital A to 16.45 in hospital AI in 1983, and from 4.51 in hospital H to 21.27 in hospital V in 1987. It would be expected that the two university hospitals would have very high ratios. When these two hospitals are removed, a definite pattern emerges with the important characteristic being the size of the hospital. Hospitals with 5,000 or fewer admissions per year average an ICU/routine care ratio of 11.01; hospitals with over 5,000 but under 10,000 admissions have an average ratio of 9.77; and hospitals with over 10,000 admissions per year have an average ratio of 9.35.

When the two smaller groups are combined and 1987 data are used, the smaller hospitals have significantly higher ratios of intensive care days to routine care days than the larger hospitals. This finding stands whether the university hospitals are included or not. That hospital size rather than case mix seems to predict ICU use runs counter to the usual hypothesis that larger hospitals have "sicker" patients. Smaller hospitals are using ICUs in different ways than larger hospitals, probably dictated by the relative availability of nursing resources.

Table 6-2: Ratio (× 100) of Intensive Care Days to Routine Medical-Surgical Days, 1983–1987, in 35 General Hospitals in Connecticut

Hospital	Ratio 1983	Ratio 1987	Rank 1983	Rank 1987
A	2.92	6.28	1	5
B	3.66	4.83	2	2
C	3.96	6.56	3	8
D	4.20	8.10	4	14
E	4.54	13.33	5	30
F	5.02	6.63	6	7
G	5.05	7.33	7	10
H	5.18	4.51	8	1
I	5.57	10.17	9	21
J	5.57	7.91	10	13
K	5.64	8.49	11	16
L	5.80	6.28	12	6
M	5.96	7.29	13	9
N	6.13	6.23	14	4
O	6.19	8.16	15	15
P	6.21	7.35	16	11
Q	6.35	7.33	17	10
R	6.39	5.76	18	3
S	6.69	10.32	19	22
T	6.77	9.85	20	20
U	7.09	11.81	21	25
V	7.17	21.27	22	35
W	7.30	9.07	23	18
X	7.46	11.77	24	24
Y	8.94	12.91	25	26
Z	8.95	7.42	26	12
AA	9.84	9.11	27	19
AB	10.24	13.28	28	28
AC	10.33	10.60	29	23
AD	11.13	14.02	30	31
AE	11.95	14.14	31	32
AF	11.99	13.14	32	27
AG	13.05	15.21	33	32
AH	13.18	15.70	34	33
AI	16.45	19.96	35	34

Source: The Connecticut Hospital Association.

Among the explanations for the overall growth pattern is the shift of cases to ambulatory care either in one-day surgery or in selected ambulatory services. Patients who get into the hospital are sicker and therefore require more intensive care. This result is consistent with other findings from case-mix analyses over the time from before to after the introduction of prospective payment.[13]

Another explanation might well have to do with the nursing shortage that began to affect hospitals in 1987. Because of shortage on the routine floors, there may be a tendency to keep patients in intensive care longer. While the shortage affects all hospital units, national data suggest that it is more serious on general medical-surgical floors than in intensive care.[14] Whatever the explanation, the effect on the cost of nursing care should not be ignored.

Intensive care is sufficiently different from care on routine floors that these two components of a patient stay must be handled separately in any analysis of nursing intensity. Draper and her collaborators suggest that there may be widespread misuse of ICU resources.[15,16] Their notion is that there are two kinds of patients in ICUs—those who are there primarily for monitoring, and who are relatively stable (and who might not require ICU time), and those who are there for therapeutic interventions. Indeed, there is a high correlation between physiological instability, as measured by the Acute Physiological Assessment/Chronic Health Evaluation (APACHE) score, and a measure of therapeutic intervention in ICUs (TISS—the Therapeutic Intervention Scoring System) in coronary care units. The relationship between APACHE and TISS in a surgical ICU holds only on the first ICU day.[17,18]

Few investigators have looked within the ICU experience to tap nursing intensity. Two recent small studies provide tantalizing suggestions for future research. One study examined care given in a general surgical ICU, the other care in a cardiac surgical ICU in a different hospital.[19,20] In neither study was there any relation between measures of physiological derangement or medical diagnosis and nursing resource requirement, as measured by TISS in the first study and by a nursing patient classification system (GRASP) in the other.

In the general surgical ICU study, 50 percent of the patients had an ICU stay of two days or less. In the cardiac surgical ICU study, the average total length of hospital stay for inlier patients was 11.8 days, of which, on the average, 9.4 days were postoperative and 3.1 were spent in the ICU. In this latter study, there was a significant negative correlation between length of ICU stay and nursing requirements in the ICU; the higher the nursing requirements, the shorter the stay.

The average daily duration of nursing care for the four highest-volume DRGs in the general surgical ICU study ranged from 18.3 to 21.5 hours. Patients on the last 12-hour shift in the unit required an average of 8.88 hours of nursing care for that shift, or more than 17 hours a day, more nursing care than is available on routine care floors. When selected DRGs were analyzed, patients over 65 years of age in DRG 149 (major small and large bowel procedures without complications) had *lower* requirements for nursing care than younger patients in the same DRG. Age may be an unstated criterion for ICU admission given the absence of protocols for ICU use in this institution.

Both studies suggested that there was considerable variation in nursing care requirements on the last ICU day. Some patients were being discharged to the routine care floors while still requiring high levels of nursing care. In fact, in the cardiac ICU study, *all* of the post-ICU days' nursing requirements were in the highest two categories of a nursing patient classification system.

Another analysis hints that, within selected DRGs, patients who spend some time in an ICU have longer total lengths of stay, higher nursing care requirements, and greater costs than other patients. Table 6-3 shows data from one hospital for selected high-volume Medicare DRGs. In all DRGs examined here both LOS and mean routine care times were greater for patients who had been in the ICU. Whether this means that "sicker" patients go to the ICU or that ICUs make people—who may not need ICU care—sicker is still an open question.

Even if two distinct groups of patients are admitted to ICUs, the difference between them is likely to be reflected more in professional fees and ancillary service use than in nursing intensity. Monitoring requires at least as much nursing time as do some of the high-technology procedures performed in ICUs. Thus relative ICU use, as measured in days of stay in special care, is a reasonable index of nursing intensity in ICUs, is easy to collect, and produces comparable information from hospital to hospital. Since ICUs use only registered nurse (RN) staffing, differences in costs of differently prepared personnel are also not an issue. Determining nursing

Table 6-3: Length of Stay and Nursing Time in All Patients and Patients with No ICU Stay

	All Discharges			Non-ICU Discharges		
DRG	*No.*	*Mean LOS*	*Mean Ns/Pt**	*No.*	*Mean LOS*	*Mean Ns/Pt**
14	323	12.45	5,567	234	10.66	4,004
89	198	8.88	3,316	176	8.14	2,660
122	140	6.89	2,488	77	5.26	1,485
125	444	4.01	1,176	407	3.64	933
127	398	8.76	3,222	340	8.03	2,593
148	131	17.74	7,801	115	17.17	6,969
174	114	6.76	2,681	102	6.28	2,203
294	115	7.61	2,418	103	7.33	2,110

*Ns/Pt = mean per case nursing minutes on routine care (non-ICU) floors.
Source: Robert B. Fetter and John D. Thompson, "Diagnosis Related Groups and Nursing Resources."

costs within ICUs is therefore simpler than measuring nursing on routine care floors.

NURSING PATIENT CLASSIFICATION

Since the development at Johns Hopkins Hospital of the concept of linking patient characteristics with nurse staffing requirements in the late 1950s, more has been written about nursing patient classification systems than about any other aspect of nursing management.[21] The literature on patient classification has been usefully reviewed by Aydelotte and Giovannetti in the United States and Canada and by Rhys Hearn in the United Kingdom.[22–24]

Classifying patients by conditions or variables that require nursing attention is complicated by the nearly infinite number of ways in which lists of patient conditions have been compiled. Giovannetti distinguishes among three general kinds of nursing patient classification methods: prototypes, task documents, and critical indicators.[25]

The prototype system is not much used now. It consists of a relatively small number of groups of "typical" patient characteristics, to which a given patient is matched. (This method may come back into favor if reliable nursing diagnoses eventually emerge.)

Task documents are lists of nursing activities applicable to a given patient. Such documents usually include activities of daily living (feeding, bathing, toileting), mobility, medications, and monitoring. The San Joaquin system (Figure 6-1) is perhaps the most widely used and simplest of these systems. It was derived from a long list of some 200 possible activities.[26] Each day (or each shift) the patient's nurse checks the box that corresponds to the patient's requirements for care on the succeeding shift or day. The column with the highest number of check marks becomes the patient's level or category of care, I through IV. I is "minimal" care. IV is "intensive"; in hospitals that use this system, it may be reserved for ICU care.

Critical indicator systems label patient conditions rather than nursing tasks (Table 6-4 is an example). In general, the listed conditions are weighted and a total score calculated. The raw score itself may be used as an index of the patient's care needs; most often, the scores are collapsed into four or more levels of care, each with a range of points, but the ranges may not be the same.

In the United States and Canada, the use of patient classification for staffing is mandated by hospital accrediting bodies. Each hospital selects its own system from the variety available, now numbering in the hundreds, or the hospital invents its own. Giovannetti and Mayer point out that there is more similarity than difference among the patient classifica-

Figure 6-1: A Task Document, San Joaquin Patient Classification System

Floor

Patient Class	I	II	III	IV
Activity independent	( )			
Bath, partial assist		( )	( )	
Position, partial assist		( )	( )	
Position, complete assist			( )	( )
Diet, partial assist		( )	( )	
Diet feed			( )	( )
I.V. add. q6 H or more or TKO		( )	( )	( )
Observe q 1–2 hrs.			( )	( )
Observe, almost constant				( )
Patient name No.		( )	( )	
Total			.5	

Comments:

Source: San Joaquin General Hospital, *San Joaquin Classification* (Stockton, CA: San Joaquin General Hospital, 1976).

tion systems, and that little increase in validity arises from adding more than the basic ADL(activities of daily living)/medication/monitoring items.[27] The major criterion for adoption of a system and the major reason for the number and variety of them is the preference of the nurses who will use the system.

Task documents are criticized both on professional and technical grounds. It is argued that nursing is more than merely the performance of tasks and that task documents are therefore an incomplete, if not actually a demeaning, operational definition of nursing practice. These kinds of patient classification systems are also faulted for reducing nursing to too few categories. Yet, tasks are what get nurses into patients' rooms; what goes on there can be captured in other ways. Critical indicator systems are criticized because patients are more individual in their characteristics than any printed list can show. Yet an exhaustive list would be so complicated it could not be useful.

All existing types of systems are alleged not to measure the "professional" component of nursing practice—the observation, assessment, and decision-making activities called "nursing process."[28] This argument parallels the controversy between internists (representing conceptual

Table 6-4: A Critical-Indicator System, Revised Rush-Medicus

Nursing Patient Classification, MED/SURG/OB-GYN/PEDS	
Assigned Weight	*Indicators*
	Assessment Observation Needs
3	Admission/transfer in
3	Discharge/transfer out
8	Confused/retarded/disoriented
2	Specimen collecting/testing
8	Respirator
8	Physiologic instability/major trauma/psychological instability
2	Intake and output
5	IV and site care
8	Monitor
6	Frequent vital signs
	Nursing Intervention Needs
4	Sensory/communication impairment
5	Examination
6	Extensive wound/skin care
6	Tube care
4	Pulmonary treatment
2	Discharge planning
4	Patient/family teaching
4	Emotional needs greater than usual
	Functional Needs
4/6	Age (0–2 yrs old = 4 pts 3–4 yrs old = 6 pts)
3	Partial immobility
6	Complete immobility
2	Bath with assistance
6	Complete/total bath
0	Up ad lib
2	Up with assistance
4	Bed rest
4	Difficult transfer/turn
2	Assist with oral/tube feeding
6	Total oral/tube feeding
2	Assist with exercise
	Special Needs
6	Isolation/isolette
4	Prepared for test/procedures
6	Assist patient off unit
151	24-hour attendance

Category I	0–15	Category III	27–49
Category II	16–26	Category IV	50+

Source: M. Sovie, et al., "Amalgam of Nursing Acuity, DRGs and Costs," *Nursing Management* 16, no. 3 (1985): 22–42.

medicine) and surgeons (representing technical medicine) over reimbursement rates that seem to favor the latter. Further, there has been
concern both in nursing and at the policy level that the proliferation of
nursing patient classification systems precludes comparative studies of
nursing requirements across institutions using different systems. No
large-scale studies have compared nursing patient classification systems.
In countries just beginning DRG-related research, it has been possible to
prescribe a uniform nursing patient classification system (as in France, for
example, which has adopted Québec's PRN system).

We suggest that the particular patient classification system used by a
given hospital is not the issue, except to the extent that its use is sanc-
tioned by the nursing staff so that reliable data are produced. There are
endless possibilities for classifying the work of nursing, using, for example, tasks (as in TISS in ICUs, for instance) or patient characteristics. In the
DRG model, however, what is of interest is the relative resources consumed, under the assumption that there is some relation between what
the patient needs and what the patient gets. What patients need is more a
matter of interest to individual institutions or even units within them, for
clinical and management decisions. Those decisions depend, appropriately, on the nursing staff's preferences for the forms in which they
want and need data. Any classification system, whether it is medical
diagnosis, APACHE, DRG, or nursing patient classification is unsatisfy-
ing to clinicians trained to consider the "whole person." But reducing
complex human beings to manageable units must still be done, and can
be accomplished without eliminating access to useful clinical information
retained in the medical record, information that can be linked to the
classification system.

The most important consideration in obtaining reliable and valid
data from patient classification is whether the nurses involved feel that
the use of the system will produce what it is intended to produce. Filling
out all those forms every day and seeing no increase in nursing staff, or
no attention to the information in other ways, and no feedback for the
effort will guarantee that nurses will eventually stop taking the system
seriously.

Patient classification is but one step on the way to linking nursing
resources to patient requirements, however. The next step—attaching a
measure of resource consumption—is the crucial one.

MEASUREMENT OF NURSING INTENSITY

To be used for staffing purposes, patient classification systems require
translation to nursing time and then to full-time equivalent nurses. The

translation of patient requirements to nursing intensity involves assigning or otherwise attaching time (minutes) to patient classification. Minutes can then be accumulated across patients to hours, divided by eight (for one full-time equivalent), and the total staffing requirement determined. That number becomes the staffing target, within a certain range, since nurses come only in whole numbers and staffing can be manipulated only in four- or eight-hour increments.

Traditional time-motion studies are the most frequently used methods of determining the time associated with nursing tasks or patient requirements. Such studies are typically conducted for a sample of patients for a few weeks, with average times calculated for tasks or indicators, and those times become part of the algorithm that converts patient classification to staffing targets. Tasks can be timed without much difficulty. Alternatively, when a new patient classification system is being put into place, patients are first classified, and then the total care to them is timed, eventually producing average times per class of patients. When time-motion studies have not been feasible, consensus of nurses on time allocation has been used to set time standards.

The simplest part of the effort is attaching direct, hands-on care time to particular patients. But a number of nursing activities do not involve direct patient contact: charting, preparing medications, arranging transfer, consulting with physicians, and so on. Further, there are activities that cannot be allocated to particular patients but must nevertheless become part of the model, if *all* of the nursing resource is to be accounted for: change of shift report, distributing supplies, stocking treatment rooms, checking narcotic counts, changing the crash cart supplies, and so on. And finally, nonpatient care time such as breaks, lunch, or off-ward conferences or meetings has to be taken into account.

The literature borrows cost-accounting terminology and sometimes defines nursing time as "fixed" and "variable." The RIMs study cited earlier used such concepts, and assigned fixed times to nursing resource groups on the assumption that patients admitted with the same cluster of variables required the same initial fixed component of nursing time. "Direct" and "indirect" times have also been defined, with "direct" time being time spent in the physical presence of the patient.

We prefer the terminology Sovie and her colleagues have used: "patient assignable" time.[29] Patient assignable time includes both activities done in the presence of the patient and activities done in the service of the patient when the nurse is not in the room. "Unit" time, then, is time that cannot be associated with particular patients, but is still patient-care time, and personal time is time that is not directly associated with patient care, such as nurses' meals. This division of time also allows for group nursing activities on certain kinds of units, such as group psychotherapy, or group instruction in baby care or breast-feeding, common in maternity services. All nursing time of all nurses can then be classified in one or another of these categories. The exercise of inventing the time algorithm is in itself instructive, as it calls attention to the variety of things nurses do (some of which they might well wish to delegate to others, if they are not in the service of individual patients).

Time standards should be service-specific. The average nursing requirements for medical-surgical, pediatric, and psychiatric patients are considerably different, and so therefore are the costs of nursing in different services (see later section).

Sovie also argues that each nursing unit should establish its own time component of the patient classification system. Hospital architecture and the size of the patient unit, as well as characteristics of patients with different conditions but the same task requirements, suggest such unit-specificity. For example, assisting a patient with a severe stroke to the bathroom on a neurological unit might well be more time-consuming than assisting a new postoperative appendectomy patient on a general surgical unit who is otherwise healthy. Feeding a baby is quite different from helping a person with an arm cast to cut food into bites. Sovie's own data show considerable variation in unit-specific times, with the lowest in the eye, ear, nose, and throat unit (0.99 hours/patient/ day) and the highest in the pediatric intensive care unit (4.41 hours/patient/ day). The unit times are treated as a constant, added to the variable patient assignable time determined from the patient classification system.[30]

The RIMs study was directed toward reimbursement and cost issues. Thus, the investigators used RN time as a standard, and then deflated LPN and aide time in proportion to the salary differential. An LPN minute was only 75 percent of an RN minute and an aide minute was still less. This maneuver simplified the cost analysis, but complicated the interpretation of data. Since *time*, rather than patient classification, is the basic unit of measurement of nursing intensity, it must be actual, rather than weighted time, so that times can be compared. Cost can be handled by actual salary differentials. Mixing the two measurements is not wise.

Decisions about *whose* time is included in the standards require some thought. In some institutions, the ward clerks are not part of the nursing budget and so their time is not contained in the standards. Some hospitals have clinical specialists who are not based on particular units, but go wherever their services are required; psychiatric liaison nurses and oncology nurse clinical specialists are cases in point. Their time may be accounted for either as part of the unit constant, which includes nursing administrative overhead, or when particular patients require the services of nurse clinical specialists, the patient's classification may be raised one level, with a resulting increase in the time and cost allocation. Whether the head nurse's time is included depends upon the particular role the head nurse assumes. It may be included as part of the unit constant, or may vary if the head nurse engages in direct patient care. In a primary nursing situation, the latter is probably more often the case.

The use of patient classification information in a primary nursing context has received little attention. Primary nursing involves the assignment of one nurse to a caseload of patients. The primary nurse designs and carries out the total care of these patients, rather than performing specific tasks (for example, giving medications or performing nursing treatments) to a whole unit, as in "functional" or "team" nursing. The primary nurse has 24-hour responsibility, authority, and accountability for the group of patients, and assigns to associate nurses the care on the off shifts.[31] Staffing standards in primary nursing require one nurse to four to six patients, a standard now nearly uniformly adopted. The literature is divided on whether LPNs can serve as primary nurses or not. Usually, institutions that have adopted primary nursing to organize care have all-RN staffs. Since staffing is fixed, it might be thought unnecessary to have a patient classification system altogether.

Since the initial application of this line of reasoning was in staffing, most of the studies of patient classification in nursing deal with predicted or projected rather than actual time given. What one is after in staffing is an estimate of nursing required in the next shift or day. Later applications of the method in hospitals that bill directly and variably for different levels of nursing provided use actual time, which can be tracked through the chart should an audit be required.

The major usefulness of patient classification in a primary nursing context presently is in tracking patient acuity, and in providing the nursing intensity information upon which a variable billing system depends. Future applications include unit-level management implications, such as assigning primary nurses to particular patients on the basis of patient requirements.

"Patient acuity" and "nursing intensity" are both important. They should be measured differently, however, because the uses to which the information might be put differ. Acuity describes patients; intensity describes nursing resources. Once patient classification and a time algorithm are in place, data can begin to accumulate, with reliance on the memory of computers, and an entire model for analysis of nursing intensity, including cost, can evolve.

THE YALE STUDY OF NURSING INTENSITY

Under the Prospective Payment System, the reimbursement hypothesis is that all patients receive the same amount of routine nursing care every day of their stay. Nursing is contained within the room and board charge assigned per diem. This hypothesis is false on the face of it. Until prospective payment forced institutions to look inside their cost accounting traditions in order to manage resources within DRG prices, there was little incentive to examine nursing resources carefully.

When the prospective payment legislation was passed, the Health Care Financing Administration (HCFA) made available contract funds through the American Nurses' Association (ANA) to begin an investigation of nursing intensity within DRGs.[32] A number of other small studies using DRGs as the framework to examine differential nursing care requirements in a small number of cases were conducted independently.[33-36] Sovie's study was the first and largest study to use nursing intensity information in one hospital merged with cost data.[37]

Table 6-5: Number of Patients, Average Nursing Hours per Case, and Average Nursing Hours per Day, by DRG: In Five Studies, 1982–1984

DRG No.	Description	Sovie			Mitchell		
		No. Pats.	Avg. Nsg. Hrs/Case	Avg. Nsg. Hrs/Day	No. Pats.	Avg. Nsg. Hrs/Case	Avg. Nsg. Hrs/Day
88	CHRONIC OBSTRUCTIVE PULMONARY DISEASE	125	47.9	4.7			
121	AMI W C.V. COMP DISCH ALIVE	91	69.6	5.2	13	109	NA
122	AMI W/O C.V. COMP DISCH ALIVE	211	56.6	5.0	12	68	NA
127	HEART FAILURE & SHOCK	206	57.0	4.4			
174	GI BLEEDING, AGE 70 CC	67	52.9	4.8			
175	GI BLEEDING, AGE <70	36	17.5	3.9			
195	CHOLECYSTECTOMY W C.D.E., AGE 70 CC	23	101.0	5.0			
197	CHOLECYSTECTOMY W/O C.D.E., AGE 70 CC	56	51.6	4.2			
209	MAJOR JOINT PROC	232	93.9	4.4	32	88	NA
210	OTH HIP/FEMUR PROC, AGE 70 CC	78	143.0	4.5	32	95	NA
219	OTH LOW EXTREM, HUMEROUS PROC, AGE 18–69	85	55.6	4.2			

NA = Not Available.

Sources: M. Sovie et al., "Amalgam of Nursing Acuity, DRGs and Costs," *Nursing Management* 16, no. 3 (1985): 22–42; M. Mitchell et al., "Determining Costs of Direct Nursing Care by DRGs," *Nursing Management* 15, no. 4 (1984): 29–32; W. Riley and V. Schaefers, "Costing Nursing

In general, all of the studies focused upon the extent to which DRG assignment did or did not predict nursing care requirements fully, and the considerable variation in nursing time within DRGs. Only one small comparison between two hospitals was made, as an incidental part of Sovie's study. In certain DRGs, she found nearly an eightfold difference in nursing costs between two hospitals in the same town. Table 6-5 shows the comparative nursing times for the DRGs included in the studies published prior to the Yale study.

The ANA study collected prospective nursing intensity data on a sample of 21 high-volume Medicare DRGs in two Wisconsin hospitals. The major methodological contributions from this study were the implication that the very high correlation between nursing resources and length of stay must be addressed and the finding of potentially different patterns of nursing resource consumption within length-of-stay groups in the same DRG.

None of these studies, however, separated intensive or special care from routine care. As we have argued earlier, such a separation is critical for proper understanding of nursing resources.

Riley			Lagona			McClain		
No. Pats.	Avg. Nsg. Hrs/Case	Avg. Nsg. Hrs/Day	No. Pats.	Avg. Nsg. Hrs/Case	Avg. Nsg. Hrs/Day	No. Pats.	Avg. Nsg. Hrs/Case	Avg. Nsg. Hrs/Day
						10	58.4	3.6
			16	125	9.1			
			19	90	8.2			
35	42	5.1						
6	28	5.1						
20	67	6.4						
						4	216.4	9.7
						6	93.4	6.6
37	49	4.8						

Services," *Nursing Management* 14, no. 12 (1983): 40–43; T. G. Lagona and M. M. Stritzel, "Nursing Care Requirements as Measured by DRG," *Journal of Nursing Administration* 14, no. 5 (1984): 15–18; J. McClain and M. Selhat, "Twenty Cases: What Nursing Cost per DRG," *Nursing Management* 15, no. 10 (1984): 27–34.

A study to develop and test models of accounting for nursing resources within DRGs was designed and conducted by the Health Systems Management Group at Yale University.[38] The purpose of the study was to devise a way to account for across-DRG variation in nursing intensity. The research also explored the possibility of using patient classification systems developed as a method for scheduling nursing staff as an approach to the measurement of nursing intensity.

Table 6-6 shows the data sets used in the project; the hospitals are labeled A through E (hospital C is actually five small hospitals, all of which used the same patient classification/nursing intensity system).[39] The hospitals all used different patient classification instruments; three of them reduced the patient characteristics to levels of care, while two of them retained the raw score. The time algorithms actually used by the hospitals assigned minutes per patient per day. Two hospitals used the information for staffing prospectively; three hospitals recorded actual times, because they were using the information for variable billing for nursing services. The total number of usable patient records was 139,498.

Missing values proved to be a problem for the attempt to analyze the nursing data from daily records. Patients going to surgery are often not put into a classification system the night before, since they are not going to be on the unit on the next shift. Newly admitted or about-to-be-discharged patients may also not be classified. More importantly, patients with very long stays, a group that may include high proportions of Medicare patients, may not be classified every day, especially if their

Table 6-6: Description of Study Sites

Hospital	Region of U.S.	Number Beds/Type	Study Year(s)	Patient Classification System	No. of Records
A	Western	400–500 Teaching	4 years 1979–1983	St. Lukes'	43,683
B	North central	400–500 Teaching	2 years 1983–1985	D. J. Sullivan	34,560
C	Northeast	226–434 Five community hospitals	9 months 1983–1984	GRASP	30,139
D	Northeast	500–750 Teaching	1 year 1982–1983	Modified Medicus	24,897
E	Northeast	500–750 Teaching	1 year 1984–1985	HANYS	22,359

Source: Robert B. Fetter and John D. Thompson, "Diagnosis Related Groups and Nursing Resources."

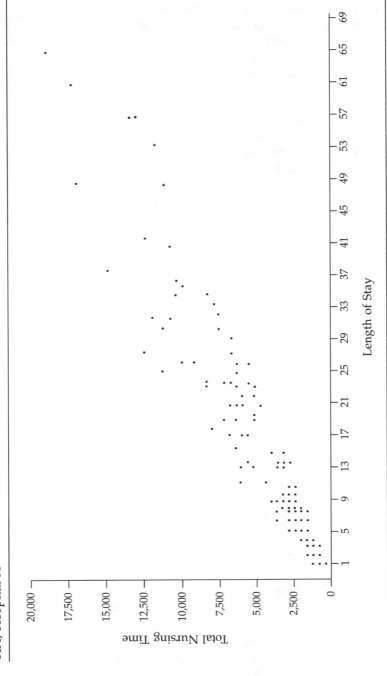

Figure 6-2: Total Nursing Time by Length of Stay, Non-ICU, DRG 14, Specific Cerebrovascular Disorders except TIA, Hospital A

Source: Robert B. Fetter and John D. Thompson, "Diagnosis Related Groups and Nursing Resources."

conditions do not change much. Therefore, conventions were adopted to impute missing information where possible.

Number of days in intensive or special care was chosen as the measurement of nursing intensity for that portion of a patient's hospital stay, following the line of reasoning described earlier. Thus the analysis concentrated on the routine care portion of the stay.

There will always be a direct, positive, and linear relationship between nursing intensity (minutes of care per patient per stay) and length of stay. Every patient gets some nursing care every day of stay, if not the same amount or in the same pattern. Figure 6-2 shows DRG 14, stroke, not a particularly good DRG in terms of its definition; the pattern of nursing intensity and length of stay can be seen clearly, as can the funnel effect of longer stays.

This form of the relation between *total* nursing time and length of stay is consistent and regular. It is possible to take advantage of this

Figure 6-3: Graphic Representation of Nursing Allocation Statistic

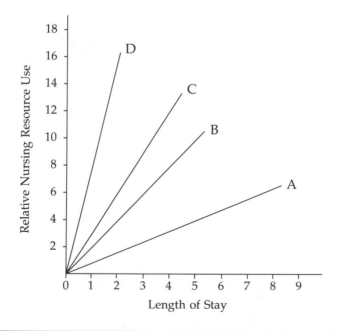

Source: Robert B. Fetter and John D. Thompson, "Diagnosis Related Groups and Nursing Resources."

correlation to construct a model of *relative* nursing intensity (one DRG relative to another) by regressing nursing time on length of stay to produce the beta weight, or slope of the line. Figure 6-3 shows the general form of the relationship. Line A would represent a DRG with relatively low requirements for nursing over relatively long lengths of stay, say hip replacement. Line D would represent a DRG with relatively high requirements for routine nursing care over shorter stays, such as, perhaps, some of the pediatric DRGs.

The beta weight can be interpreted as the increment in nursing time occasioned by one more day of stay, in minutes. Beta weights were calculated for all five data sets, for every DRG with 20 or more observations. Before proceeding further, "influential observations" were identified with a particular statistic, Cook's D.[40] These "nursing-intensity outliers" were patients whose length of stay and total nursing resource requirements were simultaneously significantly different from the rest of the cases in that DRG. These observations were eliminated from further analysis.

Table 6-7 shows selected DRGs, including those used in the ANA study, with the routine care beta weights by hospital. At first glance it would appear that there is considerable difference among hospitals in routine nursing care intensity. For example, DRG 14, stroke, has beta weights of 289, 430, 429, 220 and 376. Hospital D's weights are nearly always the lowest; hospitals B and E generally have the highest weights.

The correlations in beta weights among the hospitals can be seen in Table 6-8. The highest correlation, .62, is between hospitals A and C; the lowest, .34, between hospitals A and D. All of the correlations are statistically significant. Since there were many differences among the hospitals in size, institutional affiliation, case mix, patient classification system, time assignment and staffing mix, and use of ICU, the correlations, while modest, are not bad. The model makes it possible to compare institutions in a meaningful, case-specific way. The beta weight is a better measure of total resources consumed than the average nursing time per patient per day, since it captures the total routine care nursing resource requirement.

While data on patient days in ICU were not available, data on numbers of patients by DRG who had ICU experience was. Using the same DRGs, the differences in ICU use can be seen (Table 6-9). Even in this small sample—only nine hospitals (five data sets) and only 20 DRGs—the difference across hospitals in ICU use ranges from nearly none (0.6 percent) for DRG 39, lens extraction, to nearly 60 percent (57.9 percent) for DRG 140, angina. The DRGs with the most difference in ICU use in this sample are DRG 122 (circulatory disorders with acute myocardial infarction, no comorbidities or complications, discharged alive); DRG

Table 6-7: Weights for Selected DRGs, Routine Care Only

		\[Hospital\] A	B	C	D	E
DRG		A	B	C	D	E
14	SPEC CEREB DIS EX TIA	289	430	429	220	376
15	TIA	245	290	290	155	296
39	LENS PROCEDURES	235	221	243	157	263
88	COPD	264	291	300	196	319
89	SIMPLE PNEUM >70 CC	283	356	382	207	322
96	BRONCH & ASTHMA >70 CC	258	289	291	184	325
122	CIRC DIS AMI ALIVE	254	299	320	193	337
125	CIRC DIS EX AMI	247	263		177	314
127	HEART FAILURE & SHOCK	278	349	337	194	341
130	PVD >70 CC	256	320	302	207	319
132	ATHEROSCLEROSIS >70 CC	247	282	276		
138	CARD ARRHYTHMIA >70 CC	257	314	328	198	332
140	ANGINA	255	273	273	192	323
148	MAJOR BOWEL PROC >70 CC	300	424	384	192	323
174	G.I. HEMORRHAGE >70 CC	273	358	324	195	332
182	ESOPHG/GASTROENT >70 CC	233	289	279	161	286
243	MEDICAL BACK	225	196	231	154	285
294	DIABETES >36	229	297	312	165	311
320	KIDNEY/UTI >70 CC	274	362	374	215	313
336	TURP	257	257	276	209	307

Source: Robert B. Fetter and John D. Thompson, "Diagnosis Related Groups and Nursing Resources."

Table 6-8: Correlation Coefficients* for DRG-Specific Routine Care Nursing Weights, for DRGs with ≥ 20 Discharges, Influential Observations Removed, for Five Study Sites

	Hospital				
Hospital	A	B	C	D	E
A	1.000	.576	.621	.336	.429
B		1.000	.557	.587	.572
C			1.000	.356	.565
D				1.000	.541
E					1.000

*All r values are significant ($p < .0006$).
Source: Robert B. Fetter and John D. Thompson, "Diagnosis Related Groups and Nursing Resources."

132 (atherosclerosis in persons over 69 with comorbidities or complications); DRG 138 (cardiac arrhythmia and conduction disorders in persons over 69 with comorbidities or complications); DRG 140 (angina); and

Table 6-9: Percent of Patients without ICU Stays, Selected DRGs

	Hospital				
DRG	A	B	C	D	E
14 STROKE	75.5	72.4	86.6	90.4	90.8
15 TIA	96.7	97.4	94.5	98.6	95.7
39 LENS PROC	99.8	100	99.4	100	100
88 COPD	91.3	96.2	88.2	83.8	91.4
89 PNEUM & PLEUR >69 CC	92.6	88.9	93.0	84.1	92.7
96 BRONCH & ASTHMA >69 CC	91.5	97.2	92.4	92.1	94.1
122 CIRC DIS W AMI ALIVE	64.0	55.0	11.1	17.6	34.9
125 CIRC DIS W CATH	98.2	91.7	—	96.2	91.6
127 HEART FAILURE & SHOCK	81.3	85.4	73.7	79.4	85.2
130 PVD >69 CC	96.3	94.3	94.9	96.4	94.5
132 ATHEROSCL >69 CC	89.0	96.9	63.5	50.0	50.0
138 CARD ARRHY >69 CC	87.2	94.2	55.7	59.5	91.2
140 ANGINA	68.8	6.1	38.2	44.2	71.5
148 MAJOR BOWEL PROC >69 CC	57.4	87.8	64.6	83.3	85.0
174 G.I. HEM >69 CC	74.0	89.5	79.1	87.8	87.2
182 GASTROENT DIS >69 CC	96.8	97.8	96.2	97.4	94.8
243 MEDICAL BACK	99.4	99.3	99.2	99.1	97.9
294 CA BREAST >69 CC	94.4	89.6	92.7	97.6	89.8
320 KIDNEY/UTI >69 CC	97.8	100	95.2	100	95.9
336 TURP >69 CC	95.7	100	96.6	97.2	100

Source: Robert B. Fetter and John D. Thompson, "Diagnosis Related Groups and Nursing Resources."

DRG 148 (major bowel procedures in persons over 69 with comorbidities or complications). Four of the five DRGs are medical, and three of them and the one surgical one (DRG 148) are defined by age or complication/comorbidity. ICU use in DRG 122 is nearly six times as high in hospital A as in hospital C; ICU use in hospital D is less than half that of hospital B in DRG 132, repeating the pattern seen in Connecticut hospitals.

PEER JUDGMENT TO FORM NURSING CLUSTERS

In an effort to simplify the model and to provide a nursing weight for DRGs with fewer than 20 observations, a panel of nurse clinicians was asked to group DRGs that which would require similar amounts of care on routine floors into "clusters." The six clusters were created along the two dimensions of risk and dependency. It was assumed that patients are admitted to hospitals for nursing care either because they cannot care for themselves or because they need inpatient monitoring or treatment. Of these two factors, risk was considered the more powerful predictor of both hospital admission and nursing resource use. In general, high-risk conditions compromise or threaten one or more of the vital functions of respiration, circulation, consciousness, and higher mental processes. Often these conditions are acute or trauma-related and frequently they involve the use of high-technology medicine, which itself introduces hazards as well as benefits. Patients with high-risk conditions are found in the cardiac, pulmonary, neurologic, sepsis, hemorrhage, and extreme metabolic derangement DRGs. Additional high-risk DRGs are those with invasive procedures that require general anesthesia.

In forming the nursing clusters, the extent and estimated duration of the risk and the estimated frequency of the conditions were considered. Significant risk conditions that were predicted to persist throughout a substantial part of the hospitalization were assigned higher ranks than those conditions in which the risk was known or predicted to be short-term, such as recovery from general anesthesia after elective surgery. If a DRG included procedures or diagnoses with considerably different patient risk, the most common diagnoses or procedures determined cluster placement.

Both extremes of age may increase risk. DRGs with these variables were placed in a higher cluster than those that did not include extremes of age. Children aged 0 to 17 were considered to use approximately the same amount of nursing time as patients aged 70 or over. Patients in age-defined DRGs were ranked one cluster higher than those in their companion DRGs except when the risk of the diagnosis itself was considered a more powerful predictor of nursing time. For example, DRGs 27 to 30, which split on age, were placed in the same nursing cluster because the diagnoses in the "traumatic stupor and coma" DRGs were considered more important than age in predicting the use of nursing resources.

Patients may be physically dependent upon nurses for help with some or all of their activities of daily living because of their condition (for example, fractures), disease (such as multiple sclerosis), treatment (for example, bed rest), or some combination of these. Physical dependency increases nursing intensity; feeding, bathing, toileting, and exercising dependent patients are time-consuming activities that occur repeatedly throughout the hospital stay. DRGs were assigned to nursing clusters according to the estimated type and degree of probable patient dependency. The nursing clusters, with their assigned DRGs, can be seen in Appendix 6-A.*

Cluster 1 consisted of patients who might not even require inpatient care; typical DRGs assigned to this cluster included carpal tunnel release, abortion, and breast biopsy. Many of these patients would not even be

---

*The conceptual work to define "clusters" was done by Susan Molde, R.N., M.S.N.

admitted to inpatient care today.[41] Cluster 6 included patients with extreme requirements for nursing, and included only the severely burned patients and heart transplants. Clusters 2–5 represented relative increases in nursing intensity.

The clusters were formed conceptually, without access to data. Then, nursing weights were obtained for each cluster as the time derived through regression of nursing time on LOS using data from each of the five study sites. The cluster weights for each hospital are, therefore, beta weights. In addition, the panel was asked to assign a "typical" amount of routine nursing time (per patient per day).

The results are shown in Table 6-10. There was remarkable agreement across institutions and with the nursing panel's assigned time; except in hospital D, the cluster weights stage up from 1 to 5. The panel felt that the inclusion of all children 0 to 17 years of age in a single DRG, and the inclusion in some DRGs of both children and adults, presented a problem. Infants and toddlers generally use the most nursing time, followed by preschoolers, school-age children, and adolescents. Therefore, all pediatric DRGs and all children under 17 were removed from the data and the clusters rerun (Table 6-11). The fit for adult patients became more obvious, even for hospital D. The disproportionate effect of one high-volume DRG—childbirth—was particularly noted: adolescents require more nursing care than adults, and the volume of adolescent pregnancy in all institutions was enough to skew the results. It is possible that removing the psychiatric DRGs, which are notoriously variable in resource consumption, would further improve the homogeneity of the nursing clusters.

These analyses suggest that there is *relative* consistency across hospitals in the routine care nursing resources consumed by patients in particular DRGs, even if the actual minutes or beta weights differ. While

Table 6-10: Nursing Weights by Study Site and Assignment

| | Study Site | | | | | Assigned |
Cluster	A	B	C	D	E	Time
1	163	218	261	191	299	210
2	243	269	284	177	302	240
3	248	329	320	201	327	270
4	262	308	350	187	336	290
5	262	373	361	214	345	330
6						450

Source: Robert B. Fetter and John D. Thompson, "Diagnosis Related Groups and Nursing Resources."

Table 6-11: Nursing Cluster Weights, Adults (Age over 17) Only, by Study Site and Assignment

Cluster	Study Site					Assigned Time
	A	B	C	D	E	
1	163	214	259	264	296	210
2	244	263	290	272	311	240
3	249	323	320	289	326	270
4	262	299	351	281	335	290
5	262	367	361	301	342	330
6						450

Source: Robert B. Fetter and John D. Thompson, "Diagnosis Related Groups and Nursing Resources."

advanced age (greater than 69) has been removed from DRG definition because it no longer contributes predictive power for length of stay or cost, advanced age still may be important in nursing intensity, especially in the very old, the fastest-growing age category in the population.

The ten highest ranking DRGs (for DRGs with over 100 observations in any data set) by nursing intensity were identified. Of the 50 potential ranks (since there were ties, 52 were actually produced) there are 26 *different* DRGs. Only one, DRG 14 (stroke), appears in the top ten in all institutions. DRG 12 (degenerative disorders) appears four times; respiratory infection in children is among the top nursing-intensity DRGs in hospitals with pediatric services. The following appear three times each: surgical implantation of a permanent cardiac pacemaker in patients with heart attacks or heart failure; major bowel procedures in patients with complications; and digestive malignancy with complications or comorbidities. The majority of DRGs ranked high in nursing intensity in each hospital were medical, not surgical. The surgical DRGs included major joint procedures; major bowel procedures; stomach procedures in persons over 69 or with complications and comorbidities; and permanent pacemaker insertion in the presence of myocardial infarction, heart failure, or shock. All of these would be more common in the elderly, with increased nursing needs.

There were 119 DRGs with over 100 observations in any institution, and thus 119 possible ranks. After the data sets were made equivalent for discharges per year (to remove the effect of volume) some DRGs showed considerable differences in nursing intensity across institutions. For example, DRG 79 (respiratory infections in persons over 69 with comorbidities or complications) was highest in hospital A, but ranked 62.5 in hospital E; DRG 112 (vascular procedures) was ranked fourth in hospital C but 107th in hospital D; DRG 202 (cirrhosis) was third in hospital E but

105th in hospital D; DRG 415 (operating-room procedures for infection) was fourth in hospital D but 101st in hospital C; and DRG 451 (poisoning and toxic effects of drugs in persons aged 0–17) was highest in hospital E but ranked 103.5 in hospital A (Table 6-12). The reasons for these differences are not readily apparent by case mix or age, volume, ICU use, or differences in size among the institutions. It is possible that certain characteristics of hospitals, nurses, or physician practices may explain these variations.

For example, hospital A is in the southwestern United States, in an area known to attract large numbers of elderly persons, often with chronic lung disease. Thus, patients with respiratory infections may be treated more aggressively or may have different organisms, creating greater nursing requirements. Hospital E is in one of the poorest cities in the nation and the high nursing intensity for cirrhosis and drug overdose may be a consequence. Hospital C is five small community hospitals in which vascular procedures may represent high technology, whereas they would not be high tech in a larger medical center. The effect of physician practices (different approaches to surgery, even different relationships with nursing staff) may also be at issue.

When all DRGs were indexed to DRG 335 (trans-urethral prostatectomy: TURP) set at 1.00, and all data sets were combined, the highest nursing intensity DRGs (routine care only) are primarily trauma or pediatrics (Table 6-13).

It was apparent that the medical DRGs have the most variability in nursing resource consumption. Figures 6-4 to 6-6 show two medical DRGs, stroke and angina pectoris, and one surgical one, hernia repair, each with three different "modes" of length of stay. It appears as if there are three fairly clearly different groups of patients in the medical DRGs depending on length of stay. For two different lengths of stay

Table 6-12: DRGs by Ranked Nursing Intensity

| | *Hospital* | | | | |
DRG	*A*	*B*	*C*	*D*	*E*
79 RESP INF >69 CC	1	2	5	12.5	62.5
100 RESP SIGN >69 CC	10	8	79	26	59
112 VASC PROC	25	18	4	107	35.5
202 CIRRHOSIS	61.5	13.5	36.5	105	3
415 O.R. PROC INFECT	10.5	19.5	101	4	37
451 POISON & TOX 0–17	103.5	12	32.5	3	1

Source: Robert B. Fetter and John D. Thompson, "Diagnosis Related Groups and Nursing Resources."

Table 6-13: High-Nursing-Intensity DRGs (Indexed)

Rank	DRG Name	Index
1	EXTREME IMMATURITY, NEONATE	2.02471
2	TRAUMATIC STUPOR AND COMA <1 HR. AGE >69 AND/OR CC	1.94275
3	KIDNEY AND UTI AGE 0–17	1.84696
4	CARDIAC ARREST, UNEXPLAINED	1.80729
5	RESPIRATORY INF. AGE 0–17	1.70290
6	MAJOR CHEST PROCEDURES	1.67021
7	LARYNGOTRACHEITIS	1.61454
8	CRANIOTOMY AGE <18	1.60264
9	NEONATES DIED OR TRANSFERRED	1.55578
10	CIRCULATORY DIS., AMI, EXPIRED	1.52978
11	CRANIOTOMY FOR TRAUMA AGE >17	1.47509
12	OTITIS MEDIA & URI, AGE 0–17	1.45711
13	EAR, NOSE, THROAT MALIGNANCY	1.44722
14	BRONCHITIS, ASTHMA, AGE 0–17	1.44722
15	LYMPHOMA, LEUKEMIA, AGE 0–17	1.43858

Source: Robert B. Fetter and John D. Thompson, "Diagnosis Related Groups and Nursing Resources."

in the patients with hernia repair, however, the nursing resource uses are quite similar. The shortest length-of-stay modal group in the hernia repair DRG may be otherwise well elderly persons, having essentially one-day surgery.

Nursing care after surgery is rather well understood and regulated by medical and nursing protocols. Nonsurgical treatment of less well understood conditions requires a different variety of nursing, complicated by such associated patient conditions as age or comorbidity or even by the behaviors attendant upon uncertainty about diagnosis.

The comparisons among hospitals suggested that there is so much yet to be understood about the difference in nursing intensity (to say nothing of technical problems in comparison of data from different institutions) that any change in reimbursement policy, such as weighting DRGs by nursing intensity, would be premature. The complexity of this issue becomes even clearer when the next step in studying nursing intensity is taken—identifying and comparing costs of nursing in institutions.

COSTING NURSING SERVICES

Interest in hospital cost finding in the United States came about as a result of a much broader concern with health care costs and in response to the

Figure 6-4: Pattern of Nursing Intensity by Day-of-Stay Mode (DRG 14)

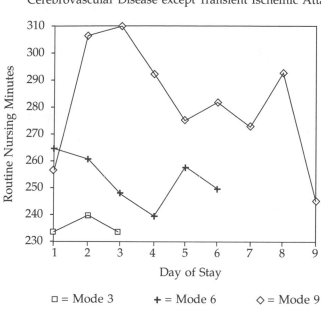

DRG 14
Cerebrovascular Disease except Transient Ischemic Attack

□ = Mode 3   + = Mode 6   ◇ = Mode 9

Source: Robert B. Fetter and John D. Thompson, "Diagnosis Related Groups and Nursing Resources."

beginning of hospital insurance. The first official cooperative effort by hospitals to devise a uniform system of keeping track of expenses and revenues appeared in 1935 in *Hospital Accounting and Statistics: A Manual for American Hospitals,* published by the American Hospital Association. The main purpose of the book was the identification and classification of accounts that would explain the basic financial position of the hospital through balance sheets and statements of income and expenses. Sensitive to the complaints of hospital administrators about a "bookkeeping" approach, the authors say on the first page of the manual:

> The accountants cannot record the skill of a nurse, the professional judgment of a pathologist, or the gratitude of a satisfied patient. But, they can record the amounts paid for nursing care or laboratory service or the amounts received from patients or governmental agencies for these and other hospital services.[42]

Figure 6-5: Pattern of Nursing Intensity by Day-of-Stay Mode (DRG 140)

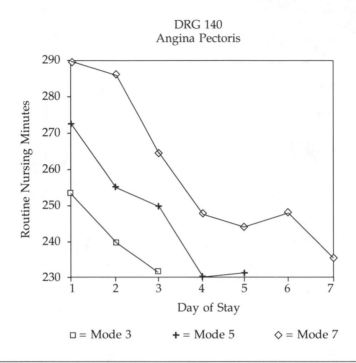

DRG 140
Angina Pectoris

□ = Mode 3   + = Mode 5   ◇ = Mode 7

Source: Robert B. Fetter and John D. Thompson, "Diagnosis Related Groups and Nursing Resources."

The manual stated that "cost per patient day" did not mean much as an acceptable unit of service. "The only service which can be expressed adequately in terms of patient days is the day rate to inpatients, usually referred to as board and room service and usually charged for by the day." The manual recommended that, if possible, the cost of "day rate services" should be determined separately from the cost of special services. Here, then, is the beginning of the distinction of "room and board" and ancillary service costs within a single hospital day.

All operating expenses were divided into (1) administrative, (2) dietary, (3) house and property, (4) professional services, and (5) general patient services. Nursing service appeared as one of the professional services along with medical and surgical service, medical records, social services, x-ray department, laboratories, operating and delivery room, pharmacy and other special professional services such as cardiography, basal metabolism, and physical therapy. Professional services were "the

Figure 6-6: Pattern of Nursing Intensity by Day-of-Stay Mode (Surgical DRG)

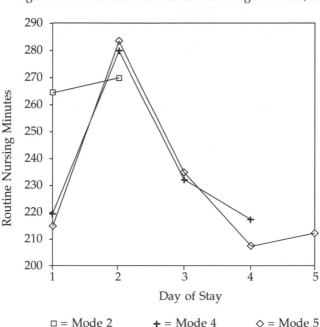

DRG 161
Inguinal and Femoral Hernia Procedure Age >69 and/or CC

□ = Mode 2   + = Mode 4   ◇ = Mode 5

Source: Robert B. Fetter and John D. Thompson, "Diagnosis Related Groups and Nursing Resources."

activities of the hospital which distinguish it from a hotel, dormitory or apartment...."

The section on nursing reflects the primary concern of accounting for nursing services in 1935—clarification of the expenses incurred for nursing services and those expended for nursing education. The commingling of hospital expenses entailed in providing nursing care and those devoted to running a nursing school were complicated by the fact that nursing care personnel also taught students and student nurses provided much, and in some hospitals most, of the nursing care to patients. In 1940, a joint committee of the American Hospital Association and the National League for Nursing Education mounted a cost-finding study of both nursing service and education.[43]

To approximate the cost of nursing service in an institution *without* a school, the study had to develop graduate nurse staffing standards for all the clinical and support divisions of the hospital. These standards were expressed as nursing care hours per patient per day, corrected for the hours of private duty nurses and not including the time of the head nurse. The staffing standard that became engraved in stone was 3.5 hours per patient per day. (Note that in the Yale study described earlier, the time assigned to cluster 1 of DRGs was 210 minutes or 3.5 hours, coming full circle.) The study did recommend separation of the costs of nursing from the rest of hospital expenses, but many of the budgeting and expense control features were not adopted as widely as were the staffing standards. The staffing goals were adopted by many hospitals even though they resulted in staff increases in the middle of a depression. Twenty years earlier a "most interesting nursing study" had been done at Mount Sinai Hospital in New York City at the request of the New York Academy of Medicine to "secure definite information as to the amount of time necessary for suitable and adequate nursing care of the average hospital patient."[44] The study found that an adequate amount of bedside nursing per average patient was 5 hours and 4 minutes per day, but 5 hours 39 minutes in pediatrics, 4 hours 57 minutes in general medicine, and 4 hours 39 minutes in the surgical service.[45]

With the introduction of sulfanilamides in the late 1930s, the role of the hospital changed to more timely diagnosis and treatment, justifying a shift in administrative attention from cost per day to cost per admission: "the significant product of a hospital is a group of recovered or improved patients, not a quantity of patient days or bed occupancy."[46] Most hospitals were charging less than their costs for room and board. Many theories have been advanced for this practice, the most likely one being that patients could compare the cost of a hospital "room" with that of a hotel, not realizing that "room and board" included many services not offered by hotels. The practice of costing and defining hospital service by this misnamed "room and board" eventually proved to be self-defeating, and can be interpreted as a deliberately confusing practice. That nursing was buried along with brooms, breakfast, and the building mortgage had consequences not only for the visibility of nursing's service, but also for the wage structures as hospitals increasingly began to compete on room and board rates, using oligopsonistic practices to artificially constrain nursing salaries.

Shortly after Medicare was passed, the American Hospital Association requested a nursing differential in per diem reimbursement. The difference in basic nursing care received by older patients was estimated at about 30 minutes of nursing care per patient per day.[47] As a consequence of this study, a differential of 8.5 percent was paid to hospitals for routine care for their Medicare patients. This differential became unnecessary when DRGs enabled patient age to be separated from case mix in determining costs of care. But the Prospective Payment System was handicapped because the expenses included in the Medicare cost report as room and board are not uniformly separated by a standard chart of accounts. The Health Care Financing Administration attempted to require hospitals to adopt a more inclusive standard chart of accounts and a more sophisticated reporting system but the attempt foundered on the recalcitrance of the American Hospital Association. Thus it is not possible to extract separate nursing expenses in routine care with any degree of comfort from the Medicare cost reports.

It has been alleged that the DRG pricing algorithm has a major flaw: that costs within each DRG are approximated by use of the average per diem costs of routine and special care services multiplied by the length of stay in each service. Lave highlighted the effect of this practice on possible price compression.[48] The assumptions that average cost per day of nursing service is the same for each DRG and that average cost per day in room and board is the same for each case (leaving only differences in intensive care to differentiate between DRGs) are quite different and could have different effects on compression of DRG prices. Thus a study was conducted to determine the average cost of various components of both routine and special care nursing.[49]

The study was carried out on the financial data from the 35 general hospitals in Connecticut, using 1984 cost reports. Operating room and ambulatory care expenses were removed first. Direct nursing costs were defined as direct salary costs for all nursing units, direct nonsalary costs for the same units, and fringe benefits for the nurses staffing the units. All personnel in the units were considered, from the head nurse to the ward clerk. The salaries of personnel assigned to or allocated from other departments in the hospital, such as housekeeping, dietary, medical records, were not considered nursing costs. These salaries are categorized as nonnursing expense. Nursing administration expenses were allocated to direct nursing expenses and the total called "nursing component expenses." The nursing component includes all of the direct nursing costs plus salaries and fringes of nursing administration. The general findings from this study appear in Table 6-14.

Direct nursing accounted for 25.44 percent of total inpatient costs; the total nursing component accounted for 27.97 percent of these same expenses. The distribution was surprisingly tight. The costs were somewhat higher than those reported by Walker and the ANA study.[50,51]

To obtain a more accurate estimate of nursing costs, an attempt was made to refine the figures by clinical service. Tables 6-15 and 6-16 break down nursing expenses per patient day by selected clinical services. The

Table 6-14: Nursing and Nonnursing Expenses per Patient Day, Routine and Special Care, All Connecticut Hospitals, 1984

	Routine Care		Special Care	
	Mean Amount	% of Room & Board	Mean Amount	% of Room & Board
Direct nursing expenses	$ 90.15	45.72%	$266.29	60.32%
Nursing component expenses	99.23	50.33	290.30	65.76
Nonnursing component expenses	98.61	49.84	151.18	34.24
Total room and board costs	$197.84	100.00%	$441.48	100.00%

Source: The Connecticut Hospital Association.

most interesting finding is the high cost of nursing in pediatrics. Further, there is considerably more difference across services than anticipated. Nursing constitutes nearly three-quarters of the costs of room and board in special care and almost half of room and board costs in the other services.

Implicit even in this allocation method is the assumption that all patients in routine care, on the average, receive the same amount of services, and that, on the average, all patients in intensive care receive the same intensity of nursing care. What is required is a refinement of the allocation process to achieve a more accurate reflection of nursing resources consumed by each patient. Such a refinement would first separate routine from special care, using number of patient days as the allocation statistic for special care, and a weighted patient day as the statistic for routine care, following the measures developed in the Yale study reported earlier.

There is another reason for costing nursing separate from the rest of the hospital expenses. There is an explosion of interest in charging for routine nursing services, as an agenda for professional nursing first articulated in testimony to the Institute of Medicine's study on nursing.[52] This movement is parallel to, but quite separate from, the interests of the government and of hospital administrators in managing nursing intensity. Three collections of papers dealing with various aspects of charging for nursing have been published under the aegis of the National League for Nursing and Sovie has summarized the research literature on this topic.[53–56]

Nursing's arguments for billing directly for nursing on routine care floors deal primarily with increased professional visibility and accountability. Further, when charges billed for nursing return in the form of payments directly for nursing services into the nursing department's

Table 6-15: Routine and Special Care Nursing Services Mean per Diem Cost and Percentage of Room and Board, Selected Clinical Services, All Connecticut General Hospitals, 1984

	Routine Adult Medical-Surgical		Special Care		Psychiatry	
	Mean Amount	% of Room & Board	Mean Amount	% of Room & Board	Mean Amount	% of Room & Board
Direct nursing salaries	$ 66.65	34.68%	$204.69	46.21%	$ 81.90	38.18%
Direct nonsalary expense	3.94	2.05	17.10	3.86	7.16	3.34
Fringe benefits	14.93	7.77	45.92	10.36	18.75	8.74
Direct nursing expenses	85.52	44.50	267.71	60.43	107.81	50.26
Nursing administration	8.86	4.61	24.20	5.46	7.57	3.53
Nursing component expenses	94.38	49.11	291.91	65.89	115.38	53.79
Nonnursing component expenses	97.80	50.89	151.10	34.11	99.11	46.21
Total room and board costs	$192.18	100.00%	$443.01	100.00%	$214.49	100.00%

Source: The Connecticut Hospital Association.

Table 6-16: Routine and Special Care Nursing Services Mean per Diem Cost and Percentage of Room and Board, Selected Clinical Services, All Connecticut General Hospitals, 1984

	Pediatrics		Maternity		NB Well		NB Sick	
	Mean Amount	% of Room & Board	Mean Amount	% of Room & Board	Mean Amount	% of Room & Board	Mean Amount	% of Room & Board
Direct nursing salaries	$121.45	37.58%	$ 67.82	32.26%	$ 68.43	42.77%	$111.21	42.98%
Direct nonsalary expense	6.44	1.99	5.86	2.79	4.77	2.98	11.86	4.58
Fringe benefits	27.21	8.42	15.20	7.23	15.46	9.66	25.15	9.72
Direct nursing expenses	155.10	47.99	88.88	42.28	88.66	55.41	148.22	57.28
Nursing administration	15.72	4.86	7.96	3.78	7.96	4.97	12.41	4.80
Nursing component expenses	170.82	52.85	96.84	46.06	96.62	60.38	160.63	62.08
Nonnursing component expenses	152.37	47.15	113.40	53.94	63.38	39.62	98.12	37.92
Total room and board costs	$323.19	100.00%	$210.24	100.00%	$160.00	100.00%	$258.75	100.00%

Source: The Connecticut Hospital Association.

account, nursing turns from a cost center to a revenue center in institutions.[57]

MANAGING NURSING INTENSITY

Nursing managers can introduce clinical innovations and management strategies when they have access to nursing intensity data that are collected over time, are broken down by hospital unit, and include DRG assignment. For example, in the Yale study, five patterns of nursing intensity across days of stay were identified. One pattern, typical of elective surgery patients, shows a peak of nursing intensity on the second day of stay, the first postoperative day. The pattern in trauma patients begins very high and then slopes down toward the end of the stay, but it never quite reaches the lowest levels, since those patients often retain disabilities requiring nursing attention. Patients in the terminal phase of illness show a pattern that begins with low levels of nursing intensity; these levels increase as the illness progresses. Some patients show essentially a flat pattern, and still other patients show no pattern at all (chronically ill elderly persons are often in this group).

Knowing that there are regularities by DRG in nursing intensity would allow nurse managers to predict staffing requirements or anticipate other necessary management decisions. For example, most elective surgery is scheduled on Mondays and Tuesdays, making Tuesdays and Wednesdays hectic on those floors. If such a pattern is detected, the staffing could be changed to relieve the pressure, or perhaps the surgical schedule could be altered to spread the work load across the week.

Provisional DRGs could be assigned upon patient admission for many patients. Knowing the relative nursing intensity (from an institution's own regressions of nursing time on length of stay by DRG) would make the allocation of resources predictable beyond simply the next shift or day. Nursing intensity could also be tracked across months of the year if there was a detectable pattern.

Patient acuity information could also be examined across time, service, or DRG, or across hospitals, to cast light on the perception that since prospective payment, patients are "sicker" than they used to be. It is possible that there are fewer "well" patient *days* spent in the hospital than there used to be; with the possible exception of AIDS and conditions that follow from newer heroic cardiac interventions in emergencies, disease itself has not changed.

Costing Nursing Services by DRG

There are many reasons why individual hospitals might wish to extend the costing of their nursing services into DRGs. Such a projection would certainly assist the nursing department in determining what portion of the hospital's DRG cost fell within their responsibility, and hospital managers who are examining the contribution to their overall DRG cost of radiology, laboratory, operating room, and pharmacy would certainly want to derive standards for so important a cost center as nursing.

It is even more imperative to separate routine and special care nursing costs from room and board costs because the remainder—"hotel cost"—is heavily weighted with fixed costs. By identifying separately the variable nursing costs, better price estimates for preferred provider organizations (PPOs) and health maintenance organizations (HMOs) could be projected, particularly if these contracts would result in an increased number of admissions by the PPOs or HMOs to that hospital. Such costing would also be valuable as a basis for strategic planning, including the selection of new services.

The early model of cost finding for nursing service did not go far enough.[58] Although this was the first model that attempted to separate nursing costs from room and board costs, the problem became somewhat more complicated by the necessity for elaborating a model that could use the Medicare chart of accounts and cost reports without breaking them up into different cost categories. The new model, seen as Figure 6-7, satisfies these requirements. It separates costs of inpatient nursing care into routine care and special services for intensive care units. These two different types of nursing costs can then be allocated to each DRG according to (1) billing for intensive care, and (2) billing by level of service for routine care. The service level can be derived from a patient classification system or accepted as one of the relative DRG values from the Yale nursing intensity study, such as the average relative value of the nursing clusters.

It must be understood that before the final nursing cost centers are derived, all nursing care given in the outpatient department must be stripped out and allocated to that department. Moreover, nursing care given in ancillary services such as the delivery room, operating room, or recovery room must be assigned to those ancillary service cost centers and included in their final cost centers.

Whether or not a hospital wishes to subdivide its routine nursing costs by clinical service, such as general medical, surgical, pediatrics, obstetrics, and psychiatry, would depend on the use to which the costing information is to be put. There are vast differences in the costs of these clinical services and if one wishes to be precise about them, even nursing unit cost figures could be derived. This latter possibility has become particularly important with the hospitalization of AIDS patients. These patients require a great deal of routine nursing time, are usually concentrated in one or two nursing units, and would be using more direct care than other patients on the floor. If the hospital has a neonatal intensive

Figure 6-7: Revised Model for DRG Costing

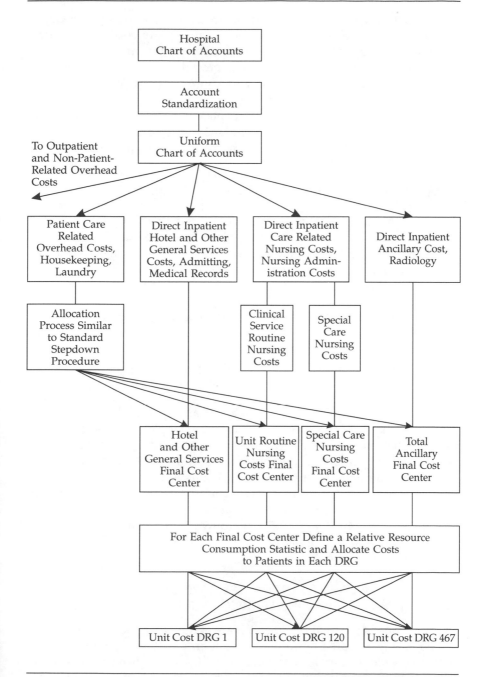

Source: Robert B. Fetter and John D. Thompson, "Diagnosis Related Groups and Nursing Resources."

care unit, it may well wish to divide its intensive care costs into neonatal and other intensive care. Many hospitals are already costing burn units separately because of the enormous requirement for nursing.

The information for such costing procedures will have to be specially derived and is most easily obtained if nursing care in routine as well as intensive care is charged for, audited, and maintained for the entire period of hospitalization. For the less explicit costing exercises, the allocation according to the Medicare standard chart of accounts will give overall routine and special care nursing costs, which can be allocated to each DRG.

Budgeting Nursing Services

Some feel that the proper way to budget for inpatient hospital care is not so much by clinical service but actually by DRGs. The exact knowledge of nursing costs would assist in the development of such budgets and in the selection of management options, such as matrix management.

The budgeting process is essentially the costing process in reverse. Nursing budgeting starts with predicting the number of cases in each DRG anticipated for the budget period. The next step is to translate costs back into nursing hours and then into full-time equivalents so that the personnel budget can be elaborated on the basis of anticipated wage increases for the coming year. The pattern of DRGs in each hospital is proving to be remarkably stable over the years. However, the budgeting process, by working back from DRGs to manpower supply and ancillary service requirements, does allow anticipated changes in treatment patterns to be incorporated. A recent example of one such change has been the increase in cesarean section and a subsequent decrease in vaginal delivery in one of the most common of all DRGs.[59] Changes in patterns in the hospital treatment of persons with AIDS are predicted. One involves shorter lengths of stay due to referral to alternative care systems, while the other predicts increased attention to the pharmaceutical problems involved with AZT (azidothymidine). Only through DRG-based costing and budgeting can these changes be predicted and managed when they come.

NURSING INTENSITY AND QUALITY
OF NURSING CARE

Examinations of the quality of health care at the patient level usually start by comparing accepted performance standards with care given, either by processes followed or by end results. DRGs have proven particularly valuable in measurements of quality of hospital care since selected standards have been derived in, for example, length of stay or utilization of specific services such as radiology or laboratory, and actual patient experience can be compared with these criteria. Early in the development of DRGs, they were conceived of as a sampling frame for selecting aberrant cases. This selection is the so-called outlier examination, and it was recommended that every outlier be examined for quality of care.

Little systematic study of outliers has ever been done, however, since prospective payment produced utilization review long before outlier status was reached. The possibilities in outlier analysis for quality assurance remain untested.

One small study examined "nursing-intensity outliers"—patients whose lengths of stay and nursing requirements were simultaneously extreme.[60] From one hospital's data for one year ($N = 22,359$), 32 patients who were nursing-intensity outliers were identified with the Cook's D statistic described earlier. There were other patients who were outliers in length of stay but whose nursing requirements were not extreme; they were not detected by the procedure. The patients fell in two distinct groups: children under 14, most of whom were under three, but none of whom was a newborn; and adults, all but two of whom were over 55. The children stayed in the hospital an average of 32 days; the adults stayed 54 days on average. Nearly half of the children were uninsured or covered by Medicaid. All but one of the children were admitted through the emergency room, as were three-quarters of the adults, but only one person, a child, was the victim of trauma. Five of the 18 adults died and six were transferred to another facility or to a nursing home. The majority of the children had diseases and disorders of the respiratory system, the nervous system, or the musculoskeletal system. The adults had nervous system or musculoskeletal conditions. Operative procedures were rare, but numerous diagnostic or therapeutic procedures were performed.

Chart review showed that between half and three-quarters of the adults had inhalation therapy, blood administration, dressings, Foley catheters, or telemetry. Half to three-quarters of the children had inhalation therapy, intubation, nasogastric tubes, drainage tubes, dressings, or telemetry. The children spent an average of 10.5 days in the ICU; the adults had little ICU time.

The children were hospitalized for acute but reversible conditions and their nursing care requirements were increased by fever, incontinence, perhaps the exigencies of poverty, and the normal physical dependence of children. The adults were chronically ill, with their care complicated particularly by depression, alcoholism and its sequelae, and incontinence. One-quarter of the adults exhibited signs of psychosis, one-third had expressive or receptive aphasia, and a third were delirious at some point in their hospital stay. The children also exhibited signs of depression, irritability, or restlessness. Infection was the most common secondary diagnosis among both age groups, but only about half of the patients with infection had it upon admission. There were also five cases of falling out of bed.

This study suggested that the adult patients were people with progressive and chronic diseases who may well have exhausted their families' resources. These are also the patients who tend to exhaust nurses' resources, people who never quite get better but never quite get worse either. The children were just plain sick, with complicated conditions.

While this study required the use of a large data set upon which to regress nursing time on length of stay to identify the "influential observations," retrospective analysis of outliers in terms of nursing variables could proceed without further methodological complexity, since at least the Medicare length-of-stay and cost outliers are available in existing data.

With increasing knowledge of the typical nursing requirements of patients by hospital and by DRG, it would be possible for institutions to identify early in a patient's hospital career the extreme need for nursing and take whatever steps are indicated. For example, Halloran has shown that the major condition that predisposes older patients, especially women, to discharge to a nursing home instead of to home is incontinence.[61] Incontinence can be treated by nurses, however, especially if its consequences in terms of quality of care are acknowledged. Concurrent review is the goal to be pursued.

Standards of care for the *utilization* of nursing services have not been developed. Three such standards can now be proposed and tested to see if the probability of poorer-quality nursing care is greater among an identified population than it is in a general hospital population.[62] The three criteria would be percentage of patients within each DRG who received any care in a special care unit; percentage of total days in special care units; and the presence of nursing-intensity outliers in the routine nursing care regression equations, discussed above.

The first two measurements are obvious and standards for special care use can be derived from national data. For quality studies, however, it is preferable that standards first be derived at the level of the individual institution, and then be tested there patient by patient. If the model proves valuable, it can be applied to interinstitutional comparisons. The monitoring of the use of special care days is a valuable quality of care inquiry apart from the nursing aspects, because when combined with existing physiological measures (such as APACHE) it may well provide an objective measurement of illness severity within a DRG.

A major observation growing out of the nursing-intensity literature is that nursing is much less driven by medical practices than has been thought to be the case. Patients may require a good deal of nursing care even though they are not being aggressively treated with high technology or drugs. And some patients who are very sick require lower amounts of nursing in part because some of the care is provided by machines. Yet most quality-assurance efforts in nursing stop with accreditation criteria, such as the presence of care plans. Under the notion that the product of the hospital is an episode of care, clearly nursing and its quality must be incorporated in any effort to understand and improve hospital services.

The Yale study of nursing intensity used nursing time as the unit of analysis, making intensity data comparable across institutions. As discussed earlier, intriguing hints of differences in nursing care were found, which if pursued might lead to quality considerations. Cooperative effort among the nursing services of various institutions would foster such analysis. The Council of Teaching Hospitals in the northeast United States has sponsored one such study; more should follow. Cross-national comparisons may also be done when hospitals in other countries adopt patient classification and time studies. Such studies are beginning in Australia and other countries.[63]

Individual hospitals might find it in their interest to conduct smaller studies of particular problems. Particularly in a time when questions are being raised about how many nurses are really needed (or available), the relationship between provision of nursing and patient outcome assumes a high priority for study.

One such study was the first inquiry into the effects of nurse staffing in 25 years or so.[64] The study took advantage of the fact that in one 400-bed hospital, there was a period of about six months on one general medicine unit in which the nurse staffing was demonstrably below the institution's own staffing standards, while staffing on another comparable unit was adequate, again by the hospital's own standards. Data for about 500 patients for the three-month period in the middle of this shortage were collected. No patients transferred in or out of either unit were included.

When the six highest-volume DRGs were analyzed, length of stay in two of them (gastrointestinal hemorrhage and stroke) was significantly higher on the short-staffed unit, after outliers had been trimmed. Further, the complication rate was higher on the short-staffed unit. Nursing intensity was also higher on the short-staffed unit, but it is unclear whether the intensity caused the short staffing or was a consequence of it. Finally, the data showed that the hospital lost $150,000 (annualized) because of lengths of stay beyond the geometric mean, an amount quite sufficient to have hired enough nurses to bring the staffing up to standard, on the assumption that nurses could be found.

CONCLUSION

This chapter began with consideration of nursing intensity within a reimbursement agenda. It is likely that the best data upon which payment decisions could be based would be data that included direct costs and charges for nursing. About 20 hospitals nationwide cost nursing services separately; in 17 more, the variable costs of nursing are reflected on the patient's bill.[65] It has been recommended that the addition of two simple items to the Uniform Hospital Discharge Data Set (UHDDS)—number of days in each level of care, and total routine nursing costs—would provide the data upon which further research and eventual decisions could be made.[66,67] The 1987 Uniform Billing form (UB 87) already provides for the entry of nursing costs; information from hospitals that presently cost or bill separately for nursing could be collected. DRG costing and budgeting of nursing resources is simply the next logical step to charging for routine nursing services.

Billing separately for nursing offers two advantages to understanding costs: clear definition of nursing costs, including allocated nursing administration (because if nursing is to be billed separately, the entire set of expenses for nursing must appear in the nursing charge), and the existence of an audit trail back to the daily patient experience. Accumulation of DRG costs for nursing services would be very simple, and in fact would represent only one further manipulation of data already being generated for other purposes.

We believe that further work on the measurement of nursing intensity and its relationship to cost should be limited to those institutions where both nursing patient classification systems and variable billing are in place. Aside from the gain in validity in such settings because of the audit trail back to the patient record, the data on each patient could be extracted easily from the UB 87 billing form, a major simplification in the data-gathering effort.

REFERENCES

1. J. D. Thompson, "The Measurement of Nursing Intensity," *Health Care Financing Review* 6, no. 2 (1984): 51.
2. L. A. Joel, "DRGs and RIMs: Implications for Nursing," *Nursing Outlook* 32, no. 1 (1984): 42–49.
3. R. P. Caterinicchio, "Relative Intensity Measures: Pricing of Inpatient Nursing Service under Diagnosis-Related Group Prospective Hospital Payment," *Health Care Financing Review* 6, no. 1 (1984): 61–70.
4. R. P. Caterinicchio, "A Debate: RIMs and the Cost of Nursing Care," *Nursing Management* 14, no. 5 (1983): 36–39.

5. P. Grimaldi and J. Micheletti, "RIMs and the Cost of Nursing Care," *Nursing Management* 13 (1982): 12–22.
6. E. Cole, testimony of the American Nurses' Association to the House Subcommittee on Health and the Environment of the Committee on Energy and Commerce, November 22, 1982.
7. North American Nursing Diagnosis Association, *Nursing Diagnosis Taxonomy* (St. Louis: North American Nursing Diagnosis Association, 1986).
8. E. Halloran, "Nursing Workload, Medical Diagnosis Related Groups and Nursing Diagnosis," *Research in Nursing and Health* 8, no. 4 (1985): 421–33.
9. E. Halloran and D. Halloran, "Exploring the DRG/Nursing Equation," *American Journal of Nursing* 85, no. 10 (1985): 1093–95.
10. M. A. Rockwell, *A Summary of Coronary Care Unit Literature* (Santa Monica, CA: The Rand Corporation, 1969).
11. E. A. Draper, "Benefits and Costs of Intensive Care," *Image—Journal of Nursing Scholarship* 15, no. 3 (1983): 90–94.
12. J. D. Thompson, "DRG Prepayment: Its Purpose and Performance," *Bulletin of the New York Academy of Medicine* 64, no. 1 (1988): 25–51.
13. Ibid.
14. Secretary's Commission on Nursing, *Interim Report* (Washington, D.C.: Secretary's Commission on Nursing, 1988).
15. Draper, "Benefits and Costs."
16. D. P. Wagner et al., "Identification of Low Risk Monitor Patients within a Medical-Surgical Intensive Care Unit," *Medical Care* 21, no. 4 (1983): 425–34.
17. W. A. Knaus et al., "APACHE—Acute Physiology and Chronic Health Evaluation: A Physiologically Based Classification System," *Critical Care Medicine* 9 (1981): 591–97.
18. L. Corcoran, "Nursing Intensity in Cardiac Surgery Patients" (master's thesis, Yale University School of Nursing, 1988).
19. A. Kiesel, "Nursing Intensity in the Surgical ICU" (master's thesis, Yale University School of Nursing, 1988).
20. Corcoran, "Nursing Intensity."
21. Thompson, "The Measurement of Nursing Intensity."
22. M. K. Aydelotte, *Nurse Staffing Methodology: A Review and Critique of Selected Literature* (Department of Health, Education, and Welfare publication no. [NIH] 73–43; Washington, D.C.: U.S. Government Printing Office, 1973).
23. P. Giovannetti, *Patient Classification Systems in Nursing: A Description and Analysis* (Department of Health, Education, and Welfare publication no. [HRA] 78–22; Hyattsville, MD: U.S. Government Printing Office, 1978).
24. E. R. Hearn, "How Many High Care Patients," *Nursing Times* 68 (1972): Part I (April 20) 472–78, Part II (April 27) 65–68.
25. P. Giovannetti and G. Mayer, "Building Confidence in Patient Classification Systems," *Nursing Management* 15 (1984): 31–34.
26. San Joaquin General Hospital, *San Joaquin Classification* (Stockton, CA: San Joaquin General Hospital, 1976).
27. Giovannetti and Mayer, "Building Confidence."
28. P. A. Prescott and C. Y. Phillips, "Gauging Nursing Intensity to Bring Costs to Light," *Nursing and Health Care* 9, no. 1 (1988): 17–22.
29. M. Sovie et al., *A Correlation Study of Nursing Patient Classification, DRGs, Other Significant Patient Variables and Costs of Patient Care* (Rochester, NY: Strong Memorial Hospital, 1984).
30. Ibid., 47.

31. M. Manthey, *The Practice of Primary Nursing* (Boston: Blackwell Scientific Publications, 1980).
32. R. C. McKibbin et al., "DRGs and Nursing Care" (Kansas City: American Nurses' Association, 1985).
33. J. McClain and M. Selhat, "Twenty Cases: What Nursing Costs per DRG," *Nursing Management* 15, no. 10 (1984): 27–34.
34. M. Mitchell et al., "Determining Costs of Direct Nursing Care by DRGs," *Nursing Management* 15, no. 4 (1984): 29–32.
35. T. G. Lagona and M. M. Stritzel, "Nursing Care Requirements As Measured by DRG," *Journal of Nursing Administration* 14, no. 5 (1984): 15–18.
36. W. Riley and V. Schaefers, "Costing Nursing Services," *Nursing Management* 14, no. 12 (1983): 40–43.
37. M. Sovie et al., "Amalgam of Nursing Acuity, DRGs and Costs," *Nursing Management* 16, no. 3 (1985): 22–42.
38. R. B. Fetter and J. D. Thompson, "Diagnosis Related Groups and Nursing Resources" (final progress report to the Health Care Financing Administration, grant no. 15-C–98500; New Haven, CT: Yale University, 1987).
39. M. Arndt and B. Skydell, "Inpatient Nursing Services: Productivity and Cost," in *Costing Out Nursing: Pricing Our Product,* ed. F. A. Shaffer (New York: National League for Nursing, 1985), 69–84.
40. D. C. Montgomery and E. A. Peck, *Introduction to Linear Regression Analysis* (New York: John Wiley & Sons, 1982).
41. Thompson, "DRG Prepayment."
42. American Hospital Association, *Hospital Accounting and Statistics: A Manual for American Hospitals* (Chicago: American Hospital Association, 1935), 1.
43. B. Pfeffercorn and C. A. Rovetta, *Administrative Cost Analysis for Nursing Service and Nursing Education* (New York: National League for Nursing and American Hospital Association, 1940).
44. E. A. Greener, "A Study of Hospital Nursing Service," *The Modern Hospital* 16, no. 1 (1921): 28–31.
45. E. H. Lewinski-Corwin, "The Hospital Nursing Situation," *American Journal of Nursing* 22, no. 4 (1922): 603–6.
46. C. R. Rorem, *A Quest for Certainty* (Ann Arbor, MI: Health Administration Press, 1982), 132.
47. J. D. Thompson et al., "Age: A Factor in Amount of Nursing Care Given," *Hospitals JAHA* 42, no. 5 (1968): 33–39.
48. J. R. Lave, "Is Compression Occurring in DRG Prices?" *Inquiry* 22 (1985): 142–47.
49. R. B. Goetzinger, "The Nursing Cost Component" (master's thesis, Yale University Department of Epidemiology and Public Health, 1986).
50. D. D. Walker, "The Cost of Nursing Care in Hospitals," in *Nursing in the '80's: Crises, Opportunities, Challenges,* ed. L. Aiken (Philadelphia: J. B. Lippincott Co., 1982).
51. McKibbin et al., "DRGs and Nursing Care."
52. Institute of Medicine, *Nursing and Nursing Education: Public Policies and Private Actions* (Washington, D.C.: National Academy Press, 1983).
53. F. A. Shaffer, ed., *Costing Out Nursing: Pricing Our Product* (New York: National League for Nursing, 1985).
54. F. A. Shaffer, ed., *Patients and Purse Strings* (New York: National League for Nursing, 1986).
55. J. C. Scherubel, ed., *Patients and Purse Strings II* (New York: National League for Nursing, 1988).

56. M. Sovie, "Variable Costs of Nursing Care in Hospitals," *Annual Review of Nursing Research* (New York: Springer Publishing Company, 1988), 131–50.

57. M. D. Sovie and T. Smith, "Pricing the Nursing Product: Charging for Nursing Care," *Nursing Economics* 4, no. 5 (1986): 216–26.

58. J. D. Thompson, R. F. Averill, and R. B. Fetter, "Planning, Budgeting and Controlling—One Look at the Future: Case-Mix Cost Accounting," *Health Services Research* 14, no. 2 (1979): 111–25.

59. F. C. Notzen, P. J. Placek, and S. M. Taffel, "Comparison of National Cesarean Section Rates," *New England Journal of Medicine* 316, no. 7 (1987): 386–89.

60. L. Talerico and D. Diers, "Nursing Intensity Outliers," *Nursing Management* 19, no. 6 (1988): 27–35.

61. E. Halloran, "Incidence and Outcomes of Urinary Incontinence Among Hospitalized Patients" (paper presented at the Yale University Hospital Administration Alumni Association, 1988).

62. J. D. Thompson, "Nursing Research and Practice Issues of the Nursing Intensity Project," in *Costing Hospital Nursing Services—Report of the Conference* (Washington, D.C.: U.S. Department of Health and Human Services, Division of Nursing, 1987), 105–36.

63. M. Cuthbert, "Measuring Nursing Intensity and Costs," in *Proceedings of the Second International Conference on the Management and Financing of Hospital Services* (New Haven, CT: Yale University, 1988).

64. S. D. Flood and D. Diers, "Nurse Staffing, Patient Outcome and Cost," *Nursing Management* 19, no. 5 (1988): 34–46.

65. S. Lampe, "Costing Hospital Nursing Services: State of the Art, A Literature Review" (background paper prepared for the Invitational Conference on Costing Nursing, Division of Nursing, U.S. Public Health Service, 1987).

66. M. Sovie, "Establishing a Nursing Minimum Dataset as a Part of the Data Requirements of DRGs," in *The Nursing Minimum Data Set,* ed. H. H. Werley and N. Lang (New York: Springer Publishing Company, 1988).

67. J. D. Thompson, "The Minimum Dataset for Nursing and the Effectiveness of Nursing Care," in *The Nursing Minimum Data Set,* ed. H. H. Werley and N. Lang (New York: Springer Publishing Company, 1988).

Appendix 6-A: DRGs in Nursing Clusters

DRGs by Cluster

		Cluster = 1	Assigned time = 210 minutes
DRG	Type	DRG Name	MDC
6	P	CARPAL TUNNEL RELEASE	1
19	M	CRANIAL & PERIPHERAL NERVE DISORDERS AGE <70 W/O CC	1
39	P	LENS PROCEDURES WITH OR WITHOUT VITRECTOMY	2
43	M	HYPHEMA	2
45	M	NEUROLOGICAL EYE DISORDERS	2
46	M	OTHER DISORDERS OF THE EYE AGE >17 W CC	2
47	M	OTHER DISORDERS OF THE EYE AGE >17 W/O CC	2

Continued

Appendix 6-A: Continued

		DRGs by Cluster	
		Cluster = 1	Assigned time = 210 minutes
DRG	Type	DRG Name	MDC
50	P	SIALOADENECTOMY	3
51	P	SALIVARY GLAND PROCEDURES EXCEPT SIALOADENECTOMY	3
56	P	RHINOPLASTY	3
61	P	MYRINGOTOMY W TUBE INSERTION AGE >17	3
62	P	MYRINGOTOMY W TUBE INSERTION AGE 0–17	3
65	M	DYSEQUILIBRIUM	3
66	M	EPISTAXIS	3
68	M	OTITIS MEDIA & URI AGE >69 &/OR CC	3
69	M	OTITIS MEDIA & URI AGE 18–69 W/O CC	3
72	M	NASAL TRAUMA & DEFORMITY	3
73	M	OTHER EAR, NOSE & THROAT DIAGNOSES AGE >17	3
74	M	OTHER EAR, NOSE & THROAT DIAGNOSES AGE 0–17	3
100	M	RESPIRATORY SIGNS & SYMPTOMS AGE <70 W/O CC	4
178	M	UNCOMPLICATED PEPTIC ULCER AGE <70 W/O CC	6
216	P	BIOPSIES OF MUSCULOSKELETAL SYSTEM & CONNECTIVE TISSUE	8
228	P	GANGLION (HAND) PROCEDURE	8
232	P	ARTHROSCOPY	8
241	M	CONNECTIVE TISSUE DISORDERS AGE <70 W/O CC	8
245	M	BONE DISEASES & SPECIFIC ARTHROPATHIES AGE <70 W/O CC	8
247	M	SIGNS & SYMPTOMS OF MUSCULOSKELETAL SYSTEM & CONN TISSUE	8
248	M	TENDONITIS, MYOSITIS & BURSITIS	8
249	M	AFTERCARE, MUSCULOSKELETAL SYSTEM & CONNECTIVE TISSUE	8
256	M	OTHER MUSCULOSKELETAL SYSTEM & CONNECTIVE TISSUE DIAGNOSES	8
262	P	BREAST BIOPSY & LOCAL EXCISION FOR NON-MALIGNANCY	9
276	M	NON-MALIGANT BREAST DISORDERS	9
283	M	MINOR SKIN DISORDERS AGE >69 &/OR CC	9
284	M	MINOR SKIN DISORDERS AGE <70 W/O CC	9
321	M	KIDNEY & URINARY TRACT INFECTIONS AGE 18–69 W/O CC	11
326	M	KIDNEY & URINARY TRACT SIGNS & SYMPTOMS AGE 18–69 W/O CC	11
329	M	URETHRAL STRICTURE AGE 18–69 W/O CC	11
332	M	OTHER KIDNEY & URINARY TRACT DIAGNOSES AGE 18–69 W/O CC	11
342	P	CIRCUMCISION AGE >17	12
343	P	CIRCUMCISION AGE 0–17	12

Continued

Appendix 6-A: Continued

		DRGs by Cluster	
		Cluster = 1	Assigned time = 210 minutes
DRG	Type	DRG Name	MDC
349	M	BENIGN PROSTATIC HYPERTROPHY AGE <70 W/O CC	12
350	M	INFLAMMATION OF THE MALE REPRODUCTIVE SYSTEM	12
351	M	STERILIZATION, MALE	12
352	M	OTHER MALE REPRODUCTIVE SYSTEM DIAGNOSES	12
359	P	INCISIONAL TUBAL INTERRUPTION FOR NON-MALIGNANCY	13
361	P	LAPAROSCOPY & ENDOSCOPY (FEMALE) EXCEPT TUBAL INTERRUPTION	13
362	P	LAPAROSCOPIC TUBAL INTERRUPTION	13
364	P	D&C, CONIZATION EXCEPT FOR MALIGNANCY	13
369	M	MENSTRUAL & OTHER FEMALE REPRODUCTIVE SYSTEM DISORDERS	13
376	M	POSTPARTUM & POST ABORTION DIAGNOSES W/O O.R. PROCEDURE	14
380	M	ABORTION W/O D&C	14
381	P	ABORTION W D&C, ASPIRATION CURETTAGE OR HYSTEROTOMY	14
382	M	FALSE LABOR	14
383	M	OTHER ANTEPARTUM DIAGNOSES W MEDICAL COMPLICATIONS	14
384	M	OTHER ANTEPARTUM DIAGNOSES W/O MEDICAL COMPLICATIONS	14
409	M	RADIOTHERAPY	17
411	M	HISTORY OF MALIGNANCY W/O ENDOSCOPY	17
412	M	HISTORY OF MALIGNANCY W ENDOSCOPY	17
421	M	VIRAL ILLNESS AGE >17	18
423	M	OTHER INFECTIOUS & PARASITIC DISEASES DIAGNOSES	18
434		SUBST ABUSE, INTOX, INDUCE MENTAL SYN EXC DEPEND &/OR OTH SYMPT TRE	20
435		SUBSTANCE DEPENDENCE, DETOX &/OR OTHER SYMPTOMATIC TREATMENT	20
447	M	ALLERGIC REACTIONS AGE >17	21
462	M	REHABILITATION	23
463	M	SIGNS & SYMPTOMS W CC	23
464	M	SIGNS & SYMPTOMS W/O CC	23
465	M	AFTERCARE W HISTORY OF MALIGNANCY AS SECONDARY DIAGNOSIS	23
466	M	AFTERCARE W/O HISTORY OF MALIGNANCY AS SECONDARY DIAGNOSIS	23
467	M	OTHER FACTORS INFLUENCING HEALTH STATUS	23

Continued

Appendix 6-A: Continued

DRGs by Cluster

Cluster = 2   Assigned time = 240 minutes

DRG	Type	DRG Name	MDC
7	P	PERIPH & CRANIAL NERVE & OTHER NERV SYST PROC AGE >69 &/OR CC	1
8	P	PERIPH & CRANIAL NERVE & OTHER NERV SYST PROC AGE <70 W/O CC	1
18	M	CRANIAL & PERIPHERAL NERVE DISORDERS AGE >69 &/OR CC	1
25	M	SEIZURE & HEADACHE AGE 18–69 W/O CC	1
32	M	CONCUSSION AGE 18–69 W/O CC	1
36	P	RETINAL PROCEDURES	2
38	P	PRIMARY IRIS PROCEDURES	2
40	P	EXTRAOCULAR PROCEDURES EXCEPT ORBIT AGE >17	2
41	P	EXTRAOCULAR PROCEDURES EXCEPT ORBIT AGE 0–17	2
42	P	INTRAOCULAR PROCEDURES EXCEPT RETINA, IRIS & LENS	2
48	M	OTHER DISORDERS OF THE EYE AGE 0–17	2
53	P	SINUS & MASTOID PROCEDURES AGE >17	3
55	P	MISCELLANEOUS EAR, NOSE & THROAT PROCEDURES	3
57	P	T&A PROC, EXCEPT TONSILLECTOMY &/OR ADENOIDECTOMY ONLY, AGE >17	3
58	P	T&A PROC, EXCEPT TONSILLECTOMY &/OR ADENOIDECTOMY ONLY, AGE 0–17	3
59	P	TONSILLECTOMY &/OR ADENOIDECTOMY ONLY, AGE >17	3
60	P	TONSILLECTOMY &/OR ADENOIDECTOMY ONLY, AGE 0–17	3
63	P	OTHER EAR, NOSE & THROAT O.R. PROCEDURES	3
70	M	OTITIS MEDIA & URI AGE 0–17	3
80	M	RESPIRATORY INFECTIONS & INFLAMMATIONS AGE 18–69 W/O CC	4
85	M	PLEURAL EFFUSION AGE >69 &/OR CC	4
86	M	PLEURAL EFFUSION AGE <70 W/O CC	4
93	M	INTERSTITIAL LUNG DISEASE AGE <70 W/O CC	4
99	M	RESPIRATORY SIGNS & SYMPTOMS AGE >69 &/OR CC	4
102	M	OTHER RESPIRATORY SYSTEM DIAGNOSES AGE <70 W/O CC	4
117	P	CARDIAC PACEMAKER REPLACE & REVIS EXCEPT PULSE GEN REPL ONLY	5
118	P	CARDIAC PACEMAKER PULSE GENERATOR REPLACEMENT ONLY	5
119	P	VEIN LIGATION & STRIPPING	5
130	M	PERIPHERAL VASCULAR DISORDERS AGE >69 &/OR CC	5

Continued

Appendix 6-A: Continued

DRGs by Cluster

Cluster = 2   Assigned time = 240 minutes

DRG	Type	DRG Name	MDC
131	M	PERIPHERAL VASCULAR DISORDERS AGE <70 W/O CC	5
133	M	ATHEROSCLEROSIS AGE <70 W/O CC	5
134	M	HYPERTENSION	5
143	M	CHEST PAIN	5
158	P	ANAL & STOMAL PROCEDURES AGE <70 W/O CC	6
162	P	INGUINAL & FEMORAL HERNIA PROCEDURES AGE 18–69 W/O CC	6
167	P	APPENDECTOMY W/O COMPLICATED PRINCIPAL DIAG AGE <70 W/O CC	6
169	P	MOUTH PROCEDURES AGE <70 W/O CC	6
177	M	UNCOMPLICATED PEPTIC ULCER AGE >69 &/OR CC	6
179	M	INFLAMMATORY BOWEL DISEASE	6
183	M	ESOPHAGITIS, GASTROENT & MISC DIGEST DISORDERS AGE 18–69 W/O CC	6
185	M	DENTAL & ORAL DIS EXCEPT EXTRACTIONS & RESTORATIONS, AGE >17	6
187	M	DENTAL EXTRACTIONS & RESTORATIONS	6
188	M	OTHER DIGESTIVE SYSTEM DIAGNOSES AGE >69 &/OR CC	6
189	M	OTHER DIGESTIVE SYSTEM DIAGNOSES AGE 18–69 W/O CC	6
190	M	OTHER DIGESTIVE SYSTEM DIAGNOSES AGE 0–17	6
199	P	HEPATOBILIARY DIAGNOSTIC PROCEDURE FOR MALIGNANCY	7
200	P	HEPATOBILIARY DIAGNOSTIC PROCEDURE FOR NON-MALIGNANCY	7
202	M	CIRRHOSIS & ALCOHOLIC HEPATITIS	7
225	P	FOOT PROCEDURES	8
227	P	SOFT TISSUE PROCEDURES AGE <70 W/O CC	8
229	P	HAND PROCEDURES EXCEPT GANGLION	8
233	P	OTHER MUSCULOSKELET SYS & CONN TISS O.R. PROC AGE >69 &/OR CC	8
234	P	OTHER MUSCULOSKELET SYS & CONN TISS O.R. PROC AGE <70 W/O CC	8
238	M	OSTEOMYELITIS	8
240	M	CONNECTIVE TISSUE DISORDERS AGE >69 &/OR CC	8
244	M	BONE DISEASES & SPECIFIC ARTHROPATHIES AGE >69 &/OR CC	8
246	M	NON-SPECIFIC ARTHROPATHIES	8
251	M	FX, SPRN, STRN & DISL OF FOREARM, HAND, FOOT AGE 18–69 W/O CC	8
254	M	FX, SPRN, STRN & DISL OF UPARM, LOWLEG EX FOOT AGE 18–69 W/O CC	8

Continued

Appendix 6-A: Continued

| | | DRGs by Cluster | |
| | | Cluster = 2 | Assigned time = 240 minutes |

DRG	Type	DRG Name	MDC
268	P	SKIN, SUBCUTANEOUS TISSUE & BREAST PLASTIC PROCEDURES	9
270	P	OTHER SKIN, SUBCUT TISS & BREAST O.R. PROC AGE <70 W/O CC	9
281	M	TRAUMA TO THE SKIN, SUBCUT TISS & BREAST AGE 18–69 W/O CC	9
308	P	MINOR BLADDER PROCEDURES AGE >69 &/OR CC	11
309	P	MINOR BLADDER PROCEDURES AGE <70 W/O CC	11
310	P	TRANSURETHRAL PROCEDURES AGE >69 &/OR CC	11
311	P	TRANSURETHRAL PROCEDURES AGE <70 W/O CC	11
312	P	URETHRAL PROCEDURES, AGE >69 &/OR CC	11
313	P	URETHRAL PROCEDURES, AGE 18–69 W/O CC	11
314	P	URETHRAL PROCEDURES, AGE 0–17	11
322	M	KIDNEY & URINARY TRACT INFECTIONS AGE 0–17	11
325	M	KIDNEY & URINARY TRACT SIGNS & SYMPTOMS AGE >69 &/OR CC	11
327	M	KIDNEY & URINARY TRACT SIGNS & SYMPTOMS AGE 0–17	11
328	M	URETHRAL STRICTURE AGE >69 &/OR CC	11
330	M	URETHRAL STRICTURE AGE 0–17	11
333	M	OTHER KIDNEY & URINARY TRACT DIAGNOSES AGE 0–17	11
338	P	TESTES PROCEDURES, FOR MALIGNANCY	12
339	P	TESTES PROCEDURES, NON-MALIGNANCY AGE >17	12
340	P	TESTES PROCEDURES, NON-MALIGNANCY AGE 0–17	12
341	P	PENIS PROCEDURES	12
348	M	BENIGN PROSTATIC HYPERTROPHY AGE >69 &/OR CC	12
356	P	FEMALE REPRODUCTIVE SYSTEM RECONSTRUCTIVE PROCEDURES	13
363	P	D&C, CONIZATION & RADIO-IMPLANT, FOR MALIGNANCY	13
368	M	INFECTIONS, FEMALE REPRODUCTIVE SYSTEM	13
373	M	VAGINAL DELIVERY W/O COMPLICATING DIAGNOSES	14
374	P	VAGINAL DELIVERY W STERILIZATION &/OR D&C	14
375	P	VAGINAL DELIVERY W O.R. PROC EXCEPT STERIL &/OR D&C	14
377	P	POSTPARTUM & POST ABORTION DIAGNOSES W O.R. PROCEDURE	14
379	M	THREATENED ABORTION	14
391		NORMAL NEWBORN	15
410	M	CHEMOTHERAPY	17
419	M	FEVER OF UNKNOWN ORIGIN AGE >69 &/OR CC	18

Continued

Appendix 6-A: Continued

		DRGs by Cluster	
		Cluster = 2	Assigned time = 240 minutes

DRG	Type	DRG Name	MDC
420	M	FEVER OF UNKNOWN ORIGIN AGE 18–69 W/O CC	18
425	M	ACUTE ADJUST REACT & DISTURBANCES OF PSYCHOSOCIAL DYSFUNCTION	19
432	M	OTHER MENTAL DISORDER DIAGNOSES	19
436		SUBSTANCE DEPENDENCE W REHABILITATION THERAPY	20
448	M	ALLERGIC REACTIONS AGE 0–17	21

		Cluster = 3	Assigned time = 270 minutes

DRG	Type	DRG Name	MDC
15	M	TRANSIENT ISCHEMIC ATTACK & PRECEREBRAL OCCLUSIONS	1
21	M	VIRAL MENINGITIS	1
22	M	HYPERTENSIVE ENCEPHALOPATHY	1
24	M	SEIZURE & HEADACHE AGE >69 &/OR CC	1
31	M	CONCUSSION AGE >69 &/OR CC	1
33	M	CONCUSSION AGE 0–17	1
34	M	OTHER DISORDERS OF NERVOUS SYSTEM AGE >69 &/OR CC	1
35	M	OTHER DISORDERS OF NERVOUS SYSTEM AGE <70 W/O CC	1
37	P	ORBITAL PROCEDURES	2
52	P	CLEFT LIP & PALATE REPAIR	3
54	P	SINUS & MASTOID PROCEDURES AGE 0–17	3
64	M	EAR, NOSE & THROAT MALIGNANCY	3
79	M	RESPIRATORY INFECTIONS & INFLAMMATIONS AGE >69 &/OR CC	4
81	M	RESPIRATORY INFECTIONS & INFLAMMATIONS AGE 0–17	4
82	M	RESPIRATORY NEOPLASMS	4
90	M	SIMPLE PNEUMONIA & PLEURISY AGE 18–69 W/O CC	4
92	M	INTERSTITIAL LUNG DISEASE AGE >69 &/OR CC	4
97	M	BRONCHITIS & ASTHMA AGE 18–69 W/O CC	4
101	M	OTHER RESPIRATORY SYSTEM DIAGNOSES AGE >69 &/OR CC	4
116	P	PERM CARDIAC PACEMAKER IMPLANT W/O AMI, HEART FAILURE OR SHOCK	5
132	M	ATHEROSCLEROSIS AGE >69 &/OR CC	5
140	M	ANGINA PECTORIS	5
145	M	OTHER CIRCULATORY SYSTEM DIAGNOSES W/O CC	5
151	P	PERITONEAL ADHESIOLYSIS AGE <70 W/O CC	6

Continued

Appendix 6-A: Continued

DRGs by Cluster

Cluster = 3

Assigned time = 270 minutes

DRG	Type	DRG Name	MDC
153	P	MINOR SMALL & LARGE BOWEL PROCEDURES AGE <70 W/O CC	6
157	P	ANAL & STOMAL PROCEDURES AGE >69 &/OR CC	6
160	P	HERNIA PROCEDURES EXCEPT INGUINAL & FEMORAL AGE 18–69 W/O CC	6
161	P	INGUINAL & FEMORAL HERNIA PROCEDURES AGE >69 &/OR CC	6
163	P	HERNIA PROCEDURES AGE 0–17	6
165	P	APPENDECTOMY W COMPLICATED PRINCIPAL DIAG AGE <70 W/O CC	6
166	P	APPENDECTOMY W/O COMPLICATED PRINCIPAL DIAG AGE >69 &/OR CC	6
168	P	MOUTH PROCEDURES AGE >69 &/OR CC	6
172	M	DIGESTIVE MALIGNANCY AGE >69 &/OR CC	6
173	M	DIGESTIVE MALIGNANCY AGE <70 W/O CC	6
181	M	G.I. OBSTRUCTION AGE <70 W/O CC	6
182	M	ESOPHAGITIS, GASTROENT & MISC DIGEST DISORDERS AGE >69 &/OR CC	6
184	M	ESOPHAGITIS, GASTROENT & MISC DIGEST DISORDERS AGE 0–17	6
186	M	DENTAL & ORAL DIS EXCEPT EXTRACTIONS & RESTORATIONS, AGE 0–17	6
204	M	DISORDERS OF PANCREAS EXCEPT MALIGNANCY	7
205	M	DISORDERS OF LIVER EXCEPT MALIG, CIRR, ALC HEPA AGE >69 &/OR CC	7
206	M	DISORDERS OF LIVER EXCEPT MALIG, CIRR, ALC HEPA AGE <70 W/O CC	7
207	M	DISORDERS OF THE BILIARY TRACT AGE >69 &/OR CC	7
208	M	DISORDERS OF THE BILIARY TRACT AGE <70 W/O CC	7
222	P	KNEE PROCEDURES AGE <70 W/O CC	8
224	P	UPPER EXTREMITY PROC EXCEPT HUMERUS & HAND AGE <70 W/O CC	8
226	P	SOFT TISSUE PROCEDURES AGE >69 &/OR CC	8
230	P	LOCAL EXCISION & REMOVAL OF INT FIX DEVICES OF HIP & FEMUR	8
231	P	LOCAL EXCISION & REMOVAL OF INT FIX DEVICES EXCEPT HIP & FEMUR	8
237	M	SPRAINS, STRAINS, & DISLOCATIONS OF HIP, PELVIS & THIGH	8
243	M	MEDICAL BACK PROBLEMS	8
250	M	FX, SPRN, STRN & DISL OF FOREARM, HAND, FOOT AGE >69 &/OR CC	8

Continued

Appendix 6-A: Continued

		DRGs by Cluster	
		Cluster = 3	Assigned time = 270 minutes

DRG	Type	DRG Name	MDC
252	M	FX, SPRN, STRN & DISL OF FOREARM, HAND, FOOT AGE 0–17	8
253	M	FX, SPRN, STRN & DISL OF UPARM, LOWLEG EX FOOT AGE >69 &/OR CC	8
255	M	FX, SPRN, STRN & DISL OF UPARM, LOWLEG EX FOOT AGE 0–17	8
259	P	SUBTOTAL MASTECTOMY FOR MALIGNANCY AGE >69 &/OR CC	9
260	P	SUBTOTAL MASTECTOMY FOR MALIGNANCY AGE <70 W/O CC	9
261	P	BREAST PROC FOR NON-MALIGNANCY EXCEPT BIOPSY & LOCAL EXCISION	9
267	P	PERIANAL & PILONIDAL PROCEDURES	9
269	P	OTHER SKIN, SUBCUT TISS & BREAST O.R. PROC AGE >69 &/OR CC	9
272	M	MAJOR SKIN DISORDERS AGE >69 &/OR CC	9
273	M	MAJOR SKIN DISORDERS AGE <70 W/O CC	9
274	M	MALIGNANT BREAST DISORDERS AGE >69 &/OR CC	9
275	M	MALIGNANT BREAST DISORDERS AGE <70 W/O CC	9
277	M	CELLULITIS AGE >69 &/OR CC	9
278	M	CELLULITIS AGE 18–69 W/O CC	9
279	M	CELLULITIS AGE 0–17	9
280	M	TRAUMA TO THE SKIN, SUBCUT TISS & BREAST AGE >69 &/OR CC	9
282	M	TRAUMA TO THE SKIN, SUBCUT TISS & BREAST AGE 0–17	9
291	P	THYROGLOSSAL PROCEDURES	10
299	M	INBORN ERRORS OF METABOLISM	10
307	P	PROSTATECTOMY AGE <70 W/O CC	11
315	P	OTHER KIDNEY & URINARY TRACT O.R. PROCEDURES	11
317	M	ADMIT FOR RENAL DIALYSIS	11
318	M	KIDNEY & URINARY TRACT NEOPLASMS AGE >69 &/OR CC	11
319	M	KIDNEY & URINARY TRACT NEOPLASMS AGE <70 W/O CC	11
320	M	KIDNEY & URINARY TRACT INFECTIONS AGE >69 &/OR CC	11
331	M	OTHER KIDNEY & URINARY TRACT DIAGNOSES AGE >69 &/OR CC	11
337	P	TRANSURETHRAL PROSTATECTOMY AGE <70 W/O CC	12
344	P	OTHER MALE REPRODUCTIVE SYSTEM O.R. PROCEDURES FOR MALIGNANCY	12

Continued

Appendix 6-A: Continued

DRGs by Cluster

Cluster = 3   Assigned time = 270 minutes

DRG	Type	DRG Name	MDC
345	P	OTHER MALE REPRODUCTIVE SYSTEM O.R. PROC EXCEPT FOR MALIGNANCY	12
346	M	MALIGNANCY, MALE REPRODUCTIVE SYSTEM, AGE >69 &/OR CC	12
347	M	MALIGNANCY, MALE REPRODUCTIVE SYSTEM, AGE <70 W/O CC	12
357	P	UTERUS & ADENEXA PROCEDURES FOR MALIGNANCY	13
358	P	UTERUS & ADENEXA PROC FOR NON-MALIGNANCY EXCEPT TUBAL INTERRUPT	13
360	P	VAGINA, CERVIX & VULVA PROCEDURES	13
365	P	OTHER FEMALE REPRODUCTIVE SYSTEM O.R. PROCEDURES	13
366	M	MALIGNANCY, FEMALE REPRODUCTIVE SYSTEM AGE >69 &/OR CC	13
367	M	MALIGNANCY, FEMALE REPRODUCTIVE SYSTEM AGE <70 W/O CC	13
371	P	CESAREAN SECTION W/O CC	14
394	P	OTHER BLOOD AND BLOOD FORMING ORGANS O.R. PROCEDURES	16
395	M	RED BLOOD CELL DISORDERS AGE >17	16
403	M	LYMPHOMA OR LEUKEMIA AGE >69 &/OR CC	17
404	M	LYMPHOMA OR LEUKEMIA AGE 18–69 W/O CC	17
405	M	LYMPHOMA OR LEUKEMIA AGE 0–17	17
413	M	OTHER MYELOPROLIF DIS OR POORLY DIFF NEOPL DIAG AGE >69 &/OR CC	17
414	M	OTHER MYELOPROLIF DIS OR POORLY DIFF NEOPL DIAG AGE <70 W/O CC	17
415	P	O.R. PROCEDURE FOR INFECTIOUS & PARASITIC DISEASES	18
422	M	VIRAL ILLNESS & FEVER OF UNKNOWN ORIGIN AGE 0–17	18
427	M	NEUROSES EXCEPT DEPRESSIVE	19
428	M	DISORDERS OF PERSONALITY & IMPULSE CONTROL	19
433		SUBSTANCE USE & INDUCED ORGANIC MENTAL DISORDERS, LEFT AMA	20
443	P	OTHER O.R. PROCEDURES FOR INJURIES AGE <70 W/O CC	21
449	M	POISONING & TOXIC EFFECTS OF DRUGS AGE >69 &/OR CC	21
450	M	POISONING & TOXIC EFFECTS OF DRUGS AGE 18–69 W/O CC	21
452	M	COMPLICATIONS OF TREATMENT AGE >69 &/OR CC	21
453	M	COMPLICATIONS OF TREATMENT AGE <70 W/O CC	21
454	M	OTHER INJURY, POISONING & TOXIC EFF DIAG AGE >69 &/OR CC	21

Continued

Appendix 6-A: Continued

DRGs by Cluster

		Cluster = 3	Assigned time = 270 minutes
DRG	Type	DRG Name	MDC
455	M	OTHER INJURY, POISONING & TOXIC EFF DIAG AGE <70 W/O CC	21
461	P	O.R. PROC W DIAGNOSES OF OTHER CONTACT W HEALTH SERVICES	23
468		UNRELATED OPERATING ROOM PROCEDURES	24

		Cluster = 4	Assigned time = 290 minutes
DRG	Type	DRG Name	MDC
5	P	EXTRACRANIAL VASCULAR PROCEDURES	1
10	M	NERVOUS SYSTEM NEOPLASMS AGE >69 &/OR CC	1
11	M	NERVOUS SYSTEM NEOPLASMS AGE <70 W/O CC	1
12	M	DEGENERATIVE NERVOUS SYSTEM DISORDERS	1
13	M	MULTIPLE SCLEROSIS & CEREBELLAR ATAXIA	1
14	M	SPECIFIC CEREBROVASCULAR DISORDERS EXCEPT TIA	1
17	M	NONSPECIFIC CEREBROVASCULAR DISORDERS W/O CC	1
26	M	SEIZURE & HEADACHE AGE 0–17	1
44	M	ACUTE MAJOR EYE INFECTIONS	2
71	M	LARYNGOTRACHEITIS	3
77	P	OTHER RESP SYSTEM O.R. PROCEDURES W/O CC	4
88	M	CHRONIC OBSTRUCTIVE PULMONARY DISEASE	4
89	M	SIMPLE PNEUMONIA & PLEURISY AGE >69 &/OR CC	4
91	M	SIMPLE PNEUMONIA & PLEURISY AGE 0–17	4
95	M	PNEUMOTHORAX AGE <70 W/O CC	4
96	M	BRONCHITIS & ASTHMA AGE >69 &/OR CC	4
98	M	BRONCHITIS & ASTHMA AGE 0–17	4
114	P	UPPER LIMB & TOE AMPUTATION FOR CIRC SYSTEM DISORDERS	5
120	P	OTHER CIRCULATORY SYSTEM O.R. PROCEDURES	5
122	M	CIRCULATORY DISORDERS W AMI W/O C.V. COMP DISCH ALIVE	5
125	M	CIRCULATORY DISORDERS EXCEPT AMI, W CARD CATH W/O COMPLEX DIAG	5
126	M	ACUTE & SUBACUTE ENDOCARDITIS	5
128	M	DEEP VEIN THROMBOPHLEBITIS	5
135	M	CARDIAC CONGENITAL & VALVULAR DISORDERS AGE >69 &/OR CC	5
136	M	CARDIAC CONGENITAL & VALVULAR DISORDERS AGE 18–69 W/O CC	5
139	M	CARDIAC ARRHYTHMIA & CONDUCTION DISORDERS AGE <70 W/O CC	5

Continued

Appendix 6-A: Continued

DRGs by Cluster

Cluster = 4   Assigned time = 290 minutes

DRG	Type	DRG Name	MDC
142	M	SYNCOPE & COLLAPSE AGE <70 W/O CC	5
147	P	RECTAL RESECTION AGE <70 W/O CC	6
149	P	MAJOR SMALL & LARGE BOWEL PROCEDURES AGE <70 W/O CC	6
150	P	PERITONEAL ADHESIOLYSIS AGE >69 &/OR CC	6
152	P	MINOR SMALL & LARGE BOWEL PROCEDURES AGE >69 &/OR CC	6
155	P	STOMACH, ESOPHAGEAL & DUODENAL PROCEDURES AGE 18–69 W/O CC	6
159	P	HERNIA PROCEDURES EXCEPT INGUINAL & FEMORAL AGE >69 &/OR CC	6
164	P	APPENDECTOMY W COMPLICATED PRINCIPAL DIAG AGE >69 &/OR CC	6
171	P	OTHER DIGESTIVE SYSTEM O.R. PROCEDURES AGE <70 W/O CC	6
175	M	G.I. HEMORRHAGE AGE <70 W/O CC	6
192	P	MINOR PANCREAS, LIVER & SHUNT PROCEDURES	7
194	P	BILIARY TRACT PROC EXCEPT TOT CHOLECYSTECTOMY AGE <70 W/O CC	7
196	P	TOTAL CHOLECYSTECTOMY W C.D.E. AGE <70 W/O CC	7
198	P	TOTAL CHOLECYSTECTOMY W/O C.D.E. AGE <70 W/O CC	7
201	P	OTHER HEPATOBILIARY OR PANCREAS O.R. PROCEDURES	7
203	M	MALIGNANCY OF HEPATOBILIARY SYSTEM OR PANCREAS	7
217	P	WND DEBRID & SKN GRFT EXCEPT HAND, FOR MUSCSKELET & CONN TISS DIS	8
219	P	LOWER EXTREM & HUMER PROC EXCEPT HIP, FOOT, FEMUR AGE 18–69 W/O CC	8
221	P	KNEE PROCEDURES AGE >69 &/OR CC	8
223	P	UPPER EXTREMITY PROC EXCEPT HUMERUS & HAND AGE >69 &/OR CC	8
235	M	FRACTURES OF FEMUR	8
242	M	SEPTIC ARTHRITIS	8
257	P	TOTAL MASTECTOMY FOR MALIGNANCY AGE >69 &/OR CC	9
258	P	TOTAL MASTECTOMY FOR MALIGNANCY AGE <70 W/O CC	9
263	P	SKIN GRAFT &/OR DEBRID FOR SKN ULCER OR CELLULITIS AGE >69 &/OR CC	9
264	P	SKIN GRAFT &/OR DEBRID FOR SKN ULCER OR CELLULITIS AGE <70 W/O CC	9

Continued

Appendix 6-A: Continued

DRGs by Cluster

Cluster = 4   Assigned time = 290 minutes

DRG	Type	DRG Name	MDC
265	P	SKIN GRAFT &/OR DEBRID EXCEPT FOR SKIN ULCER OR CELLULITIS W CC	9
266	P	SKIN GRAFT &/OR DEBRID EXCEPT FOR SKIN ULCER OR CELLULITIS W/O CC	9
271	M	SKIN ULCERS	9
287	P	SKIN GRAFTS & WOUND DEBRID FOR ENDOC, NUTRIT & METAB DISORDERS	10
293	P	OTHER ENDOCRINE, NUTRIT & METAB O.R. PROC AGE <70 W/O CC	10
296	M	NUTRITIONAL & MISC METABOLIC DISORDERS AGE >69 &/OR CC	10
297	M	NUTRITIONAL & MISC METABOLIC DISORDERS AGE 18–69 W/O CC	10
301	M	ENDOCRINE DISORDERS AGE <70 W/O CC	10
305	P	KIDNEY, URETER & MAJOR BLADDER PROC FOR NON-NEOPL AGE <70 W/O CC	11
306	P	PROSTATECTOMY AGE >69 &/OR CC	11
323	M	URINARY STONES AGE >69 &/OR CC	11
324	M	URINARY STONES AGE <70 W/O CC	11
336	P	TRANSURETHRAL PROSTATECTOMY AGE >69 &/OR CC	12
355	P	NON-RADICAL HYSTERECTOMY AGE <70 W/O CC	13
370	P	CESAREAN SECTION W CC	14
372	M	VAGINAL DELIVERY W COMPLICATING DIAGNOSES	14
378	M	ECTOPIC PREGNANCY	14
388		PREMATURITY W/O MAJOR PROBLEMS	15
392	P	SPLENECTOMY AGE >17	16
393	P	SPLENECTOMY AGE 0–17	16
396	M	RED BLOOD CELL DISORDERS AGE 0–17	16
397	M	COAGULATION DISORDERS	16
402	P	LYMPHOMA OR LEUKEMIA W OTHER O.R. PROC AGE <70 W/O CC	17
416	M	SEPTICEMIA AGE >17	18
417	M	SEPTICEMIA AGE 0–17	18
418	M	POSTOPERATIVE & POST-TRAUMATIC INFECTIONS	18
424	P	O.R. PROCEDURE W PRINCIPAL DIAGNOSES OF MENTAL ILLNESS	19
426	M	DEPRESSIVE NEUROSES	19
430	M	PSYCHOSES	19
437		SUBSTANCE DEPENDENCE, COMBINED REHAB & DETOX THERAPY	20
439	P	SKIN GRAFTS FOR INJURIES	21
440	P	WOUND DEBRIDEMENTS FOR INJURIES	21

Continued

Appendix 6-A: Continued

DRGs by Cluster

Cluster = 4   Assigned time = 290 minutes

DRG	Type	DRG Name	MDC
441	P	HAND PROCEDURES FOR INJURIES	21
442	P	OTHER O.R. PROCEDURES FOR INJURIES AGE >69 &/OR CC	21
445	M	MULTIPLE TRAUMA AGE 18–69 W/O CC	21
451	M	POISONING & TOXIC EFFECTS OF DRUGS AGE 0–17	21

Cluster = 5   Assigned time = 330 minutes

DRG	Type	DRG Name	MDC
1	P	CRANIOTOMY AGE >17 EXCEPT FOR TRAUMA	1
2	P	CRANIOTOMY FOR TRAUMA AGE >17	1
3	P	CRANIOTOMY AGE <18	1
4	P	SPINAL PROCEDURES	1
9	M	SPINAL DISORDERS & INJURIES	1
16	M	NONSPECIFIC CEREBROVASCULAR DISORDERS W CC	1
20	M	NERVOUS SYSTEM INFECTION EXCEPT VIRAL MENINGITIS	1
23	M	NONTRAUMATIC STUPOR & COMA	1
27	M	TRAUMATIC STUPOR & COMA, COMA >1 HR	1
28	M	TRAUMATIC STUPOR & COMA, COMA <1 HR AGE >69 &/OR CC	1
29	M	TRAUMATIC STUPOR & COMA, COMA <1 HR AGE 18–69 W/O CC	1
30	M	TRAUMATIC STUPOR & COMA, COMA <1 HR AGE 0–17	1
49	P	MAJOR HEAD & NECK PROCEDURES	3
67	M	EPIGLOTTITIS	3
75	P	MAJOR CHEST PROCEDURES	4
76	P	OTHER RESP SYSTEM O.R. PROCEDURES W CC	4
78	M	PULMONARY EMBOLISM	4
83	M	MAJOR CHEST TRAUMA AGE >69 &/OR CC	4
84	M	MAJOR CHEST TRAUMA AGE <70 W/O CC	4
87	M	PULMONARY EDEMA & RESPIRATORY FAILURE	4
94	M	PNEUMOTHORAX AGE >69 &/OR CC	4
104	P	CARDIAC VALVE PROCEDURE W PUMP & W CARDIAC CATH	5
105	P	CARDIAC VALVE PROCEDURE W PUMP & W/O CARDIAC CATH	5
106	P	CORONARY BYPASS W CARDIAC CATH	5
107	P	CORONARY BYPASS W/O CARDIAC CATH	5
108	P	OTHER CARDIOVASCULAR OR THORACIC PROC, W PUMP	5
109	P	CARDIOTHORACIC PROCEDURES W/O PUMP	5

Continued

Appendix 6-A: Continued

DRGs by Cluster

Cluster = 5   Assigned time = 330 minutes

DRG	Type	DRG Name	MDC
110	P	MAJOR RECONSTRUCTIVE VASCULAR PROC W/O PUMP AGE >69 &/OR CC	5
111	P	MAJOR RECONSTRUCTIVE VASCULAR PROC W/O PUMP AGE <70 W/O CC	5
112	P	VASCULAR PROCEDURES EXCEPT MAJOR RECONSTRUCTION W/O PUMP	5
113	P	AMPUTATION FOR CIRC SYSTEM DISORDERS EXCEPT UPPER LIMB & TOE	5
115	P	PERM CARDIAC PACEMAKER IMPLANT W AMI, HEART FAILURE OR SHOCK	5
121	M	CIRCULATORY DISORDERS W AMI & C.V. COMP DISCH ALIVE	5
123	M	CIRCULATORY DISORDERS W AMI, EXPIRED	5
124	M	CIRCULATORY DISORDERS EXCEPT AMI, W CARD CATH & COMPLEX DIAG	5
127	M	HEART FAILURE & SHOCK	5
129	M	CARDIAC ARREST, UNEXPLAINED	5
137	M	CARDIAC CONGENITAL & VALVULAR DISORDERS AGE 0–17	5
138	M	CARDIAC ARRHYTHMIA & CONDUCTION DISORDERS AGE >69 &/OR CC	5
141	M	SYNCOPE & COLLAPSE AGE >69 &/OR CC	5
144	M	OTHER CIRCULATORY SYSTEM DIAGNOSES W CC	5
146	P	RECTAL RESECTION AGE >69 &/OR CC	6
148	P	MAJOR SMALL & LARGE BOWEL PROCEDURES AGE >69 &/OR CC	6
154	P	STOMACH, ESOPHAGEAL & DUODENAL PROCEDURES AGE >69 &/OR CC	6
156	P	STOMACH, ESOPHAGEAL & DUODENAL PROCEDURES AGE 0–17	6
170	P	OTHER DIGESTIVE SYSTEM O.R. PROCEDURES AGE >69 &/OR CC	6
174	M	G.I. HEMORRHAGE AGE >69 &/OR CC	6
176	M	COMPLICATED PEPTIC ULCER	6
180	M	G.I. OBSTRUCTION AGE >69 &/OR CC	6
191	P	MAJOR PANCREAS, LIVER & SHUNT PROCEDURES	7
193	P	BILIARY TRACT PROC EXCEPT TOT CHOLECYSTECTOMY AGE >69 &/OR CC	7
195	P	TOTAL CHOLECYSTECTOMY W C.D.E. AGE >69 &/OR CC	7
197	P	TOTAL CHOLECYSTECTOMY W/O C.D.E. AGE >69 &/OR CC	7
209	P	MAJOR JOINT & LIMB REATTACHMENT PROCEDURES	8

Continued

Appendix 6-A: Continued

DRGs by Cluster

Cluster = 5   Assigned time = 330 minutes

DRG	Type	DRG Name	MDC
210	P	HIP & FEMUR PROCEDURES EXCEPT MAJOR JOINT AGE >69 &/OR CC	8
211	P	HIP & FEMUR PROCEDURES EXCEPT MAJOR JOINT AGE 18–69 W/O CC	8
212	P	HIP & FEMUR PROCEDURES EXCEPT MAJOR JOINT AGE 0–17	8
213	P	AMPUTATION FOR MUSCULOSKELETAL SYSTEM & CONN TISSUE DISORDERS	8
214	P	BACK & NECK PROCEDURES AGE >69 &/OR CC	8
215	P	BACK & NECK PROCEDURES AGE <70 W/O CC	8
218	P	LOWER EXTREM & HUMER PROC EXCEPT HIP, FOOT, FEMUR AGE >69 &/OR CC	8
220	P	LOWER EXTREM & HUMER PROC EXCEPT HIP, FOOT, FEMUR AGE 0–17	8
236	M	FRACTURES OF HIP & PELVIS	8
239	M	PATHOLOGICAL FRACTURES & MUSCULOSKELETAL & CONN TISS MALIGNANCY	8
285	P	AMPUTAT OF LOWER LIMB FOR ENDOCRINE, NUTRIT, & METABOL DISORDERS	10
286	P	ADRENAL & PITUITARY PROCEDURES	10
288	P	O.R. PROCEDURES FOR OBESITY	10
289	P	PARATHYROID PROCEDURES	10
290	P	THYROID PROCEDURES	10
292	P	OTHER ENDOCRINE, NUTRIT & METAB O.R. PROC AGE >69 &/OR CC	10
294	M	DIABETES AGE >35	10
295	M	DIABETES AGE 0–35	10
298	M	NUTRITIONAL & MISC METABOLIC DISORDERS AGE 0–17	10
300	M	ENDOCRINE DISORDERS AGE >69 &/OR CC	10
302	P	KIDNEY TRANSPLANT	11
303	P	KIDNEY, URETER & MAJOR BLADDER PROCEDURES FOR NEOPLASM	11
304	P	KIDNEY, URETER & MAJOR BLADDER PROC FOR NON-NEOPL AGE >69 &/OR CC	11
316	M	RENAL FAILURE	11
334	P	MAJOR MALE PELVIC PROCEDURES W CC	12
335	P	MAJOR MALE PELVIC PROCEDURES W/O CC	12
353	P	PELVIC EVISCERATION, RADICAL HYSTERECTOMY & RADICAL VULVECTOMY	13
354	P	NON-RADICAL HYSTERECTOMY AGE >69 &/OR CC	13
385		NEONATES, DIED OR TRANSFERRED	15
386		EXTREME IMMATURITY OR RESPIRATORY DISTRESS SYNDROME, NEONATE	15

Continued

Appendix 6-A: Continued

DRGs by Cluster

Cluster = 5   Assigned time = 330 minutes

DRG	Type	DRG Name	MDC
387		PREMATURITY W MAJOR PROBLEMS	15
389		FULL TERM NEONATE W MAJOR PROBLEMS	15
390		NEONATE W OTHER SIGNIFICANT PROBLEMS	15
398	M	RETICULOENDOTHELIAL & IMMUNITY DISORDERS AGE >69 &/OR CC	16
399	M	RETICULOENDOTHELIAL & IMMUNITY DISORDERS AGE <70 W/O CC	16
400	P	LYMPHOMA & LEUKEMIA W MAJOR O.R. PROCEDURE	17
401	P	LYMPHOMA OR LEUKEMIA W OTHER O.R. PROC AGE >69 &/OR CC	17
406	P	MYELOPROLIF DISORD OR POORLY DIFF NEOPL W MAJ O.R. PROC & CC	17
407	P	MYELOPROLIF DISORD OR POORLY DIFF NEOPL W MAJ O.R. PROC W/O CC	17
408	P	MYELOPROLIF DISORD OR POORLY DIFF NEOPL W OTHER O.R. PROC	17
429	M	ORGANIC DISTURBANCES & MENTAL RETARDATION	19
431	M	CHILDHOOD MENTAL DISORDERS	19
444	M	MULTIPLE TRAUMA AGE >69 &/OR CC	21
446	M	MULTIPLE TRAUMA AGE 0–17	21
458	P	NON-EXTENSIVE BURNS W SKIN GRAFT	22
459	P	NON-EXTENSIVE BURNS W WOUND DEBRIDEMENT & OTHER O.R. PROC	22
460	M	NON-EXTENSIVE BURNS W/O O.R. PROCEDURE	22
471	P	BILATERAL OR MULTIPLE MAJOR JOINT PROCS OF LOWER EXTREMITY	8

Cluster = 6   Assigned time = 450 minutes

DRG	Type	DRG Name	MDC
103	P	HEART TRANSPLANT	5
456		BURNS, TRANSFERRED TO ANOTHER ACUTE CARE FACILITY	22
457	M	EXTENSIVE BURNS	22

Cluster = .

DRG	Type	DRG Name	MDC
438		NO LONGER VALID	20
469		PRINCIPAL DIAGNOSIS INVALID AS DISCHARGE DIAGNOSIS	24
470		UNGROUPABLE	24

Source: Robert B. Fetter and John D. Thompson, "Diagnosis Related Groups and Nursing Resources."

7

Cost-Variance Analysis

Audrey L. Fetter, Edward A. Harms, and Robert B. Fetter

The concepts of product-line management and case-mix cost accounting discussed in Chapters 4 and 5 provide the foundation for an analysis of variations in hospital costs over time. "Cost-variance analysis" can be used to examine differences between budgeted and actual expenditures or changes in hospital costs from one period to another. A cost-variance analysis determines the relative contributions of three separate factors to the observed differences or changes: (1) the case mix of the hospital, (2) the practice patterns of the hospital's medical staff, and (3) the operating efficiency of the hospital's departments.

This chapter illustrates the technique of cost-variance analysis, first by describing a hypothetical analysis of a firm's budgeted versus actual expenditures for labor, and then by presenting a case study involving one of the departments of a university teaching hospital. The case study analyzes changes in departmental costs over a three-year period and assigns responsibility for specific changes to the hospital administration or the medical staff.

This chapter also discusses an additional application of the product-line model, the selection and design of hospital products. The chapter concludes with a description of barriers to the implementation of product-line management and case-mix accounting systems.

LABOR COST EXAMPLE

Suppose a facility uses 1,000 hours of labor during a given period when only 900 hours had been budgeted on the basis of past experience.

Adapted from Audrey L. Fetter, "Cost Measurement and Control in a Hospital Patient Service Department: A New Approach" (master's essay, Department of Epidemiology and Public Health, Yale University, 1980).

Suppose also that the actual cost per hour was $5.00, while the budgeted cost per hour was $5.50. The net result is a spending excess of $50 for labor (Table 7-1). Since both the number of hours and the price per hour for labor varied from the budgeted amounts, the +$50 cost variance is composed of an *unfavorable* efficiency variance of $550 (more hours were used than expected) and a *favorable* price variance of $500 (the price paid per hour was less than expected). Although the net result is an unfavorable variance of +$50, this two-factor analysis shows that, from a managerial perspective, two different processes were responsible for the variance.

The analysis may be extended to three factors by considering, in addition, the volume of production (Table 7-2). In the present example, 500 units were budgeted compared with 525 units that were actually produced.

It can be seen that a three-factor cost-variance analysis proceeds by successively holding two factors constant and considering the difference between "standard" and actual amounts of the third factor. Volume variance is computed by holding hours and unit price at standard. Efficiency variance is calculated by holding volume at actual and unit price at standard and varying the hours per unit. Price variance is determined in an analogous fashion.

The cost-variance analysis reveals a series of problems and a picture rather different from what might be inferred by simply looking at the $50 variance between expected and actual spending. Algebraically, there will usually be a residual term (labeled "interaction") as a consequence of the particular factors chosen as constant. This term is that portion of the total variance not explained independently by the three given factors.

CASE STUDY

This case study examines year-to-year cost variations in the department of diagnostic radiology of an 800-bed university teaching hospital.[1] This department consisted of five cost centers, each with a separate budget. The budgets contained line items for direct expenses: salaries, general supplies, services, maintenance, and cost transfers. The two cost centers that performed the more common general radiographic procedures were included in the study.[2] Data from fiscal years 1976, 1977, and 1978 were analyzed.

A list of all departmental procedures and their relative value units was obtained for each of the three years. The general radiographic procedures were divided into two procedural categories: group I included

Table 7-1: Two-Factor Analysis of Labor Cost Variance

Hours		Price ($)		Variance	
Actual	Budget	Actual	Budget	Amount ($)	Type
1,000	900	5,000 ($5.00/hr.)	4,950 ($5.50/hr.)	+ $ 50	Total
Actual hours @ standard cost Standard hours @ standard cost			5,500 4,950	+ $550	Efficiency
Actual hours @ actual cost Actual hours @ standard cost			5,000 5,500	− $500	Price

routine examinations and group II included more sophisticated procedures (those requiring a radiologist's direct involvement and the use of
special equipment and contrast media).

Film purchases and technicians' salaries accounted for a large share
of the department's operating costs, and these are the expenses that have
been analyzed (Table 7-3).[3] Various cost adjustments were necessary
before costs could be assigned to resources. Departmental costs were
classified as fixed, variable, or semivariable and separated into inpatient
and outpatient costs. (See Chapter 5.)

Table 7-2: Three-Factor Analysis of Labor Cost Variance

Hours		Price ($)		Volume		Variance	
Actual	Budget	Actual	Budget	Actual	Projected	Amount ($)	Type
1,000	900	5,000 ($5.00/hr.)	4,950 ($5.50/hr.)	525	500	+ 50	Total
Actual volume @ standard hours @ standard price = 525 × 1.8 × 5.50 = 5,200 Budgeted volume @ standard hours @ standard price = 500 × 1.8 × 5.50 = 4,950						+250	Volume
Actual volume @ actual hours @ standard price = 525 × 1.9 × 5.50 = 5,486 Actual volume @ standard hours @ standard price = 525 × 1.8 × 5.50 = 5,198						+288	Efficiency
Actual volume @ standard hours @ actual price = 525 × 1.8 × 5.00 = 4,725 Actual volume @ standard hours @ standard price = 525 × 1.8 × 5.50 = 5,198						−473	Price
						− 15	Interaction

Cost variances have been examined at three levels (Figure 7-1). At the macro (departmental) level, changes in case mix show up as changes in overall utilization of resources. At the micro-costing level, case-mix changes show up as changes in utilization of procedures. At the DRG level, the effects of case mix are displayed explicitly.

Macro Level

The macro-level analysis separates total department cost variances into components due to changes in factor prices, changes in resource utilization, and changes in patient volume (price, efficiency, and volume variance respectively). The data at this level are based on cost information easily obtained from departmental cost budgets.

The combined film and technician V and technician VI labor costs for 1976, 1977, and 1978 were $422,700, $433,943, and $444,782, respectively (Table 7-3). The percentage changes in cost from year to year are quite small ($11,243 or 2.77 percent from 1976 to 1977 and $10,839 or 2.5 percent from 1977 to 1978). Without further analysis, these changes might be dismissed as managerially inconsequential. However, the $11,243 variance between 1976 and 1977 will be further analyzed.

First we consider the effect of changes in labor cost and film cost together with the units of each resource utilized. The total cost change is the sum of the changes due to factor price changes plus the change in film and labor utilization. Table 7-4 shows the results based on this calculation. Variance in cost is now expressed in terms of the effect of changes in cost from one year to the next at a constant level of service.

From this table one can determine the effect of the change of cost per unit resource (inflation or price change) and the change in the amount of resources used (departmental utilization change) on total costs. The figure shows the inflationary effect of increased costs partially offset by the

Table 7-3: Overall Labor and Film Cost Changes, Radiology Department

1976 Cost		1977 Cost		1978 Cost
$422,700		$433,943		$444,782
	1976–1977 Change		1977–1978 Change	
	$11,243		$10,839	
	2.7%		2.5%	

Source: Audrey L. Fetter, "Cost Measurement and Control in a Hospital Patient Service Department: A New Approach."

Figure 7-1: Model of Departmental Cost Variance Analysis

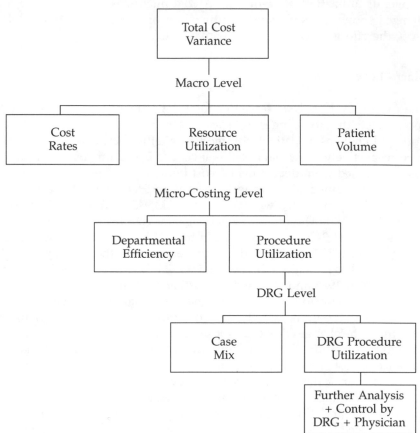

purchase of fewer resources, the total cost increase of 2.7 percent being a result of the 6.3 percent increase in unit cost (price inflation) and the 3.7 percent cost decrease due to use of fewer resources.

Note that the changes associated with departmental utilization (number of units consumed) cannot be analyzed further at this point. The cost decrease could reflect a number of factors: a decrease in the number of patients treated, an increase in the efficiency of labor or film utilization, fewer tests given per patient, or a case mix requiring fewer procedures.

The next step in the analysis is to account for the effect of patient volume on the change in resource use. Adding in the patient volume factor, the change in total costs of operating the department of radiology

Table 7-4: Accounting for Changes in Prices and Resource Utilization (1976 to 1977)*

Factor of Production	Technician V	Technician VI	Film	Total
Cost change due to:				
Cost/unit of input	$11,828	$3,745	$11,152	$26,725
	8.4%	3.6%	6.3%	6.3%
Units of resources utilized	$1,894	($8,943)	($8,433)	($15,482)
	1.3%	(8.5%)	(4.8%)	(3.7%)
Total cost change	$13,722	($5,198)	$2,719	$11,243
	9.8%	(4.9%)	1.5%	2.7%

*Parentheses indicate negative quantities.
Source: Audrey L. Fetter, "Cost Measurement and Control in a Hospital Patient Service Department: A New Approach."

is expressed as the sum of the changes due to price changes at a constant level of output (1976), changes in volume of patients, and changes in units of labor and film utilized per patient (Table 7-5).

Of the $15,482 cost decrease attributed to changes in the utilization of resources (Table 7-3), $4,163 was due to a decrease in number of patients from one year to the next (Table 7-5). The effect of changes in patient volume had been hidden in the utilization term in Table 7-4.

The analysis thus far has revealed that inflation has caused significant cost increases, which have been partially offset by a decrease in the

Table 7-5: Accounting for Changes in Patient Volume (1976 to 1977)*

Factor of Production	Technician V	Technician VI	Film	Total
Cost change due to:				
Cost/unit of input	$11,828	$3,745	$11,152	$26,725
	8.4%	3.6%	6.3%	6.3%
Units of resources utilized at constant (1976) patient volume	$3,376	($7,985)	($6,710)	($11,319)
	2.4%	(7.6%)	(3.8%)	(2.7%)
Number of patients	($1,482)	($958)	($1,723)	($4,163)
	(1.1%)	(0.9%)	(1.0%)	(1.0%)
Total cost change	$13,722	($5,198)	$2,719	$11,243
	9.8%	(4.9%)	1.5%	2.7%

*Parentheses indicate negative quantities.
Source: Audrey L. Fetter, "Cost Measurement and Control in a Hospital Patient Service Department: A New Approach."

number of patients treated and a decrease in the number of resources used to treat those patients. Questions, however, still remain. Was the department efficient in its use of resources? Did the cost of individual procedures vary over time? Did the number of procedures per patient vary from one year to the next? These questions cannot be answered without further investigation of the factors that influence departmental utilization.

Micro-Costing Level

The micro-costing level of analysis further analyzes the resource consumption findings of the macro-level study, providing a link between the procedures performed and the resources utilized in the department. First, the number of units of each type of resource required to perform a single procedure must be determined. When totaled over all procedures performed by the department, the amount of resources required to provide the observed level of service can be predicted.

When consecutive years are compared, the results can be analyzed in terms of changes in the procedures provided and the resources required by those procedures. Comparisons between predicted and observed resource utilization can be used to assess the department's ability to respond to the differing levels of service demanded of it.

Unlike information at the macro level, information at the micro-costing level is not routinely collected at most hospitals. However, the degree of analysis it permits is worth the effort and cost involved in obtaining the information, at least for the major ancillary service departments.

Formulas (see Appendix 7-A) can be applied to the macro-level data that add the variables of utilization of resources by procedure and average number of procedures per patient. Cost variance can now be expressed in terms of four factors:

— *Rate:* the effect of changes in cost of labor and film at a constant level of services

— *Patient volume:* the changes in cost attributed to changes in number of patients, with current-year cost used for all other terms

— *Departmental efficiency:* the effect of changes in the resources available for use in the department and those utilized

— *Procedure utilization:* the effect of changes due to changes in the number of procedures performed per patient; costs, departmental efficiency, and volume are held constant at the current level (1976)

The department resource utilization term from the macro-level analysis is broken down into change due to two components: (1) resources available compared with resources required, and (2) the number of procedures per patient. Component 1 is the department efficiency term. It is the result of management decisions and is, therefore, under the control of hospital administration. Component 2 is the procedure utilization term. It is the result of procedures ordered per patient and is, therefore, under the control of physicians.

The results of micro-costing analysis study, comparing the first to the second year, are shown in Table 7-6. Tables 7-4, 7-5, and 7-6 are actually the same except for the measure of resource utilization, which has been progressively refined in each table.

Table 7-6 indicates a 2.6 percent increase in the ratio of resources available for use to resources actually used to perform the procedures. This increase indicates that there has been an increase in the cost of utilizing the labor resources and a slight decrease in utilization of film entirely independent of changes in the unit cost of these resources. This indicates a decrease in departmental efficiency with respect to labor.

Changes in operating efficiency can have significant implications for the department head. A decrease in efficiency could denote carelessness in the use of films or staffing beyond the needs of the departmental services. On the other hand, a decrease in efficiency might be warranted, for example, when an increase in staffing results in a small cost increase

Table 7-6: Accounting for Resource/Procedure Use per Patient (1976 to 1977)*

Factor of Production	Technician V	Technician VI	Film	Total
Cost change due to:				
Cost/unit of input	$11,828	$3,745	$11,152	$26,725
	8.4%	3.6%	6.3%	6.3%
Ratio of resources available	$10,338	$1,626	($829)	$11,135
to resources needed	7.3%	1.5%	(0.5%)	2.6%
Number of procedures per	($6,962)	($9,611)	($5,881)	($22,454)
patient	(4.9%)	(9.1%)	(3.3%)	(5.3%)
Number of patients	($1,482)	($958)	($1,723)	($4,163)
	(1.1%)	(0.9%)	(1.0%)	(1.0%)
Total cost change	$13,722	($5,198)	$2,719	$11,243
	9.8%	(4.9%)	1.5%	2.7%

*Parentheses indicate negative quantities.

Source: Audrey L. Fetter, "Cost Measurement and Control in a Hospital Patient Service Department: A New Approach."

along with a substantial improvement in service quality. It is up to the department head to balance the benefits of change against cost.

The increase in resource utilization (2.6 percent) has been more than offset by a 6.3 percent reduction in the total cost of procedures actually performed. Only a portion of this decrease, 1 percent, is the result of fewer patients. This shows that physicians have ordered fewer tests per patient, resulting in a decreased cost per patient for diagnostic radiology procedures. At this point administrators may want to know specifically which procedures or physicians have produced this change.

The decrease in the utilization of diagnostic tests resulted in a total cost decrease of $22,454. Table 7-7 illustrates how those procedures, with a significant change in resource utilization from the previous period, have contributed to the overall reduction in resource costs. The decreased utilization of procedure 204000 (intravenous pyelogram), for example, has resulted in a dramatic decrease in the cost of film and technician salary. Comparing such data over several years will help indicate whether these variations reflect long-term changes in the patterns of diagnostic tests ordered by physicians or temporary aberrations.

The type of information found in Table 7-7 could be used by an administrator to establish communication with the medical staff regarding utilization. The physicians will be able to identify which changes are permanent and, possibly, determine reasons for the variations. This exchange of information will familiarize the medical staff with the effect of diagnostic decisions on hospital costs.

The staff may pose some questions, however, that at this point would be difficult or impossible to answer. Is it possible that the patients

Table 7-7: Procedures with >5% Cost Variance by Resource (1976 to 1977)*

Procedure	Technician V	Technician VI	Film	Total
208000	$ 00	$6,421	$3,277	$ 9,698
202110	1,448	00	1,622	3,070
203100	00	(752)	(394)	(1,146)
.	.	.	.	.
.	.	.	.	.
.	.	.	.	.
201000	(2,021)	00	(952)	(2,973)
204000	00	(12,794)	(6,529)	(19,323)
Total (13 procedures)	($6,962)	($9,611)	($5,880)	($22,454)

*Parentheses indicate negative quantities.

Source: Audrey L. Fetter, "Cost Measurement and Control in a Hospital Patient Service Department: A New Approach."

being treated during these two periods needed fewer tests? In other words, does the mix of cases treated in the last three years account for the decrease in the number of tests per patient? If the hospital is treating patients whose illnesses are less severe, then it would be expected that diagnostic procedures per patient would decrease. The case-mix influence, then, must be accounted for if a true evaluation of the variance in cost is to be made.

DRG Level

The DRG-level analysis accounts for case mix by analyzing patients in terms of DRGs, associating the procedures performed by the department with the DRGs utilizing those procedures. In this way, the demand for services placed on the department can be analyzed in terms of the relative number of patients in each DRG (the case mix) and the patterns of care received by those patients (DRG procedure utilization). The patterns of care may then be further analyzed in terms of the treatment pattern of individual physicians.

The case-study data thus far indicate an overall decrease in costs associated with a decrease in the density of procedures per patient. It has not been determined if some, or all, of this decrease is associated with a change in the mix of patients treated. Classification of patients into DRGs, based on resource utilization, makes it possible to isolate those changes in cost that were caused by changes in the mix of patients treated. It is then possible to compute variance through formulas (see Appendix 7-B) that express variance in terms of five contributing factors: the four factors listed earlier (factor costs, patient volume, departmental efficiency, and procedure utilization) and a fifth factor, case mix. The case-mix factor may be defined as the contribution to the total variation in costs due to changes in case mix, when costs, departmental efficiency, resource utilization, and patient volume are held at current-year levels (1976 in the present example).

Table 7-8 indicates that there has been a change to a less expensive mix of cases treated. Thus, the DRG-level analysis has shown that the decrease in the number of procedures performed per patient is not as significant as might have been inferred from the micro-costing-level analysis, which did not consider case mix.

The study hospital showed a significant shift to a less expensive case mix over the three-year period of the study. This shift, however, did not explain all of the decreased utilization of diagnostic procedures. Physicians also ordered fewer diagnostic procedures for their patients, thereby decreasing the operating costs of the department. The data allow a realistic evaluation of the effect of changes in physician utilization patterns on

Table 7-8: Accounting for Case Mix and DRG Procedure Utilization (1976 to 1977)*

Factor of Production	Technician V	Technician VI	Film	Total
Cost change due to:				
Cost/unit of input	$11,828	$ 3,745	$11,152	$26,725
Ratio of resources available to resources needed	10,338	1,626	(829)	(11,135)
Number of procedures per patient type	(5,803)	(8,614)	(4,969)	(19,386)
Case mix	(1,159)	(997)	(912)	(3,068)
Number of patients	(1,482)	(958)	(1,723)	(4,163)
Total cost change	$13,722	($5,198)	$ 2,719	$11,243

*Parentheses indicate negative quantities.
Source: Audrey L. Fetter, "Cost Measurement and Control in a Hospital Patient Service Department: A New Approach."

hospital costs and a determination of which DRGs were most affected by these changes.

The next step in the DRG-level analysis would depend on the purpose of the analysis. Reports can be generated that summarize cost changes from 1976 and from 1977 to 1978 by source of control (Tables 7-9 and 7-10). Most likely, administration will want to act upon the information in areas where it has control, either direct or indirect. This information will allow department heads to operate their departments with explicit targets for increased efficiency and procedure resource utilization. The chief executive officer, together with the marketing department, can discuss the implications of a significant change in the number of patients and formulate strategies accordingly.

As an example of what may prove to be a management concern, Tables 7-9 and 7-10 show two important factors that contributed to the changes from 1976 to 1978. First, costs for labor and film should actually have decreased over the three-year period because of changes in patient volume, case mix, and physicians' orders. Furthermore, film utilization improved, indicating additional savings. But, second, the utilization of labor, and especially technician VI labor, showed significant unfavorable cost changes. It appears that even though demand for procedures was dropping because of a combination of factors, labor costs were not decreasing commensurately. Furthermore, there was evidently a shift of available labor from technician V to technician VI (Promotions in lieu of wage raises?), resulting in an apparent shortage of the lower grade and a

Table 7-9: Source of Cost Changes (1976 to 1977)*

	Total Cost Change	Cost/Unit of Input	Units of Input/ Unit of Output	Outputs/ Patient Class	Case Mix	Volume
			Cost Change Due to:			
Technician V	$13,722	$11,828	$10,388	($5,803)	($1,159)	($1,482)
	9.8%	8.4%	7.3%	(4.1%)	(0.8%)	(1.1%)
Technician VI	($5,198)	$3,745	$1,626	($8,614)	($997)	($958)
	(4.9%)	3.8%	1.5%	(8.2%)	(0.9%)	(0.9%)
Film	$2,719	$11,512	($829)	($4,969)	($912)	($1,723)
	1.5%	6.3%	(0.5%)	(2.8%)	(0.5%)	(1.0%)
Total	$11,243	$26,725	$11,135	($19,386)	($3,068)	($4,163)
	2.7%	6.3%	2.6%	(4.6%)	(0.7%)	(1.0%)
Controlled by		Inflation/ Management	Management	Physicians	Planning and marketing physicians' services	

*Parentheses indicate negative quantities.
Source: Audrey L. Fetter, "Cost Measurement and Control in a Hospital Patient Service Department: A New Approach."

Table 7-10: Source of Cost Changes (1977 to 1978)*

	Total Cost Change	Cost/Unit of Input	Units of Input/ Unit of Output	Outputs/ Patient Class	Case Mix	Volume
			Cost Change Due to:			
Technician V	($19,529)	$12,573	($21,684)	($2,064)	($6,204)	($2,150)
	12.6%	8.1%	(14.0%)	(1.3%)	(4.0%)	(1.4%)
Technician VI	$42,285	$4,469	$55,938	($8,765)	($7,092)	($2,265)
	43.4%	4.5%	56.1%	(8.8%)	(7.1%)	(2.3%)
Film	($11,917)	$8,897	($7,544)	($3,159)	($7,418)	($2,673)
	6.6%	5.0%	(4.2%)	(1.8%)	(4.1%)	(1.5%)
Total	$10,839	$25,939	$26,710	($14,008)	($20,714)	($7,088)
	2.5%	6.0%	6.2%	(3.2%)	(4.8%)	(1.6%)
Controlled by		Inflation/ Management	Management	Physicians	Planning and marketing physicians' services	

*Parentheses indicate negative quantities.
Source: Audrey L. Fetter, "Cost Measurement and Control in a Hospital Patient Service Department: A New Approach."

very significant surplus of technician VI labor. This is clearly a management problem of some importance and needs to be understood. Without this kind of analysis, the 2.7 percent and 2.5 percent total cost increases recorded over the period might have been dismissed as inconsequential.

Some factors lie outside the control of administration, yet their implications are no less important. Inflation cannot be changed, but administrators must account for it and its effect on future prices. Case mix cannot be altered, but an analysis of changes in the distribution of cases among the DRGs over a period of time can significantly affect long-range planning. The physicians' utilization of procedures cannot be controlled by administration, but, with detailed information on procedure utilization, administrators can work together with physicians to control unnecessary costs.

Analysis of physician utilization can proceed in one of two ways, by DRG or by procedure. Table 7-11 presents an analysis of DRG cost variance (5 percent or more from previous period) due to changes in the utilization of procedures per patient. Analyzing changes in DRG costs can be essential in an environment of prospective payment, where reimbursement is set at a fixed rate regardless of cost.

The first DRG in the table, DRG 232 (arthroscopy), shows a significant cost increase. Identification of this variance makes it possible to search for causes of the cost increase by analyzing the procedures used in DRG 232 and the physicians who ordered them.

Table 7-11: DRGs with >5% Cost Variance Due to Change in Utilization of Procedures (1976 to 1977)*

DRG	Technician V	Technician VI	Film	Total
232	$ 346	$1,605	$ 1,096	$ 3,047
229	274	396	496	1,167
373	434	108	507	1,050
.	.	.	.	.
.	.	.	.	.
.	.	.	.	.
127	(565)	(239)	(765)	(1,570)
348	(722)	(309)	(539)	(1,570)
330	(812)	(419)	(757)	(1,988)
321	(883)	(342)	(1,077)	(2,302)
Total (16 DRGs)	($5,803)	($8,614)	($14,969)	($19,384)

*Parentheses indicate negative quantities.
Source: Audrey L. Fetter, "Cost Measurement and Control in a Hospital Patient Service Department: A New Approach."

Table 7-12: Procedures with >5% Cost Variance by Resource Accounting for Case Mix (1976 to 1977)*

Procedure	Technician V	Technician VI	Film	Total
208000	$ 00	$6,815	$3,478	$10,294
202110	1,094	00	1,226	2,320
.	.	.	.	.
.	.	.	.	.
.	.	.	.	.
207000	(612)	00	(303)	(916)
207400	(680)	00	(248)	(928)
.	.	.	.	.
.	.	.	.	.
.	.	.	.	.
201000	(1,741)	00	(820)	(2,561)
204000	00	(12,142)	(4,968)	(18,353)
Total (20 procedures)	($5,803)	($8,614)	($5,968)	($19,385)

*Parentheses indicate negative quantities.
Source: Audrey L. Fetter, "Cost Measurement and Control in a Hospital Patient Service Department: A New Approach."

Table 7-12 presents an analysis of the cost variance of specific procedures (5 percent or more from previous period) as a result of changes in the average number ordered per patient. Table 7-12 is similar to Table 7-7, the only difference being the exclusion of the case-mix factor (by eliminating the "case-mix term" in the equation of Appendix 7-B). Note that when the case-mix factor is excluded, procedure 208000 shows an even larger increase in utilization cost. This shows that the number of nephrotomographs with intravenous pyelogram increased by a greater amount than the severity of patient illness demanded; that is, the severity of patient illness demanded less utilization of this procedure than was apparent from the analysis at the departmental level. Analysis at the DRG level (that is, accounting for the effect of case mix on cost) has permitted a more accurate evaluation of the financial implications of the ordering practices of physicians.

The significant deviation in cost of procedure 208000 can be investigated further. Table 7-13 illustrates how the increased utilization of this procedure has increased the cost of several DRGs.

DRG 232 appears to be the DRG most obviously affected, in both DRG and procedure analysis. Altogether, 151 DRGs in the study had cost increases due to the increased utilization of procedure 208000, suggesting an increasing popularity for this procedure. Variance data from the fol-

Table 7-13: DRGs with >2% Cost Variance Due to Change in Utilization of Procedure 208000 (1976 to 1977)

DRG	Technician V	Technician VI	Film	Total
232	00	$434	$221	$656
333	00	325	166	491
242	00	182	93	274
11	00	101	92	273
8	00	178	91	269
210	00	174	89	263
48	00	160	81	241
328	00	141	72	213

Source: Audrey L. Fetter, "Cost Measurement and Control in a Hospital Patient Service Department: A New Approach."

lowing fiscal years will help indicate whether the growth in popularity was warranted and if it will continue.

Table 7-14 lists data from the following year, indicating whether the use of procedure 208000 has leveled off. The table suggests that this level of use is now fairly standard practice in three of the DRGs. However, five of the DRGs, which showed the largest cost increase due to the rise in utilization of procedure 208000, now show a decrease in cost almost equal to last year's increase. This decrease suggests that the level of use in fiscal year 1977 was unwarranted.

Such an observation, however, is unfair to make without the input of the medical staff. It is now possible to involve the medical staff in an analysis of the variance in costs over time. Given the opportunity to see

Table 7-14: Selected DRGs with Cost Variance Due to Change in Utilization of Procedure 208000 (1977 to 1978)*

DRG	Technician V	Technician VI	Film	Total
232	00	$ 371	$ 119	$ 490
333	00	(182)	(58)	(241)
242	00	(222)	(71)	(293)
11	00	353	133	466
8	00	(123)	(39)	(162)
210	00	(131)	(42)	(173)
48	00	(111)	(36)	(147)
328	00	220	60	290

*Parentheses indicate negative quantities.
Source: Audrey L. Fetter, "Cost Measurement and Control in a Hospital Patient Service Department: A New Approach."

what effect their diagnostic ordering patterns have on hospital patient costs, physicians will be able to judge their medical practices against costs. This introduces a means of forming a bridge between administrator and physician, enabling them to work together to contain those costs.

ADDITIONAL APPLICATIONS OF CASE-MIX ACCOUNTING AND PRODUCT-LINE MANAGEMENT

Product-line management and case-mix accounting can be extended to other areas of hospital production besides cost control: product selection and design, process selection, facility location, and quality control. Product-line selection will be discussed to exemplify the possibilities of analysis with a product-oriented focus.

In manufacturing companies, decisions on what goods to produce are based on the firm's primary task and areas of distinctive competence. Potential products are screened to eliminate those that are unworkable, that is, those that are incompatible with the firm's resources (managerial/ technical skills and physical facilities). Financial studies and marketing analyses are often performed as part of the screening.

Product selection in the hospital setting would also begin by defining a hospital's task and areas of distinctive competence. "Areas of distinctive competence" refers to the types of cases requiring services for which the medical staff have the skills and the hospital has the resources to provide. Screening a hospital's "products" or DRGs would include an evaluation of the following:

— Personnel skill available and required to provide high quality products
— Equipment available versus equipment required to deliver services
— Costs and revenues by DRG to determine where the hospital is competitive
— Needs of the population in the service area (through market studies)
— Physician specialties as a means of determining the kinds of services that are being provided and the needs of patients

One possible result of such a process might be an agreement among a small group of hospitals to specialize in certain services that require a particular level of expertise or a large additional capital investment, such as a burn unit or a neonatal unit. Each hospital could then "produce," in addition to general services, the DRGs for which it has particular competence.

Product-oriented management and accounting has important implications in light of the federal government's decision in October 1983 to pay hospitals a fixed rate per DRG for providing services to Medicare patients. This Prospective Payment System allows a hospital to keep the difference if the treatment of a patient costs less than the fixed DRG rate that is paid to the hospital by Medicare; if the hospital's costs for providing services exceed the rate, the hospital must absorb the loss. The system necessitates cost analysis. Hospitals have a clear incentive to minimize costs and maximize the efficiency and effectiveness of their services. Accurate information pertaining to the costs of treating different types of cases (DRGs) is becoming critical to a hospital's financial viability.

BARRIERS TO IMPLEMENTATION

There are several barriers to the implementation of case-mix accounting and product-line management. First, the time and effort involved in incorporating and learning this new approach are considerable. There is a tendency to put off change as long as possible.

Second, case-mix analysis may be viewed as a depersonalization of health care services. It represents one of the many factors in the changing image of the hospital, from shelter for the sick and needy to technical center for the acute and insured. To some opponents, the place for case-mix accounting is in business, not health care. Opponents argue that the sick must be treated as individuals, not as numbers—that is, the sick must be "cured," not given a DRG number and a "bundle of services." Aggregating patients into product lines is seen as too "technocratic," creating an assembly-line approach to health care and diminishing the physician's moral and ethical obligation to the patient.

The counterargument is that the "impersonal" information derived from case-mix analysis—percentages, averages, cost-to-charge ratios—can benefit the individual patient in a very personal way. Improved effectiveness and efficiency of a service benefits more than just the hospital; the individual patient who will receive and pay for that service also profits, directly or indirectly. A patient benefits from the higher level of accountability of those responsible for the patient's care. Also, the monitoring of patient care according to agreed-upon norms of practice results in a higher awareness of what is actually taking place in a hospital and, with it, a higher quality of care. Thus, with the appropriate use of case-mix analysis, both the hospital and the patient receive the ultimate benefits.

ENDNOTES

1. The department of diagnostic radiology was selected because (1) the direct cost for operating this department is a substantial proportion of the cost of operating the hospital, (2) radiologic procedures are performed over a wide range of DRGs, and (3) the rise in diagnostic procedures had a significant impact on hospital costs.
2. The multidimensional imaging services provided made it necessary to limit the scope of the project to the area of general radiography.
3. Four line items (salaries, film, medical-surgical supplies, and pharmaceutical) accounted for 87 percent or more of the combined budgets for the two cost centers in the study. Two levels of technicians (V and VI) were identified as the only personnel directly involved in administering tests in these two cost centers. The technician VI level requires more experience and has a higher salary range. Information was provided with the number of staff-minutes required for administering each test by both personnel classifications.

SELECTED BIBLIOGRAPHY

Berman, H. J., and Weeks, L. E. *The Financial Management of Hospitals.* Ann Arbor, MI: Health Administration Press, 1976.

Klarman, H. E. "Increase in the Cost of Physician and Hospital Services." *Inquiry* 8, no. 1 (1976): 22–36.

Levine, H. S. "A Small Problem in the Analysis of Growth." *Review of Economics and Statistics* 42 (1960): 225–28.

Shuman, L. J., et al. *Manual for Implementing Radiology Micro-Costing.* Systems Management Engineering and Operations Research, Department of Industrial Engineering, University of Pittsburgh, 1972.

Silvers, J. B., and Prahad, C. K. *Financial Management of Health Institutions.* Flushing, NY: Spectrum Publications Inc., 1974.

Thompson, J. D.; Averill, R. F.; and Fetter, R. B. "Planning, Budgeting and Controlling—One Look at the Future: Case-Mix Cost Accounting." *Health Services Research* 14, no. 2 (1974): 111–25.

APPENDIX 7-A:
MICRO-COSTING FORMULAS

Total departmental costs can be expressed as:

$$T = \sum_{ik} C_i F U_{ik} P_k \qquad \text{or} \qquad T = \sum_{ik} C_i F U_{ik} (P_k/N) N$$

where

U_{ik} = utilization of resource i in procedure k
P_k = number of procedures k
P_k/N = average number of procedures k per patient

The factor F is the ratio of the actual hospital resources available to the total resource requirements as predicted by the micro-costing study and can be expressed by:

$$F = U_i / \sum_k U_{ik} P_k$$

Variations in cost can now be expressed by the formulas:

$$\Delta C = \sum_{ik} \Delta C_i F U_{ik} (P_k/N) N \qquad \text{(Rate)}$$

$$+ \sum_{ik} C_i \Delta F U_{ik} (P_k/N) N \qquad \text{(Departmental Efficiency)}$$

$$+ \sum_{ik} C_i' F' \Delta U_{ik} (P_k/N) N \qquad \text{(Procedure Resource Utilization)}$$

$$+ \sum_{ik} C_i' F' U_{ik}' \Delta (P_k/N) N \qquad \text{(Procedure Utilization)}$$

$$+ \sum_{ik} C_i' F' U_{ik}' (P/N) \Delta N \qquad \text{(Patient Volume)}$$

APPENDIX 7-B:
DRG-COSTING FORMULAS

Total departmental costs can be expressed as:

$$T = \sum_{ikj} C_i F U_{ik} P_{kj} M_j N$$

where

$N =$ Number of patients in DRG j

$P_{kj} =$ Average number of procedures k performed per patient in DRG j

$M_j = N_j/N$

$\quad =$ fraction of patients in DRG j

Variations in cost can be expressed as:

$$\Delta T = \sum_{ikj} \Delta C_i F U_{ik} P_{kj} M_j N \qquad \text{(Rate)}$$

$$+ \sum_{ikj} C_i' \Delta F U_{ik} P_{kj} M_j N \qquad \text{(Departmental Efficiency)}$$

$$+ \sum_{ikj} C_i' F' \Delta U_{ik} P_{kj} M_j N \qquad \text{(Procedure Utilization)}$$

$$+ \sum_{ikj} C_i' F' U_{ik}' \Delta P_{kj} M_j N \qquad \text{(DRG Utilization)}$$

$$+ \sum_{ikj} C_i' F' U_{ik}' P_{kj}' \Delta M_j N \qquad \text{(Case-Mix Term)}$$

$$+ \sum_{ikj} C_i' F' U_{ik}' P_{kj}' M_j' \Delta N \qquad \text{(Patient Volume)}$$

Part III

Use of DRGs for Financing
Patient Care

8

Structure of a DRG-Based Prospective Payment System

Richard F. Averill and Michael J. Kalison

In April 1983 Congress enacted legislation to create the Medicare Prospective Payment System (PPS). PPS represented the most radical change in hospital payment methods since the creation of the Medicare system. Prior to PPS, Medicare paid hospitals under a cost-based system, essentially paying hospitals for whatever they spent. There were many reasons why major reforms in the cost-based Medicare hospital payment system were necessary.[1]

— Under cost-based payment, there were no incentives for hospitals to operate efficiently.

— During the three years prior to PPS Medicare payments to hospitals increased on average by 19 percent, which was nearly three times the average overall rate of inflation.

— The Medicare hospital deductible was increasing at a rate corresponding to the inflation in hospital expenditures, causing a burden on Medicare beneficiaries.

— Since the majority of Medicare expenditures were for hospital care, the rapid rate of increase in hospital costs was endangering the solvency of the Medicare Trust Fund.

— The funding of the expenditures for hospital inflation was jeopardizing the ability of Medicare to fund other needed health programs.

— Under cost-based payment, Medicare was paying up to sixfold differences across hospitals for comparable services.

— The reporting requirements of the cost-based system were some of the most burdensome in the federal government.

The primary approach to reform of the Medicare hospital payment system focused on establishing prospective payment rates for hospital payment. In 1972 Congress authorized the Health Care Financing Administration (HCFA) to institute state prospective-payment demonstration projects. In any prospective payment system, hospitals are provided with an explicit set of payment rates. In general, the payment rates have four essential characteristics:

1. The payment rates are established in advance and are fixed for the fiscal period to which they apply.

2. The payment rates are not automatically determined by the hospital's past or current actual cost.

3. The prospective payment rates are payment in full.

4. The hospital retains the profit or suffers a loss resulting from the difference between the payment rate and the hospital cost.

Thus, the payment rate received by a hospital will remain unchanged regardless of the hospital's overall cost experience. This risk generates a strong financial incentive for hospitals to control costs.

Between 1972 and 1983, numerous alternative forms of prospective payment systems were implemented by states as demonstration projects. During this period Connecticut, Maryland, Massachusetts, New Jersey, New York, Rhode Island, Washington, and Wisconsin implemented prospective payment systems. As a result of these demonstration projects, several general conclusions were reached:[2]

— Prospectivity itself was effective in reducing the rate of increase in hospital costs.

— All state systems required consideration of hospital case mix.

— Failure to adequately address the case-mix issue results in an active appeals process.

— Small rural hospitals frequently required special exceptions unless case mix was explicitly recognized in the payment system.

— Prospective payment rates were established through use of actual hospital costs for a base year.

— Successful systems had a firm legal basis and strict enforcement, and could not be manipulated by the hospitals.

— Individual hospital budget review systems were often managed by exception and were complex to administer.

— All systems had some inherent undesirable incentives that required the insertion of countermeasures.

The results of the demonstration projects were very positive. They demonstrated that there were alternatives to cost-based hospital reimbursement that were feasible for implementation and could contain hospital costs.

HCFA established specific goals for Medicare payment system reform on the basis of this experience with a cost-based system and with the demonstration sites. As different system designs were considered, certain criteria were used to evaluate the alternatives.[3] A satisfactory system had to:

— be easy to understand and simple to administer

— be capable of being implemented in the near future

— ensure predictability of government outlays

— help hospitals gain predictability of their Medicare revenues

— establish the federal government as a prudent buyer of services

— assure that Medicare expenditures for inpatient hospital services were no greater than those that would have been incurred if the system of retrospective cost reimbursement had been continued

— provide incentives for hospital management, flexibility, innovation, planning, and control

— reduce the cost-reporting burden on hospitals

— continue to assure beneficiary access to quality care

— prohibit hospitals from charging beneficiaries anything for services other than statutorily defined coinsurance and deductibles

Under these criteria, the system selected as the basis for the Medicare PPS was patterned after the New Jersey demonstration project. The unit of payment was established as the case. Predetermined payment rates were established for patients in each DRG. The rates were considered payment in full and were not negotiable. The DRG payment rates were based on actual cost from a base year, and were trended forward by a hospital market-basket price index.

The basic concept of prospective DRG rates seems extremely simple. However, numerous individual design components of a DRG prospective payment system can significantly affect the incentives and effectiveness of the system. Indeed, while both Medicare and the state of New Jersey pay hospitals on the basis of prospective DRG rates, the two systems are quite different in many aspects of actual implementation. This chapter will examine each design component of a DRG-based prospective payment system, and the actual alternatives implemented by Medicare and the state of New Jersey will be compared. In addition, the expansion of prospective payment systems to include price flexibility, physician payment, severity of illness, and quality of care will be discussed. The chapter will conclude with some policy recommendations regarding future directions of prospective payment systems.

DESIGN OF A DRG-BASED PROSPECTIVE
PAYMENT SYSTEM

All-Payer versus Individual-Payer

The premise underlying any prospective system is that hospitals will respond to the financial incentives inherent in the system and begin to deliver care more cost-effectively. With hospital care delivered in a more cost-effective manner, lower hospital costs can be achieved without reducing the quality of care.

To realize such cost reductions, the incentives must be communicated to the medical community. Physicians control the utilization of the vast majority of hospital resources and, therefore, are critical to any effort at cost control. However, if the incentives for cost control exist only for a single payer, and hospitals continue to be financially rewarded by other payers for using more bed days and ancillary services, then the development of an integrated cost-control strategy by an individual hospital will be extremely difficult. A hospital cannot expect its physicians to behave differently for different payers. Unless the incentives are uniform across payers, a hospital will have difficulty determining and implementing a strategy to respond to the incentives.

If diverse payment practices exist among payers, there will undoubtedly be opportunities for manipulating the payment system. With a focus on gamesmanship, hospitals will look to accountants and lawyers to respond to the payment environment rather than to improved management systems and improved utilization practices by their medical staffs. Failure to establish DRG payment rates across all payers could jeopardize the success of the system, not because prospective rates by DRG are not an effective payment framework, but because the incentives in the system are confused and, therefore, are difficult to communicate to the hospital and medical communities.

Perhaps the most fundamental difference between the Medicare and New Jersey systems is that in New Jersey the DRG rates apply to all payers (including Medicare), whereas in the Medicare system the DRG rates apply only to Medicare patients. While an all-payer system presents a more uniform set of incentives to hospitals, it also places more responsibilities on the payers. Since in an all-payer system virtually all sources of revenue are controlled by the DRG payment rates, there is a greater obligation on the part of the payers to insure that the DRG payment amounts are both adequate and fair.

Regulation versus Contract: The Fundamental Difference

In addition to the all-payer distinction, the New Jersey and Medicare DRG prospective payment systems differ in the basic nature of their relationship with the hospitals. The New Jersey system is a regulatory system with certain legal obligations to hospitals. The Medicare system is basically a contractual relationship between Medicare and each hospital in which either party has the option to terminate the contract.

New Jersey state legislation obliges the state "to provide for the financial solvency of a hospital which is properly utilized and which delivers, effectively and efficiently, appropriate and necessary health care services of a high quality required by its mix of patients."[4] Since in the New Jersey system all payers are covered, so are costs such as bad debts, which are considered a legitimate cost of doing business. It is simply an obligation that payers are not free to ignore under a closed system where the failure to recognize such costs would cause system leakage and, ultimately, bankruptcy.

On the other hand, state regulation is not considered insurance against bad decisions. Similarly, regulation does not provide protection against losses in volume. Only services that the public continues to need remain covered by the legal framework. Taken as a whole, however, the system does create a relationship between performance and bottom line. From a hospital point of view, having discharged their obligation to perform efficiently, the regulated hospitals obtain an affirmative legal right to be treated fairly.

The relationship of Medicare to the hospital community is founded on a contract, that is, a provider agreement. Thus, for example, if Medicare is thought of as an insurance company run for the benefit of the elderly, it is not surprising that the only payment made for costs such as uncompensated care is for those bad debts attributable to deductibles and coinsurance that are related to covered services consumed by its beneficiaries; or that the program has claimed the right to restrict its payment for malpractice premium expense to only that portion of paid malpractice losses attributable to its beneficiaries.[5] Under a contractual theory there need be no relationship whatsoever between superior operational performance and bottom line success. Naturally, certain providers will profit handsomely under this kind of freedom.

By viewing itself as an insurance company merely representing its beneficiaries (the elderly and the poor), government also frees itself from certain affirmative regulatory burdens, thus obtaining the freedom to act in its own economic interest. Consider, for example, Medicare acting as a preferred provider organization, making the national price per DRG a maximum, and awarding volume in exchange for discounts.

There are, of course, limitations to the contract-versus-regulation dichotomy. For example, Medicare is not free to act in a totally arbitrary manner. Moreover, because of its size and influence in the marketplace, it is unlikely that Medicare would be permitted total freedom to drive bargains. The contract-versus-regulation distinction has had a fundamental influence on the manner in which New Jersey and Medicare have implemented their respective DRG prospective payment systems and is an important concept to understand when evaluating evolution of both systems.

Financial Elements and Adjustment Factors

The computation of the DRG payment amount can differ significantly depending on the financial elements included in the DRG rate and the adjustment factors incorporated into the calculation.

Uncompensated Care. Medicare does not recognize the hospital costs associated with uncompensated care. Thus, the Medicare DRG payment rates do not include any provision for payments towards the hospital's cost of indigent care. In the New Jersey system medical indigence and bad debts, less any offsetting grants, are apportioned to the DRG payment rates of a hospital, provided that the hospital enforces adequate collection practices. Since medical indigence is viewed as a statewide problem and not an individual hospital problem, these costs are allocated among all the payers, including Medicare. More recently, the state has implemented an uncompensated-care trust fund.

Working Capital. Medicare does not recognize the hospital costs associated with having sufficient working capital available. In the New Jersey system, hospitals in financial difficulty at the start of the system were given a one-time working cash infusion. On an ongoing basis, hospital DRG rates include an allowance for working capital. Payers who provide prompt payment receive a discount from the established DRG payment rates.

Fixed/Variable Costs. In the Medicare system, all costs with the exception of capital and direct medical education costs are considered variable and included in the DRG rates. In the New Jersey system, the reimbursement rate is separated into fixed and variable components. Costs related to patient care, such as nursing and laboratory costs and the cost of major movable equipment, are considered variable and are reimbursed by the DRG. Costs not related to patient care, such as general administration and malpractice insurance, are considered fixed costs and are reimbursed on a lump-sum basis after review through a peer group comparison. In the New Jersey system approximately one-third of the costs are considered fixed and two-thirds are considered variable.

Volume Variability. In the Medicare system, there is full volume variability. Hospital revenue will increase or decrease without limit depending on changes in patient volume. The New Jersey system includes an adjustment designed to moderate the full effect of changes in patient volume on patient revenue.

Equalization of Labor Costs. Both the Medicare and the New Jersey systems recognize that labor costs can vary significantly by geographic region. Both systems adjust the DRG payment amounts for the relative cost of labor in the hospital's labor market.

Effects of Teaching Programs. Hospitals with medical education programs tend to incur higher patient care costs. These higher costs are primarily the result of the performance of additional testing and procedures as part of teaching. In addition, the presence of interns and residents tends to place additional demands on hospital staff, demands that lead to higher staffing levels. Both the Medicare and the New Jersey systems recognize the indirect costs associated with teaching programs. Medicare provides a percentage add-on to the DRG rates based on the size of a hospital's teaching program. The New Jersey system computes the standard DRG payment amounts for three separate peer groups of hospitals corresponding to major teaching, minor teaching, and nonteaching hospitals.

Inflation Update Factor. In both the Medicare and the New Jersey system, the standard base DRG payment rates are updated annually for the effect of inflation on hospital costs. Since the inception of the Medicare Prospective Payment System, the inflation update factor has been primarily a politically established number intended to achieve specific budgetary results. Thus, the Medicare update factor has not reflected actual hospital inflation. The rationale behind providing less than actual hospital inflation is that the original base DRG payment amounts reflected hospital actual cost after decades of cost-based payment. Therefore, the original base rates were established too high, with the result that hospitals made high profits in the initial years of the Medicare Prospective Payment System. Further, as hospitals improved the accuracy of their medical records coding, higher DRG payments were paid to hospitals as a result of more accurate DRG assignment.

Outliers. Outliers are atypical patients who can be assigned to a DRG but have an extremely high or an extremely low cost or length of stay relative to most patients in the same DRG. Such atypical patients can be very expensive to treat and must be recognized as exceptions in the calculation of the DRG payment amounts. Failure to provide additional payments for high-cost outliers would have several undesired consequences. Hospitals would have to absorb large losses when treating outlier cases. If a small hospital encountered several outlier cases, its financial viability could be threatened. If hospitals were able to identify, prior to admission, the cases that were likely to become outliers, there would be incentive for hospitals to refuse to admit these patients. The Medicare system recognizes only high-cost and length-of-stay outliers and provides additional per diem payments to hospitals for patients exceeding the outlier threshold. Approximately 2 percent of Medicare patients are considered outliers. The New Jersey system has both high and low outliers. The outlier thresholds in New Jersey are much more restrictive than those in Medicare; approximately 35 percent of the patients in New Jersey are classified as outliers. Low outliers are paid on a per diem basis and high outliers have an additional per diem payment added to the DRG case payment amount. Since New Jersey has an all-payer system, the high percentage of outliers is, in part, a reaction to the need to protect self-pay patients from paying DRG amounts that are significantly higher than the actual hospital charges.

The description of financial elements and adjustment factors in the New Jersey prospective payment system is based on the implementation of the system between 1980 and 1988. Because New Jersey was the first DRG prospective payment system, many of the features of the system were implemented to protect hospitals from the unknown impact of the transition from cost-based to prospective payment. In fiscal year 1989 the state of New Jersey planned significant modifications of the payment system that were to include the elimination of the fixed/variable and volume-variability methodology.

Capital Cost and the Role of Regional Planning

Both the Medicare and New Jersey prospective payment systems exclude the cost of capital from the prospective DRG rates. Capital-related costs are reimbursed under both systems on a reasonable-cost basis. A cost-based approach to capital reimbursement creates many undesirable incentives:

— Capital payments are linked directly to facilities used to deliver patient care. Accordingly, hospitals may be reluctant to close down underutilized parts of facilities because under the current payment scheme, such closure would result in the forfeiture of depreciation and interest payments. Because payment is based on cost, there is no incentive for hospital management to control the underlying cost of the project.

— Because hospitals are paid for borrowed funds at prevailing interest rates, there is no incentive to select the most economically appropriate financial mix (debt/equity), or to delay borrowing at times of exceptionally high interest rates, a phenomenon not applicable to most other industries.

— During the early years of debt financing, depreciation often exceeds principal, thus providing a cash cushion. These "excess" funds can be used to subsidize management inefficiency. As the financing matures, the balance between depreciation and interest may shift, creating an incentive to refinance debt.

Continuing the cost pass-through policy as applied to capital contradicts the economic incentives that would otherwise apply were capital costs included within the prospective DRG payment framework. Indeed, a perverse incentive is created to substitute capital for labor, whether or not appropriate.

The economic impact of continuing to treat capital in a manner inconsistent with the treatment of other inputs is not harmless. For example, the New Jersey prospective payment system, with its capital pass-through, was proposed and enacted into law in 1979. Between 1974 and 1981, while prospective payment was beginning to exert pressure on noncapital expenditures, the New Jersey health planning system approved $1.5 billion in capital expenditures (per capita, more than all but three states).[6]

The surge in capital spending in New Jersey furnishes a particularly disturbing example of the power of perverse financial incentives. Since the implementation of prospective payment for operating costs, the New Jersey hospital system went from undercapacity to overcapacity as a result of a decline in occupancy of approximately 20 percent. Yet, despite the drop in demand, the capital pass-through created an unintended incentive for hospitals to increase and maximize capital spending. The experience in New Jersey suggests that the failure to include capital in the prospective payment framework can produce potentially unnecessary capital investment in spite of declining utilization resulting from prospective payment for operating costs and comprehensive centralized planning.

Removing the artificial distinction between capital and noncapital inputs will make the rate structure more internally consistent, thereby encouraging hospital managers to consider the full range of potential operational trade-offs. Incorporating the capital component into prospectively determined rates will also give hospitals the incentive to make capital investment decisions that are more sensitive to real market conditions, such as deferring new construction when interest rates are high, substituting more cost-effective alternatives such as modernization, or eliminating unneeded projects altogether. Perhaps most importantly, linking capital to real volume creates the financial preconditions for eliminating unneeded or inefficient facilities. Within a financial environment marked by "scarce resources," devoting capital resources to unneeded or inefficient facilities can only compromise the financial health of the facilities that are needed and efficient. Conversely, promoting the financial health of needed and efficient facilities will occur naturally under a prospective capital payment system sensitive to both volume and patient case mix.

There are various methods for adding capital to prospectively determined rates, including a fixed amount or fixed percentage add-on.[7,8] The net effect of adding a fixed percentage to each DRG would be to increase every hospital's total DRG payments by the selected percentage. However, a patient undergoing coronary bypass surgery cannot be expected to require the same kinds and amounts of resources (including capital resources) as a patient facing an uncomplicated appendectomy. A refinement of the DRG add-on approach would treat capital on a DRG-specific basis (cost-based pricing), which would return to the hospital the appropriate amount of capital for each kind of case it treats. As a result, the total DRG payment for each hospital would be increased by different amounts depending on each facility's case mix. This approach recognizes that hospitals have different overall capital requirements because of case-mix variations.

Including capital in the prospective DRG rates will send an important message to providers at the decision-making level. On the assumption that capital costs are properly allocated, the correct amount of capital will be returned to each provider, given its own case mix. As providers study the various components that make up each DRG rate, they can be expected to respond to the demands of real volume and case mix. Thus, a successful service that the public demands will generate, over time, the amount of capital resources necessary to replicate that service, while an unsuccessful service will be naturally terminated. Since quality tends to vary with volume, the increased specialization promoted by more precise capital allocation should result in improved patient care. Although exceptions will always be required to deal with situations such as "sole community provider," where market forces are unable to produce the desired result, in the general environment prospective capital payment will reward hospital management that prudently manages capital resources. In the end, it will increase sensitivity to real demand, encourage hospitals to specialize in whatever they do best, and sensitize management to the same kinds of market considerations that the rest of American industry has always been obliged to respect.

With capital payments incorporated into the prospective DRG rates the role of planning would be significantly altered. In the environment of cost-based reimbursement, health planning agencies were developed as a "gatekeeping" device, a last line of defense before Medicare assumed its commitment. Under this financial framework, health planning agencies focused primarily on new capital investment. A variety of statistics were examined, including bed counts, length of stay, projected occupancy, projected cost, and so forth. Although well-intended, in reality the planning process sometimes diverted hospital management away from consideration of the impact of real market forces. Considerable energy was often devoted to finding and developing the set of projections that would favorably influence the planning agency.

With capital incorporated into the prospective DRG rates, planning agencies will no longer need to monitor investment in equipment. Since equipment will be incorporated into the rate per case, there are natural incentives for management to behave in a prudent business fashion. Planning agencies will also no longer need to monitor investment in plant. If the capital pass-through is eliminated, cautious market forces will automatically temper the overoptimism that supports unrealistic volume projections, even if management acts imprudently. Rather than duplicate these financial incentives, thereby fostering potentially inconsistent investment results, planning agencies should seek to fully understand the imperatives of prospective payment, to let the natural incentives work without interference, and to complement the financial framework. For example, such agencies might collect information regionally in order to assist the public, hospital management, and the financial markets in making proper decisions. Even though theoretical, a periodic inventory of the plans of all of the providers in a region might be helpful in assessing new investment.

A residual role for planning agencies involves assuring "access." As providers make investment decisions in a manner consistent with the financial incentives of prospective payment, some areas, such as inner

cities, may be left underserved. Such changes must be carefully monitored and attention focused on these problems. Nevertheless, simply
defining "access" as a planning issue would leave these agencies vulnerable to the same charge of ineffectiveness that was directed at them
previously. Access is essentially a financing problem; if the money is
there, the care will be provided. Thus, the main objective of the planning
agency would be refocused on developing those data sets that are most
helpful, and providing this information to financing sources in a timely
way. In general, planning agencies should avoid intervening where prospective payment provides natural financial incentives. Rather, planning
agencies should seek to complement prospective payment by developing
information helpful to the public, the industry, and the financial markets,
and by focusing on those areas, such as deteriorating access, where
prospective payment provides no incentive safeguards.

Appeals

The regulatory process is distributed between rules and exceptions. As a
general statement, rules (such as the inflation adjustment) are more efficient because they operate automatically. However, no regulatory system
has yet been invented that operates totally without the need for human
intervention and, in this regard, appeals processes are necessary. In both
the New Jersey and Medicare systems, independent appeals commissions
that are generally guided by principles of administrative law have been
established. The Medicare system has two commissions, the Provider
Reimbursement Review Board (PRRB) and the Prospective Payment Assessment Commission (ProPAC). The PRRB has general jurisdiction over
appeals by hospitals arising under PPS. In the Medicare system, there are
certain restrictions on what can be heard by the courts should an appeal
from an adverse decision be taken. For example, there is no administrative or judicial review of "the establishment of diagnosis-related groups,
of the methodology for the classification of discharges, within such
groups, and of the appropriate weighting factors thereof...."[9] Once
national DRG rates are established and hospital-specific costs are removed from the rate-setting equation, the significance of the types of
appeals traditionally heard by the PRRB is unclear. On the other hand, the
issues related to medical practice and technology that ProPAC must
evaluate will probably increase in importance. However, the decisions of
ProPAC are only recommendations and are not binding on Medicare.
Thus, under the Medicare system, the opportunity for an individual
hospital to appeal its payment is extremely limited.
    In the New Jersey system, there is the Hospital Rate Setting Com-
mission (HRSC), whose responsibilities include evaluating hospital-

specific rate appeals. For example, DRG appeals are designed to address "[a]ny issue concerning differences in an institutional course of action or in patterns of medical practice, affecting a Diagnosis Related Group or group of Diagnosis Related Groups, which is likely to affect one or more institutions."[10] As an example of this general class of appeals, a New Jersey hospital appealed to the HRSC for consideration of the costs associated with a new piece of advanced diagnostic equipment, a Dyna Camera.[11] As physicians utilized the technology over a period of time, they were able to increase the level of diagnostic certainty that could be obtained in a certain percentage of cases. By relating the equipment to DRGs the hospital and its physicians were able to detect a gradual shift from surgical to nonsurgical management as physicians were able to avoid exploratory surgery in certain instances. Since nonsurgical treatment is less risky and generally less costly than surgical treatment in the relevant group of cases, the demonstration persuaded the HRSC to provide additional funds to the hospital. As another example of this type of appeal, a hospital observed that in the DRG for strokes, the hospital's length of stay was shorter but its costs were higher than the statewide standard.[12] Virtually all of the excess cost was caused by the incremental expense involved in running a special stroke program. The special stroke program not only provided higher quality of care but also gave two additional economic benefits to the health care system: shortened length of stay, which freed up capacity; and fewer subsequent readmissions, which lowered overall system cost.

Thus, the New Jersey system provides for appeals by individual hospitals relative to the payment amounts of individual DRGs, whereas the Medicare system provides virtually no options for such appeals.

Phase-in of the DRG Rates

The establishment of a single DRG rate across all hospitals would cause major shifts in the aggregate payment levels of many hospitals.[13] This result should not be surprising. After years of cost-based reimbursement, the relative performance of hospitals varies significantly. In light of such variation, hospitals must be given the opportunity to adapt to a prospective payment system.

A phase-in process of the DRG payment rates is necessary not only to reduce the chance of an individual hospital's experiencing extreme profits or losses during the initial years of the system, but also to place an emphasis on financial rewards for improved productivity. With a single DRG rate across hospitals, some hospitals would receive a large amount of additional revenue in the initial year, not because they responded to the prospective incentives and improved productivity, but because the initial standard included hospitals whose performance under cost-based reimbursement resulted in relatively high costs. The hospitals receiving significant additional revenue would have little motivation to seek new productivity.

While it is reasonable to reward historical efficiency in the initial year, this reward should not be excessive. A phase-in period provides the historically efficient hospital with only a modest reward in the initial year unless it achieves additional productivity gains. Conversely, a phase-in process moderates the financial penalties for the historically less efficient hospitals. This condition allows time for the less efficient hospital to concentrate on improving productivity without having to contend with a major financial crisis.

The change to an incentive-based prospective payment system represents a major change in the way hospitals have to be managed. Such a change requires a reasonable period of time. The ultimate standard rate by DRG should reflect hospital performance after hospitals have had the opportunity to mature under the system. A phase-in of the DRG standard provides that opportunity.

Medicare developed a four year phase-in of the DRG payment rates. During the phase-in period, Medicare payments to hospitals were determined by a combination of national and regional DRG rates and hospital-specific actual costs. The percentage of hospital payment derived from the DRG rate portion increases in each successive year of the phase-in. At the end of the phase-in, except for adjustments such as wage indices and teaching status, every hospital will receive from Medicare the same payment for each DRG. Thus, Medicare at the end of the phase-in will have, in essence, established a single national set of DRG payment rates.

The basic philosophical argument for a national DRG rate is that the average price per case in each DRG should be the same across hospitals. A national DRG rate would provide a uniform standard set of payments across all hospitals. Thus, at least in theory, each hospital would have an equal opportunity to earn and retain a profit. Efficient hospitals would be able to achieve the maximum reward commensurate with their actual level of performance. Inefficient hospitals would be penalized to a degree commensurate with their performance, thereby supplying the funds required to reward the efficient. National DRG rates would serve a key judicial axiom, namely, that the public should not be obliged to subsidize inefficiency.

Conversely, failure to move to a national rate would permanently deprive hospitals with superior performance of the profits they are entitled to and would continue to subsidize the inefficient. What is perhaps most important, the failure to reward the efficient fully could ultimately destroy the motivation of all providers to improve.

Three basic arguments are used against the implementation of national DRG rates:

— Hospitals should not be held accountable for costs that are legitimately beyond their control.

— Costs per case within some DRGs vary substantially.

— The public good is best served when hospitals focus on improving their own relative performance.

Each of these arguments must be given serious consideration before a national set of DRG rates is adopted. During the initial years of the phase-in, the hospital's-actual-cost portion of hospital payment helped account for hospital cost differences related to location that were largely beyond the control of individual institutions. Such differences include unemployment rates, regional market-basket prices, population density, indigent caseload, scope of services, utility costs, transportation costs, and the need to maintain access to care.

Failure to give proper consideration to costs legitimately beyond the control of the provider would be "arbitrary." In enacting PPS, Congress directed HCFA not to ignore many of the uncontrollable factors noted above. The establishment of a single set of national rates would intensify the need to evaluate and adjust for such factors, probably on an individual basis. However, even if such potential adjustments are adequate, the more adjustments that are added to a prospective payment system, the more difficult it will be to manage and understand. At a minimum, the effort of evaluating, constructing, and updating such adjustments would require a substantial effort by Medicare, in addition to increasing the complexity of PPS.

Patients in each DRG should experience similar costs. "Similar costs" means that the costs incurred are relatively consistent across patients in each DRG. Nevertheless, some variation in cost will exist among patients. In other words, the definition of each DRG is not so specific that every patient is identical, but rather that the level of variation is known and predictable. While the precise cost of a particular patient cannot be predicted by knowing the DRG, the average cost of a group of patients in a DRG can be predicted accurately. Thus, the cost or payment amount for a DRG represents a statistical average with a certain level of inherent variability.

The degree of variability in cost within a DRG differs across the individual DRGs. DRGs that represent patients with well-established treatment protocols, such as tonsillectomy patients, display very low levels of variability in the cost per patient. On the other hand, DRGs that represent patients for whom the treatment protocol is not well established, such as patients with inflammatory bowel disease, display high levels of variability in the cost per patient. In essence, the variability in the cost per patient reflects the clinical consensus or lack of consensus on the treatment protocol for the patients in each DRG. For example, surgical patients consistently exhibit a lower variability in the cost per patient than medical patients. This lower variability reflects the fact that the decision to perform surgery defines the treatment protocol relatively precisely. Thus, the confidence with which national DRG rates can be established varies across DRGs.

Cost variations within DRGs across regions can arise when location factors produce different local inpatient prices, for example, or can result from differences in medical practice patterns. Practice patterns vary substantially across the regions of the country. For example, patients in the same DRG may have very different average lengths of stay in different areas. Such differences raise the basic question of whether practice-pattern differences are a legitimate reason for providing different levels of payment to hospitals. The answer to this question will likely vary depending on the DRG involved.

For an uncomplicated appendectomy or cataract extraction, one may assert with a high degree of confidence that any regional differences in practice patterns are not legitimate reasons to provide different levels of payment. However, for patients with myeloproliferative diseases or metabolic disorders, the confidence that practice-pattern differences are not legitimate is not as high. As a basic rule, great care must be taken before driving diverse practice patterns to a standard course of treatment through the payment mechanism.

One of the arguments for a single national DRG rate was that the public should not be obliged to subsidize inefficient hospitals, and efficient hospitals should be given the maximum rewards consistent with their own levels of performance. It can also be argued that the public good is better served by encouraging each individual hospital to improve on its own relative performance than by imposing a single national DRG rate. Establishing prospective rates that reflect at least a portion of the local, historical norm places the emphasis on encouraging regional, area-wide hospital improvement. As each institution implements positive change relative to its past performance, the overall effectiveness of the hospital system is improved.

A single national DRG rate would shift money among hospitals, causing a potentially unmanageable financial crisis to the inefficient while at the same time furnishing excess dollars to the efficient who, because of their superior performance, probably have the least need for the additional payment. Providing additional money to an efficient hospital for merely maintaining the status quo may leave the hospital with no motivation to increase efficiency. On the other hand, the financial pressure on an inefficient hospital can improve the quality of care and services. The effect on patients treated in hospitals experiencing financial difficulties must be closely monitored.

In recognition of the arguments against a single set of DRG rates, the state of New Jersey did not establish a phase-in that would lead to a single set of statewide DRG rates. Instead, the New Jersey system relies on a blending of the average statewide cost in a DRG and the individual hospital's actual cost in the DRG. The basis for the blending is the coefficient of variation (CV) of the statewide per case cost distribution for each DRG. The CV is computed by dividing the standard deviation of the per case cost distribution in a DRG by the mean cost in that DRG. DRGs in which a high proportion of patients have costs close to the average have a low CV; DRGs in which a substantial proportion of patients have costs that differ significantly from the average have a high CV.

The basic formula for determining a hospital's payment rate for a DRG would be to multiply the hospital's actual cost in a DRG by the CV, and to add that product to the product of the state DRG rate and (1 − CV). For example, consider the two DRGs shown in Table 8-1.

The payment for DRG A would be computed as (0.8 × $1500) + (0.2 × $1000), resulting in a payment of $1400. The use of the CV provides an objective means of phasing in a statewide rate by DRG. The CV has the property that as diverse practice patterns move toward a standard course of treatment and more hospitals move toward an optimal level of operating efficiency, the CVs will automatically become lower, and more of the statewide DRG rates will be used in determining hospital payment rates. Thus, the CV provides a natural means of moving toward a single statewide DRG rate. Further, as DRGs are improved by including factors such as patient severity, the CV will continue to decrease. Practically, New Jersey will never move to a single statewide rate, since the CV will never become zero. Thus, Medicare and New Jersey have taken very different approaches to the phase-in of the DRGs. Medicare moves to single national rate over a defined period of time and New Jersey maintains some diminishing recognition of hospitals' actual costs.

EXPANSION OF PROSPECTIVE PAYMENT SYSTEMS

Price Flexibility

Both Medicare and the New Jersey system provide virtually no price flexibility. In the New Jersey system a payer can request a discount on the DRG rates. Such a discount is allowed only if the payer can demonstrate

Table 8-1: Computation of a Hospital's Payment Rate for Two Hypothetical DRGs

DRG	Coefficient of Variation	Hospital Cost	State Rate	Computation	Hospital Payment
A	0.8	$1,500	$1,000	(0.8 × $1,500) + (0.2 × $1,000)	$1,400
B	0.4	$2,500	$2,000	(0.4 × $2,500) + (0.6 × $2,000)	$2,200

that its payment practices result in quantifiable economic benefits that directly result in a lower cost of providing care (for example, prompt-payment practices that lower the hospital's cost of working capital). However, in both systems, hospitals must accept the PPS payment amounts as payment in full. A hospital may neither increase nor decrease the PPS payment amounts. Thus, price has been removed as a consideration in the consumer (patient) decision-making process.

The practical effect of this policy is to eliminate opportunities for price competition.[14,15] Prior to DRGs meaningful price competition was simply not possible because pricing information was incomprehensible to the consumer. However, the DRG payment rates provide consumers with a basis for price comparison.

The availability of a DRG price list, coupled with excess hospital capacity and increased cost awareness on the part of consumers, has created the conditions necessary to have a real competitive market in the hospital industry. Maintaining a centrally determined set of DRG prices without any price flexibility will inevitably create artificial incentives. Some hospitals will continue to provide specific types of services longer than the market would have allowed, while at the same time other hospitals will be denied the opportunity to use price discounts as a means of attracting additional patients. Since real changes in the health care system usually result from shifts in patient volume, it is important to allow price competition in a prospective payment system in order to induce shifts in patient volume. In general, administrative judgment should be substituted for the market only when the market fails to function.

Price flexibility can provide significant financial benefits to patients. Although the DRG payment amounts are accepted by hospitals as payment in full, the patient can still have significant liability. For example, in fiscal year 1988, Medicare beneficiaries had to pay a deductible of $534 plus a daily coinsurance for hospital stays that exceeded 60 days. The availability of price flexibility should result in a reduction in beneficiaries' out-of-pocket expenses. Moreover, if patients were attracted to hospitals with high-volume programs, an additional benefit should result. Studies have demonstrated that quality of care improved with volume. Thus, patients attracted to high-volume programs by price discounts may also be receiving a higher quality of care.

The availability of direct financial benefits to the patient is a critical element of an effective competitive framework. Without direct financial incentives, the patient would have no motivation to select one hospital over another. A fundamental assumption of any competitive proposal is that a significant number of patients will behave as informed consumers and will select hospitals based on price (that is, the out-of-pocket expense to the patient).

Under a more flexible system hospitals would be allowed to discount the standard DRG prices for specific DRGs, or across all DRGs. Such discounts would not be limited to the amount of the patient's deductible. At the beginning of each fiscal year, hospitals would submit their DRG-specific discount schedules. The discount schedule would remain in effect for the entire fiscal year. In subsequent fiscal years, a hospital would be able to increase or decrease its discounts or eliminate them entirely. The provision of discounts would be at the hospital's discretion, and no hospital would be required to provide a discount. Hospitals willing to trade price for volume would have a greater opportunity to attract patients by offering substantial discounts as part of their marketing strategy. With excess capacity and the economies of scale that result from increased volume, such a discount strategy could result in a significant improvement in the financial performance of a hospital. Hospitals would be able to publicize the availability of such discounts and the associated direct financial benefits to the patient. For example, if a hospital wanted to increase its cardiac surgery volume, it could focus its discount strategy on the cardiac surgery DRGs. Or a hospital could provide a uniform discount across all DRGs. Indeed, hospitals could even compete regionally or nationally for patients. For a specific program, such as cardiac surgery, a hospital could provide a discount that would eliminate the entire deductible and also provide transportation to the hospital at no cost to the patient.

Institutional marketing strategies vary, and, in this regard, some hospitals may wish to market their services as extremely high in quality, or to offer some VIP-type services. In the same way that the providers could discount, they could also be allowed to place a premium on certain DRGs, or across all DRGs. The full cost associated with any premium above the standard DRG payment rates would be the responsibility of the patient. The expansion of price flexibility to include not only discounting but also premiums has the danger that many hospitals might seek to impose a premium and thus significantly increase the cost to the patient.

However, in the current economic climate, it is unlikely that many hospitals would be willing to risk being labeled a high-cost hospital unless they could clearly demonstrate to the beneficiaries the additional value provided. Thus, with the exception of a few major teaching hospitals, few hospitals would attempt to add a premium based strictly on their quality of care. However, some hospitals may wish to add a premium for VIP services.

An example of how competition among hospitals might evolve can be illustrated by a comparison with the airline industry. There are no-frills airlines that attempt to provide basic transportation at the lowest cost with no extra services. Often associated with low fares are such inconveniences as off-peak departure times or restrictions on cancellation. Alternatively, there are full-service airlines with a complete range of services, frequent flights, and no restrictions on cancellation. For the full-service airlines there is also the option, at a significant premium, for first-class service. Customers choose the airline and service level that best suits their personal preferences.

Under a competitive framework hospitals may position themselves similarly. For example, some hospitals may market themselves as providing basic hospital services. Early-morning admissions, multiple patients per room, and family assistance with routine nursing services during the recuperative period might all be required to obtain the lower price. A hospital providing a traditional level of hospital services might require none of these restrictions and would not discount the PPS price. There could also be the equivalent of first-class service, in which private rooms, many hotel-type amenities, and options for extended recuperative times would be available at a premium price.

Neither Medicare nor the New Jersey system allows any form of price flexibility. Indeed, under the Department of Justice interpretation of section 1877 of the Social Security Act (42 U.S.C. section 1320a-7b), the waiver of the Part A deductible or coinsurance constitutes a federal crime. Although the Medicare and New Jersey systems have achieved significant cost savings, competitive market forces should be introduced as a means of achieving the next generation of cost savings.

Physician Payment

The costs associated with physician services provided to inpatients are excluded from the prospective DRG rates in both the Medicare and New Jersey systems. Hospital prospective payment creates strong financial incentives to reduce hospital bed-day utilization and the use of ancillary and other hospital services. To respond effectively to the inherent incentives contained in PPS, hospital management must reduce operating expenses in concert with physicians' reducing the average resource utilization per patient. Since physicians control, for the most part, the amount and type of resources utilized in the treatment of patients, any attempt to reduce the average cost per patient must address physician practice patterns. The current practice of reimbursing physicians on the basis of a portion of the actual, customary, prevailing, or reasonable charge for a service is in conflict with the incentives in hospital prospective payment. Physician reimbursement on this basis provides physicians with incentives to provide more services and consume more resources when treating patients. The physician community must not experience an incentive structure in conflict with that of the hospital. Otherwise, the full potential of prospective payment may not be realized. Thus, a prospective payment system for inpatient physician costs needs to be developed.

There are two basic approaches to developing a prospective payment system for physicians. In the first approach a fixed price would be established that reflects the relative value of the physician services required in the rendering of specific services. Three possible scenarios for determining the value of these services have been suggested: (1) establish a scale based on prevailing charges, (2) determine the production costs (physician time requirements and overhead adjusted for specialty training) associated with each service and base a fee scale on those findings, or (3) create competitive market forces among physicians in a geographic area by encouraging them to submit the amount they would charge to render a specific service. For each of these models, physicians would receive fees only in the amount established by the relative value scale for the service rendered.

The second approach to establishing a physician prospective payment system for services rendered to inpatients would be to develop for each DRG a physician-payment component. The prospective DRG payment rates for physicians can be determined in basically the same manner as the DRG payment rates for hospitals. Using historical charge data, the average physician's fee by DRG can be computed and adjusted for area wage differences to establish a prospective payment rate. Using this approach, payments for physician services would reflect the actual case mix of a physician. The use of DRGs for physician payment would require that the DRG definitions be revised to adjust explicitly for patient severity. Paying a set amount per hospitalization would for the first time provide physicians with a strong financial incentive to render their services efficiently and effectively.

Under a DRG-based hospital prospective payment system for physician reimbursement, there are several options for the rendering of payment. Among the various options, two alternatives provide the most feasible approaches. One approach would bundle the physician DRG payment with the hospital DRG payment rate. When the hospital submitted a discharge abstract and bill for a patient, the combined payment would be remitted to the hospital. The hospital would then be responsible for reimbursing the physicians that treated the patient. Hospitals could then elect to contract with certain physician groups to provide treatment, negotiate with individual members of their medical staff to determine the amount of reimbursement the physician would receive, or simply pass the payment through directly to the physicians that treated the patient. The creation of an all-inclusive inpatient DRG payment rate would offer the benefits of streamlining the billing process, provide an easier method for consumers and purchasers of health care services to determine in advance the cost of the services to be provided, and provide hospitals with the financial leverage to insure that standards of care are maintained by their medical staffs.

Another approach is to pay the medical staff as an organized entity for physician services. The medical staff, through its corporate structure and bylaws, would create mechanisms whereby it could receive payments directly from the fiscal intermediaries and then disburse them to individual physicians for services rendered. Similar to Independent Practice Association (IPA) models, this approach would place the medical staff "at risk" for the efficiency of its members. The failure of individual physicians to provide efficient, effective care would result in financial losses for all of the members. The medical staff could withhold payment for physicians who are poor performers and financially reward its members when performance achieves expectations. Paying the medical staff versus individual physicians spreads the financial risk across all members, thereby preventing the chance that individual physicians could suffer significant financial losses due to variations in patient severity.

Severity of Illness

The original formulation of the DRGs intentionally limited the patient attributes used in the definition of the DRGs to routinely collected items. If there are patient characteristics that are not routinely collected (for example, blood pressure) but that systemically affect the amount and type of hospital resources used by particular types of patients, then failure to include these characteristics in the DRG definitions could cause inequities in the DRG payment system. Further, if DRGs were used as the basis for physician payment, then the importance of explicitly recognizing patient severity in the DRG structure increases.

Since the inception of the PPS, there has been a persistent questioning of whether the DRGs adequately account for the severity of illness of particular types of patients. The concept of severity of illness has, in general, been used to refer to the extent of a particular disease in an individual patient. For example, a patient with a gastrointestinal (GI) bleed and with a hematocrit less than 26 on average would be expected to present more treatment difficulty for the physician or present a higher risk of mortality. The GI bleed patient with a hematocrit less than 26 is said to be more severely ill than a GI bleed patient with a hematocrit above 26. In essence, the rationale behind the concept of severity of illness is that simply identifying that a patient has a particular diagnosis is an insufficient description of the patient. To describe a patient fully, additional information on how the disease is manifesting itself in the patient is necessary.

Most schemes for measuring severity of illness require the collection of a substantial amount of detailed information on each patient, such as laboratory results, which are currently not collected on the Uniform Billing form UB 82. On the basis of the additional information, a patient is then assigned to a severity level, typically a numerical rank, such as 1 through 4. Most proposals for incorporating severity of illness into PPS have focused on developing separate payment amounts for each of the severity levels for each DRG, thereby increasing the number of payment categories in PPS approximately fourfold.[16] The implementation of any of the severity measures currently available would require substantial additional data collection with associated costs. In order to justify the additional cost and effort necessary to incorporate a severity measure into the DRGs, four issues need to be carefully evaluated: (1) auditability, (2) credibility, (3) severity differences across hospitals, and (4) impact on the distribution of payments across hospitals.

The information used to determine the amount of payment under PPS must be objective and readily verifiable. Medicare requires a random sample of claims from hospitals to be audited in order to verify the accuracy of the information used to determine payment. If highly subjective measures are used in the definition of the severity measure, then it will be difficult and time-consuming for Medicare to audit the information reliably. Even the information currently used to assign a DRG has some degree of subjectivity and, therefore, causes some problems from an audit perspective. For example, the DRGs require the specification of the principal diagnosis, which is the diagnosis that after evaluation of the patient is determined to have caused the admission to the hospital. For patients with multiple diagnoses, the determination of the principal diagnosis can be subject to interpretation. Given the audit difficulties presented by such a well-defined and straightforward concept as principal diagnosis, any severity-of-illness measure used in a prospective payment system must be based on only objective, readily obtainable information.

The development of the DRGs included the participation of more than 100 physicians. The DRG definitions are publicly available and open to scrutiny and criticism by all interested parties. The large-scale participation in the development of the DRGs and the multiple revisions of the DRG definitions as a result of public suggestions have provided the DRGs with a degree of credibility and acceptance that would otherwise not have been possible. Not all of the severity measures currently available have allowed a public evaluation of the development process and the formal logic and definitions. In order to be credible, all aspects of any severity system used for payment must be available for public evaluation. Only with thorough testing and rigorous evaluation can any severity measure gain the acceptance and credibility necessary to be used in the DRGs.

An evaluation of the need for a severity measure must take into account the intended use of the severity measure. The basic role of the DRGs—and, potentially, the role of severity measures—is to provide a framework for identifying an equitable amount of payment for the different types of patients treated by hospitals. Prospective payment by DRG is based on averaging. Thus, the amount of payment for an individual patient may be either high or low. However, on average over a group of patients in the same DRG, the payment should be equitable.

A common misconception about DRG payments is that no patients should have a cost higher than the payment amount or stay longer than the average length of stay for the DRG. The definition of the patients in each DRG is not so precise that every patient is identical. There are variations across patients within a DRG, due to severity of illness and other factors, that cause the resource needs of patients within the DRG to vary. It is expected that there will be patients whose costs exceed or fall below the payment amount. So long as the variations in resource needs are random and not associated with particular types of hospitals, there will be no inequities in the system. For example, suppose acute myocardial infarction (AMI) patients with a Killip score of 3 or 4 were more costly to treat. If these patients went only to certain hospitals, then the payment system would be inequitable if it did not pay a higher amount for these patients. On the other hand, if these patients were randomly distributed among all hospitals treating AMI patients, then there would be no need to identify them as a separate DRG. Each hospital would treat a certain percentage of AMI patients with a Killip score of 3 or 4 and on average the payment amount would be equitable. Since payment levels in PPS are essentially determined by allocating available funds to the DRGs and then in turn to hospitals, the addition of a severity factor in PPS would not increase overall payments but merely reallocate available funds among hospitals. The issue of severity is not a budgetary question but an allocation question.

Both the New Jersey and Medicare systems currently provide additional payment to teaching hospitals through the use of a teaching adjustment factor. The teaching factor was incorporated to compensate teaching hospitals for the indirect cost of teaching (that is, more services being provided to patients as part of the teaching process) and, since teaching hospitals would be expected to treat the more severely ill patients, to compensate teaching hospitals for any deficiencies in the DRGs with respect to severity of illness. The addition of a severity-of-illness factor to PPS would be expected to increase payments to teaching hospitals and decrease payments to nonteaching hospitals. If such a reallocation of payments occurred, then the teaching factor would need to be reevaluated and possibly reduced. If the net result of adding a severity factor to PPS is to reduce the teaching adjustment factor a commensurate amount, then the cost of collecting the severity information might not be justified. For a severity factor to be valuable it must result in an allocation of payments across hospitals that is more equitable than the allocation currently achieved by the combination of the DRGs and the teaching adjustment factor.

Given that there are patient characteristics that measure a patient's severity of illness and that meet the four listed criteria, a method of incorporating the severity measure into the DRGs must be developed. As mentioned previously, the most commonly proposed method would be to establish additional payment categories for each severity level for each DRG. However, other alternatives need to be considered. While the existing DRGs did not explicitly incorporate severity into their definition, they did attempt to reflect the severity of a patient's condition by identifying significant complications and comorbidities. In general, patients are assigned to a different DRG if they have a significant complication or comorbidity. For some types of patients, however, the presence of complications or comorbidities did not systematically affect the amount and type of hospital resources utilized. For example, patients hospitalized for a carpal tunnel release were not found to have their use of hospital resources significantly affected by the presence of complications or comorbidities. All patients hospitalized for carpal tunnel release are in the same DRG primarily because this is an elective surgery that would not, in general, be performed if the patient were in poor condition. Thus, any measure of severity has to be evaluated to identify precisely the types of patients for whom severity is an important determinant of hospital resources.

Quality of Care

The establishment of prospective DRG payment rates provides a measure of the amount of payment that would be fair compensation to hospitals for treating patients in each DRG. While the DRG prospective payment rates provide an indication of a fair price for the services rendered, they provide no indication of the quality of the services. Some hospitals may have fewer complications, fewer readmissions, lower mortality rates, and, in general, better patient outcomes. Clearly, from a payer and patient perspective, the hospitals with better outcomes are a preferable, and, in the long run, a more cost-effective alternative. When price is removed as a differentiator of hospitals, the quality of the services rendered becomes the primary discriminator among hospitals. The incentives under prospective payment are for hospitals to provide fewer inpatient services and to discharge patients as quickly as possible. Thus, under prospective payment quality of care is of great concern.

In the Omnibus Budget Reconciliation Act of 1986, Congress required HCFA to begin to develop criteria for measuring quality of care as well as procedures for identifying and correcting problems in quality of care.[17] As tools for measuring quality of care become available, prospective payment systems will need to determine whether the quality assessment results can be incorporated into the payment mechanism. One obvious alternative would be to lower the DRG payment amounts in DRGs in which hospitals had poor quality-of-care performance and perhaps increase the payment amounts to hospitals with good quality-of-care performance. However, great care must be taken before imposing such penalties. If a hospital is provided less payment because of a quality problem, then it may not have the funds to correct the problem, and quality may deteriorate further. Another alternative would be to prohibit hospitals from treating patients in whose treatment the hospital is not meeting quality-of-care standards. The difficulty with a prohibition approach is the selection of the threshold at which the prohibition would be enforced. Suppose it was decided that a hospital with a mortality rate of more than 10 percent above the established standard for AMI patients would be prohibited from treating AMI patients. If there were two neighboring hospitals, one 11 percent above the standard, and one 10 percent above the standard, then the 11 percent hospital would be prohibited from treating AMI patients while the 10 percent hospital could continue to treat AMI patients. Such dramatic differences in penalties are difficult to justify by such small differences in performance. Further, the imposition of prohibitions, by harming the hospital's reputation, could reduce admissions to such a degree that the viability of the hospital could be jeopardized. A third alternative would be simply to publish the quality measures and allow the consumer (patient) to choose among hospitals.

While quality measures as a component of a prospective payment system must be introduced only with great care, the use of such measures is the logical next step in the evolution of prospective payment systems. Not only must the question of how much to pay be answered, but also the question of what is being purchased must be addressed. Neither the Medicare nor the New Jersey system has any direct links between quality assessment and the prospective payment amounts.

CONCLUSION

Hospital prospective payment by DRG began in New Jersey in 1980 and has been the basis of Medicare payment since 1983. A broad range of system design issues shape the precise nature of a DRG prospective payment system. These issues range from basic financial issues, such as computation of the annual inflation factor, to system flexibility issues, such as the ability of hospitals to discount the established DRG prices. By most standards, DRG prospective payment has been successful in slowing the growth in hospital costs. However, many of the details of the implementation of DRG prospective payment systems still reflect the original uncertainty of the impact of a switch from cost-based payment to prospective payment. Now that there is sufficient direct implementation experience, the approach to DRG prospective payment needs to be expanded as follows:

— If necessary, an adjustment for patient severity should be added to the DRG definitions to insure that all patient attributes affecting hospital costs are accounted for by the DRGs.

— Capital costs should be included in the DRG payment amounts.

— All physician costs associated with an inpatient hospital stay should be included in the DRG payment amounts.

— The DRG inflation update factor should be computed on the basis of a predefined algorithm and be independent of political manipulations.

— The establishment of a single set of national DRG payment rates should be implemented cautiously in order to insure that legitimate regional differences in cost are adequately taken into consideration.

— Hospitals should be allowed to discount the standard DRG payment amounts in order to encourage competition.

— States in which multiple major payers are paying under prospective DRG systems must actively coordinate payment amounts to hospitals to insure that legitimate hospital costs (such as cost of indigent care) are not excluded from the DRG payment rates by all the major payers.

— Objective quality-of-care measures should be evaluated in establishing the DRG payment rates for a hospital.

Prospective payment by DRG represents a significant advance over cost-based reimbursement because it creates the opportunity for hospitals to profit from performance. In general, the evolution of prospective payment by the DRG must be directed toward a system in which the DRG payment amounts are more comprehensive (capital, physician costs, etc., are included in the rates), the DRG payment amount across payers is coordinated (for example, the cost of indigent care is not excluded by all payers), and price and quality competition across hospitals is allowed and encouraged. The future direction of prospective payment systems by DRG should evolve toward a more comprehensive system with cross-payer coordination at the state level but with the flexibility to allow price and quality competition among hospitals.

REFERENCES

1. R. Schweiker, "Hospital Prospective Payment for Medicare" (Report to Congress; Washington, D.C.: U.S. Department of Health and Human Services, 1982).
2. Ibid.
3. Ibid.
4. N.J.S.A. 26:2H-2(1)
5. See *Hadley Memorial Hospital, Inc., d/b/a Hadley Regional Medical Center, et al.* v. *Schweiker,* U.S. Court of Appeals, Tenth Circuit, no. 80–1806, September 13, 1982.
6. Governor's Advisory Committee on Capital Expenditure for Healthcare Facilities, "Making Less Do More—Capital Policy for New Jersey Hospitals" (Trenton, NJ: State of New Jersey, 1984).
7. M. Kalison and R. Averill, "Building Capital into Prospective Payment," *Business and Health* (June 1985): 34–37.
8. M. Kalison and R. Averill, "Regulation vs. Contract: The Future of Capital under PPS," *Healthcare Financial Management* monograph series (1984).
9. U.S. Congress, Social Security Act, section 1878(g)(2) and section 1886(d)(7).
10. N.J.A.C. 8:31B-3.58(b).
11. R. Shakno, *Physician's Guide to DRGs* (Chicago: Pluribus Press, 1983).
12. Department of Health, State of New Jersey, "A Prospective Payment System Based on Patient Case-Mix for New Jersey Hospitals 1976–8" (Seventh quarterly report under contract no. 600-0022; Baltimore: Health Care Financing Administration, U.S. Department of Health, Education, and Welfare, 1977).

13. R. Averill and M. Kalison, "Are National DRG Rates the Best Choice for PPS?" *Healthcare Financial Management* (August 1985): 62–66.
14. R. Averill and M. Kalison, "The Next Step: Introducing Competitive Pricing into PPS," *Healthcare Financial Management* (August 1986): 58–62.
15. R. Averill and M. Kalison, "The Challenge of 'Real' Competition in Medicare," *Health Affairs* (Fall 1986): 47–57.
16. S. Horn et al., "Severity of Illness within DRGs: Impact on Prospective Payment," *American Journal of Public Health* 75 (1985): 1195–99.
17. U.S. Congress, Second Omnibus Budget Reconciliation Act (PL 99-509).

9

Experience with a DRG-Based Prospective Payment System

Stuart Guterman, Paul W. Eggers, Gerald Riley,
Timothy F. Greene, and Sherry A. Terrell

$\mathbf{M}$edicare's Prospective Payment System (PPS) is designed to
change hospital behavior by directly altering the economic incentives
facing hospital decision makers. Hospitals' responses to these incentives
can, in turn, be expected to have a far-reaching effect on other groups of
institutions and individuals that provide, consume, and pay for health
care. Medicare beneficiaries are obviously affected by the new payment
system, as the quality of the care that they receive, their access to the care
that they need, and their out-of-pocket costs for care provided both in the
hospital and in other settings are, in part, determined by hospitals'
responses to PPS incentives.

Other payers for inpatient hospital services may also be affected, as
they attempt to avoid a potential shifting of hospital costs from Medicare
patients to their own patients and as they respond to the example set by
the PPS cost-containment approach. Among other providers of health
care, physicians may be affected both as practitioners within the inpatient
setting and as providers of potential substitutes for inpatient care, and
providers of posthospital subacute care may feel the effects of PPS
through an increase in the volume and complexity of services demanded
from them.

This chapter presents a summary of the findings of research on the
impact of PPS on these major groups of actors in the health care system. In

Adapted from Stuart Guterman, Paul W. Eggers, Gerald Riley, Timothy F. Greene, and
Sherry A. Terrell, "The First Three Years of Medicare Prospective Payment: An Overview,"
Health Care Financing Review 9, no. 3 (April 1988): 67–77. HCFA Pub. No. 03263. Office of
Research and Demonstrations, Health Care Financing Administration. Washington, D.C.,
U.S. Government Printing Office.

addition, since the maintenance of the fiscal solvency of the Medicare Hospital Insurance Trust Fund was the primary impetus for the enactment of PPS, the effect of the new payment system on the Medicare program itself is examined.

ATTRIBUTING OBSERVED EFFECTS

One of the major problems in evaluating PPS is that of attribution. It is difficult to draw strong causal inferences about the effects of the new system because of the rapidly changing nature of the health care sector. Many changes are occurring that might plausibly account for effects of the sort anticipated under prospective payment. For instance, PPS is but one of many public and private initiatives to control the cost of health care. Also, the rapidly increasing supply of physicians is likely to be an important influence on the effectiveness of efforts to contain health care costs. Thus, both desirable and undesirable effects that might be consistent with expectations about PPS may actually be caused by other factors, or, most likely, be the joint product of PPS and several other factors.

These considerations require that a great deal of caution be exercised in attributing positive or negative effects to one or another of the many changes occurring in the health care sector. However, although the attribution of effects is clearly a major concern of efforts to evaluate PPS, the lack of conclusive evidence of causality need not imply that policy conclusions cannot be drawn. PPS has as its objective the accomplishment of certain desirable changes in the health care system. To the extent that those changes are, in fact, observed, the Medicare program and its beneficiaries can be judged to be better off under the new system, regardless of whether this improvement may be conclusively attributed to any one policy. To the extent that undesirable effects are observed, a problem may be indicated, again, irrespective of the ability to attribute these effects to any one policy.

Thus, it may not be necessary to know with certainty that PPS is the cause of the observed changes to be able to conclude that some policy response is necessary. What is necessary, however, is to distinguish clearly between those problems that can and should be dealt with explicitly through PPS and those that, although they may be equally important, must be dealt with through other policy avenues.

DATA SOURCES

The major source of data for this chapter is the Medicare Statistical System. The Health Care Financing Administration (HCFA) collects a rich body of data associated with the utilization and cost of inpatient hospital services and other in-hospital and ambulatory care services covered by Medicare.

Additional sources of data for the PPS evaluation are provided by HCFA-supported contract and grant research activities. These activities have provided many of the analyses of the impact of PPS as well. Finally, where appropriate, sources of data outside of HCFA are used, including other government agencies, such as the National Center for Health Statistics, and sources in the private sector, such as the American Hospital Association.

In analyzing the impact of PPS during its third year (fiscal year 1986), an attempt has been made to incorporate the most recent data available at the time that the analyses were conducted. For some of these analyses, at least preliminary data on fiscal year 1986 were available. For many of the analyses, however, including many of the hospital-level analyses and most of the beneficiary-level analyses, data were not yet available for fiscal year 1986. Fiscal year 1985 data were therefore used in these analyses.

IMPACT ON HOSPITALS

The hospital industry has undergone tremendous change in recent years. An unprecedented decline in admissions has been observed for both Medicare and non-Medicare patients. This, combined with the steep decline in average length of stay for Medicare patients as hospitals came under the new system, has resulted in declining inpatient volumes. Despite a decrease in the number of inpatient beds, occupancy rates are at an all-time low, leading to increased competition among hospitals to attract patients.[1] However, the decline in inpatient volume has not been uniformly distributed across hospital types. It has been concentrated among small hospitals, putting those hospitals in a particularly disadvantageous position.[2]

The decline in length of stay under PPS has been achieved through shorter stays across the board, rather than efforts aimed specifically at patients who have the longest stays (and are, presumably, the most severely ill).[3] The correlation between the financial pressure imposed by PPS and steepness of declines in length of stay provides another indication that PPS has been effective in encouraging hospitals to change the way that they provide inpatient care.[4]

The dramatic declines in average length of stay under PPS may be leveling off, however. Among PPS cases only (not including New York and Massachusetts), there has been little change since the first year of prospective payment. This may reflect an unexpectedly strong initial response to the PPS incentive to shorten lengths of stay. It may also be attributed to the fact that, since utilization review has diverted many of the less severely ill patients from inpatient to outpatient and other ambulatory care, there has been an increase in the average severity of illness among those Medicare patients who are admitted to the hospital.

Hospitals, on average, received Medicare payments that were considerably higher than the corresponding costs in the first two years under PPS, although the trend seems to have begun turning downward in the third year. The distribution of these payment margins is uneven, with urban hospitals faring better than rural hospitals, large hospitals better than small hospitals, and teaching hospitals better than nonteaching hospitals. Recent changes in the PPS payment rules may have reduced some of the unevenness in the distribution of payment margins across hospital groups, but this unevenness suggests that distributional issues will become increasingly important as average margins fall.

Data on hospitals' overall financial performance indicate that they fared well in general during the early years of PPS.[5,6] However, the gap between those hospitals that are doing well and those that are not appears to be becoming wider, mostly because of the increase in total margins at the high end of the range. A comparison of hospitals at the top of the distribution with those at the bottom indicates that urban and proprietary hospitals, as well as regional referral centers, are disproportionately represented among those with large margins, and sole community hospitals are disproportionately represented among those at the lower end of the range.[7]

In response to the rapidly changing environment facing the hospital industry, hospital administrators report undertaking initiatives in several areas in an attempt to control costs and increase the viability of their institutions.[8] These changes include structural changes (such as eliminating beds and converting them to more efficient uses), changes in the use of both labor and nonlabor inputs (such as staffing reductions, skill-mix reconfigurations, and group purchasing), and organizational changes (such as the hiring of more business-oriented managers and the initiation of interfacility cost-sharing arrangements).

Finally, the overall rate of investment reported in the Medicare cost reports for the first year of PPS indicates a somewhat slower rate of investment in fixed assets. However, these data most likely reflect investment decisions made several years before the implementation of prospective payment; it will take more time to see the effect of PPS on this aspect of hospital behavior. Moreover, the intensity of fixed assets per bed has increased, indicating that the decrease in patient volume has outstripped the effective reduction in the growth of capital stock. The diffusion of new technology does not appear to have been affected by PPS; many services that have not yet reached some critical level of availability have continued to grow, both in the number of areas in which they are available and in the number of hospitals in each area in which they are available.[9]

IMPACT ON MEDICARE BENEFICIARIES

The Medicare population experienced declines in the overall use of hospital care in both 1984 and 1985. However, the nature of the decline in 1985 differed greatly from that of the 1984 decline. In 1984, there were sharp decreases in length of stay, evidenced uniformly across beneficiary groups—the aged, the disabled, and those with end-stage renal disease (ESRD)—and across demographic groups within beneficiary category. In 1985, average lengths of stay fell only slightly, but discharge rates were less consistent. Among the aged, a moderate decline in 1984 was followed by a much larger decline in 1985. Among the disabled, a large decline in 1984 was followed by a more moderate decline in 1985. The ESRD population experienced an increase in their discharge rate in 1984 and a small decline in 1985. As a result, the net decline in total days of care since the beginning of PPS was similar for the aged and disabled populations. The decline among ESRD beneficiaries was much smaller than for the other two groups.

Although there have been declines in discharge rates among all age groups of the aged, the rate of decline has been lowest among people 85 or older. Since the beginning of PPS, decline in discharges has been considerably less in this latter group than among persons aged 65 to 69. If PPS is reducing access to hospital care, it seems that it has not resulted in a relative deterioration of access to care for this most vulnerable group. On the other hand, to the extent that older beneficiaries are at greater risk of premature discharges, there is some potential cause for concern. Length-of-stay reductions were greatest for the oldest group. Because the need for subacute posthospital care is greatest for older persons, length-of-stay reductions could pose greater problems for this group.

Among the disabled, the youngest age group had a large decline in discharge rate in 1984. In 1985, this group had an increase in discharges that partially counteracted the previous year's decrease and resulted in a net change since the beginning of PPS comparable to that for other age groups. This seems to indicate a general instability in discharge rates from one year to the next and highlights the caution that should be taken in interpreting results for any single year.

Hospital mortality rates for the Medicare population increased between fiscal year 1984 and fiscal year 1985. The fact that total population-based mortality did not change during this time and that there was a large decline in admission rates strongly suggests that hospital-based mortality has been affected by the distribution of cases across diagnoses or DRGs. Adjusting the fiscal year 1985 mortality rates according to the disease- or DRG-specific risk of mortality in fiscal year 1984 accounts for about one-half of the increase in hospital mortality. An analysis of changes in mortality rates based on a variant of the disease staging methodology developed by SysteMetrics, Inc., suggests that most, if not all, of the remaining increase in mortality can be explained by the mix of cases across risk groups.[10]

The impact of PPS on beneficiary liability can be examined here only from the relatively narrow perspective of Medicare-covered services, because of the lack of data on other out-of-pocket expenses for Medicare beneficiaries. This is an unfortunate limitation, since much of the potential financial burden resulting from changes in the way health care is delivered is related to these noncovered services. The most apparent impact of PPS is in the dramatic reduction in the liability per beneficiary for inpatient coinsurance days. There has also been a decline in the rate of growth of other components of beneficiary liability for hospital services that was caused by the decrease in both the rate of admissions and the average length of hospital stays for Medicare beneficiaries. Other factors behind this trend include changes in the rules for payment of physicians and a decline in the general rate of inflation.

IMPACT ON POSTHOSPITAL CARE

The use of home health agency (HHA) services has increased rapidly among Medicare beneficiaries in recent years. This increase in utilization began before the implementation of PPS and has continued since, although at a slower rate. The percentage of beneficiaries using HHA services following hospitalization has increased for all age groups and across states. The utilization of skilled nursing facility (SNF) services increased following the implementation of PPS, after a period of no increase from 1981 to 1983.

It appears likely that the increase in SNF utilization is related to PPS, but attribution of the increase in HHA utilization is not clear. A time series analysis conducted for HCFA indicated a small effect of PPS on HHA utilization and a larger effect on SNF use.[11]

These findings do not suggest widespread problems with access to posthospital care under PPS. A few of the studies cited do raise, however, a question about access to SNF care for the most severely ill and the impaired elderly. SNF utilization by these two groups appears to have declined following PPS, contrary to the overall trend for Medicare beneficiaries. These findings are preliminary, however, and are based on small samples. Further research to analyze this issue is under way.

IMPACT ON OTHER PAYERS

During the period of implementation of PPS, many changes have occurred in the markets for health insurance and health care services. Although government expenditures for hospital care grew more slowly in 1985 than did expenditures in the private sector, overall private health insurance premiums grew more during 1983–86 than did private health insurance benefit payments.

PPS appears to have had different effects on each payer. State Medicaid programs have increasingly responded to budget pressures by adopting prospective inpatient hospital payment systems in general and DRG-based systems in particular.[12] Medicaid DRG-based systems are clearly modeled on the federal Medicare system.

Blue Cross plans moved from retrospective to prospective primary methods of hospital payment between 1981 and 1985.[13] Although these changes cannot be conclusively attributed to PPS, there were statistically significant declines in inpatient utilization growth rates, increases in outpatient utilization growth rates, and decreases in payment growth rates for Blue Cross subscribers under 65 between the pre-PPS and post-PPS periods.[14]

The PPS period was also characterized by increased cost-containment activity by commercial insurers; shifts to alternatives, such as self-insurance; and growth of alternative payment systems, such as health maintenance organizations (HMOs) and preferred provider organizations (PPOs).[15] However, there is no strong evidence for attributing these changes to PPS.

IMPACT ON OTHER PROVIDERS

Ambulatory care continues to be the fastest-growing segment of the health care industry. Outpatient revenue per visit has grown at an accelerated rate since PPS, although the increase in the rate of growth is not statistically significant. Both Medicare and non-Medicare outpatient visits declined slightly during the first year of PPS and increased during the second year, but Medicare visits increased by a substantially greater percentage.

Both medical and surgical services provided under Medicare supplemental medical insurance appear to be shifting away from the inpatient setting toward office and outpatient settings.[16] The percent of reasonable charges for surgery in outpatient settings has increased faster than the percent of procedures performed, indicating that more complex procedures are being performed outside of the hospital.

Since the implementation of PPS, the supply of post-acute-care providers has increased. Some of this increase may be attributable to the increased demand for postacute care brought about by the earlier hospital discharge of Medicare patients. It also results, in part, from demographic factors (including the aging of the population), changes in states' Medicaid eligibility and reimbursement policies, and, in the case of home health care, changes in home health coverage under Medicare and efforts to use home- and community-based services wherever possible to avoid premature or inappropriate institutionalization.

The number of Medicare-certified SNFs increased in the period following PPS. A study of nursing homes in ten states indicated that, in homes that served a large number of Medicare patients prior to PPS, the needs of patients for subacute care increased in the post-PPS period. It appears that these "high-Medicare" homes made room for more patients needing subacute care by transferring patients with more chronic long-term care conditions and numerous functional limitations to the more traditional nursing homes.[17]

The number of HHAs also increased during this time period. Although part of this increase is believed to have been caused by changes in Medicare home health coverage legislated in the Omnibus Budget Reconciliation Act of 1980, the increase may also be attributable to the implementation of PPS and state Medicaid policies.

Home health care patients in the post-PPS period had increases in their needs both for subacute care and for more functional and chronic long-term care.[18] Although this trend may have been partly attributable to the implementation of PPS, it also may have resulted from the diversion of patients from nursing homes that occurred because of increased preadmission screening and case-management programs.

In the period immediately following the implementation of PPS, HHAs increased their average staffing levels. However, the average number of staff has since decreased to below the 1982 level; the probable reason for this change is an increase in the number of small HHAs, rather than a decrease in the size of existing HHAs. At the same time that the average HHA staff size was decreasing, the proportion of HHAs offering various types of services was increasing.

The supply of both swing beds and hospices, both relatively new programs, increased substantially since PPS was implemented. It is not possible to say to what extent this growth was the result of PPS. We do know that both of these programs tend to be concentrated within certain geographical areas.

IMPACT ON MEDICARE PROGRAM
OPERATIONS AND EXPENDITURES

By fiscal year 1986, 48 states and the District of Columbia were under prospective payment, including some 84 percent of all hospitals participating in Medicare. In addition, Puerto Rico was brought under the nationwide system in fiscal year 1988. The number of hospitals and units that have been certified to be excluded from prospective payment is growing, while research is being conducted on how best to include these hospitals under PPS.

In order to monitor the appropriateness, necessity, and quality of care under PPS, 54 professional review organizations (PROs) have been established. These PROs have been reviewing medical records in an attempt to detect problems in the way that medical care is provided to Medicare beneficiaries and billed to the program. A "SuperPRO" has been established to review the performance of the PROs.

Data on PRO denial rates indicate, however, that there is wide variation in the stringency of PRO review. SuperPRO data also indicate that there is wide variation in the success of PROs in detecting problems from medical records. The fiscal intermediaries (FIs), whose primary responsibility is the processing and paying of Part A claims, are also responsible for coverage determinations and some medical/utilization review functions. There is wide variation in FI denial rates, which affects Medicare payments for skilled nursing and home health care as well as hospital care.[19]

These findings may lead to several alternative conclusions: they may reflect differences in local health care practice; they may reflect differences in the stringency of local PRO or FI review; or they may reflect differences in the level of performance of the local review entities. In any case, it does not appear that such local variation is consistent with the objectives of a nationwide system such as PPS.

PPS appears to have slowed the rate of increase in Medicare inpatient hospital benefit payments. Although this increase still exceeds the general rate of inflation, it represents a downturn in the rapid growth of inpatient hospital payments that was seen as a major threat to the solvency of the Medicare Trust Fund.

Outpatient hospital payments are increasing at a real rate far greater than their growth rate immediately prior to the implementation of the Tax Equity and Fiscal Responsibility Act of 1982 (TEFRA). This may indicate that some of the savings on inpatient services under PPS are being spent on outpatient services. Physician payments have increased at a somewhat slower real rate under PPS than before TEFRA, but this slight decrease may have resulted from the Medicare physician fee freeze that was in effect for much of the early PPS period.

Skilled nursing payments have constituted a steadily decreasing share of total Medicare benefit payments since early in the history of the program. Skilled nursing payments have increased under PPS at a slower rate even than inpatient hospital payments, but, when compared with the decrease in the pre-TEFRA period, this slow increase may indicate a relative upturn. The share of home health payments has increased rapidly over the years, however. The real rate of increase in home health payments under PPS is slightly higher than it was in the pre-TEFRA period. That the combined share of skilled nursing and home health payments has increased under PPS may be a response to the expected increase in the demand for posthospital subacute care, but it is difficult to tell from payment data alone.

The overall level of Medicare benefit payments is increasing at a slower rate under PPS because of a sharp decline in the growth of Medicare hospital insurance payments, although Medicare supplemental medical insurance payments are increasing at a somewhat faster real rate than before TEFRA. Total Medicare benefit payments per enrollee have increased at a real rate that is only about three-quarters of its pre-TEFRA growth rate.

CONCLUSIONS

The data presented in this chapter support several conclusions about PPS in its first three years.

First, the new system has been implemented fairly smoothly; essentially all of the hospitals that were intended to be covered by prospective payment are included in the system. Moreover, two of the four states that were originally waived from participation had joined the nationwide payment system by the end of fiscal year 1986.

Second, the implementation of PPS does appear to be affecting the way that hospitals operate. The average length of stay is down (although it appears to be leveling off), the rate of increase in Medicare costs is down, and practice patterns appear to be changing.

Third, hospitals in general appear to have reaped the benefits of their cost-cutting behavior in the form of large operating margins, although more recent data show that these margins have decreased somewhat and some hospitals have not done as well as others.

It also seems clear that the change in hospital behavior is having an effect now, and will probably have an increasing effect on the other actors in the health care system—Medicare beneficiaries, other payers for inpatient hospital services, and other health care providers. As time passes, these effects will become clearer, both because the parties involved will have had a chance to develop further their responses to the new health care environment and because health services researchers both within and outside of the government will have had additional opportunity to develop data sources and analytic methods that will enable them to assess the impact of the system more accurately.

ACKNOWLEDGMENTS

The authors would like to thank the many people who have been and continue to be involved in the evaluation of PPS. In particular, contributions to this chapter were derived from material prepared by Jerry Cromwell, Greg Pope, Ann Hendricks, and Marty Gaynor of Health Economics Research, Inc.; John Conklin and David Klingman of Syste-Metrics, Inc.; and Larry Forgy, Judy Williams, and Andrea Hassol of Abt Associates, Inc. Contributing staff from HCFA's Office of Research included Larry Kucken of the Division of Beneficiary Studies and Judy Sangl, Marni Hall, Terry Kay, John Petrie, and Deborah Williams of the Division of Reimbursement and Economic Studies.

Many additional people within and outside of HCFA have contributed their labor, data, and comments to the PPS evaluation effort; although they are not named here, their contributions are greatly appreciated.

REFERENCES

1. American Hospital Association, *National Hospital Panel Survey Report* (Chicago: American Hospital Association, 1979, 1980, 1981, 1982, 1983, 1984, 1985, 1986).
2. J. Cromwell, "Hospital Management and Cost Control" (Working paper; Needham, MA: Health Economics Research, Inc., May 1987).
3. G. Pope, "Analysis of Changes in Variation of Length-of-Stay and Cost per Discharge among Urban Hospitals" (Working paper; Needham, MA: Health Economics Research, Inc., May 1987).
4. J. Feder, J. Hadley, and S. Zuckerman, "How Did Medicare's Prospective Payment System Affect Hospitals?" *New England Journal of Medicine* 317, no. 14 (1987): 867–73.
5. A. Hendricks, "Hospital Profits in TEFRA and PPS-1" (Working paper; Needham, MA: Health Economics Research, Inc., May 1987).
6. D. Kidder, "The Impact of PPS on Hospital Costs, Efficiency, and Financial Viability" (Working paper; Cambridge, MA: Abt Associates, Inc., May 1987).
7. A. Hendricks, "Hospital Profits in TEFRA and PPS-1."
8. J. Cromwell, "Hospital Management and Cost Control."

9. M. Gaynor, "Investment and Service Adoption under PPS" (Working paper; Cambridge, MA: Abt Associates, Inc., May 1987).

10. J. Conklin and R. Houchens, "PPS Impact on Mortality Rates: Adjusting for Case Mix Severity" (Working paper; New York: SysteMetrics/McGraw Hill, May 1987).

11. R. J. Schmitz, "An Overview of Post-Hospital Care Utilization" (Working paper, Cambridge, MA: Abt Associates, Inc., July 1987).

12. J. Singer, S. Karon, S. Pendleton, and S. Bachman, "The Effects of Medicare PPS on Medicaid Programs" (Working paper; Waltham, MA: Brandeis Health Policy Research Consortium, December 1986).

13. R. Scheffler and J. Gibbs, "Blue Cross Primary Method of Hospital Payment and Alternative Delivery Strategies: Other Factors Affecting the Impact of the Prospective Payment System on the Private Sector" (Working paper; Chicago: Blue Cross and Blue Shield Association, June 1987).

14. R. Scheffler and J. Gibbs, "Blue Cross Utilization and Payment Rates before and after Prospective Payment: December 1986 Update" (Working paper; Chicago: Blue Cross and Blue Shield Association, December 1986).

15. H. Korda, "Competition and the Response of Alternative Health Plans (AHPs): Impact of the PPS on AHPs and Their Availability to Medicare and Non-Medicare Beneficiaries" (Working paper; Cambridge, MA: Abt Associates, Inc., June 1987).

16. U.S. Department of Health and Human Services, "Impact of Prospective Payment on Physician Charges under Medicare," *Health Care Spending Bulletin* no. 86-02 (Baltimore: Bureau of Data Management and Strategy, Health Care Financing Administration, 1986).

17. P. Shaughnessy, A. Kramer, and M. Pettigrew, "Findings on Case Mix and Quality of Care in Nursing Homes and Home Health Agencies" (Working paper; Denver: University of Colorado Center for Health Services Research, July 1987).

18. L. Forgy and J. Williams, "Preliminary Analysis of Mediqual Data" (Working paper; Cambridge, MA: Abt Associates, Inc., May 1987).

19. A. Hassol, "Medicare Program Operations: Denial Rates among Fiscal Intermediaries and Peer Review Organizations" (Working paper; Cambridge, MA: Abt Associates, Inc., April 1987).

See also:

U.S. Department of Health and Human Services. *The Impact of the Medicare Hospital Prospective Payment System: 1984 Annual Report.* Report to Congress; Health Care Financing Administration (HCFA) publication no. 03231. Washington, D.C.: HCFA, August 1986.

———. *The Impact of the Medicare Hospital Prospective Payment System: 1985 Annual Report.* Report to Congress; Health Care Financing Administration (HCFA) publication no. 03251. Washington, D.C.: HCFA, August 1987.

Part IV

International Use of DRGs

10

Development and Application of DRGs in Other Countries

George R. Palmer, Jean L. Freeman, and
Jean-Marie Rodrigues

A considerable interest in DRGs in countries other than the United States has been developing rapidly in recent years. DRG projects are currently being conducted in 17 European countries, as well as in Australia, Canada, and Korea, with a view to their use for national, regional, and institutional budgeting and for internal hospital management.[1] The attention devoted by all these countries to the measurement of case mix has been stimulated by the concerns of governments about the escalation of hospital expenditures and the demand for hospital bed utilization in a period of increasing pressure to restrict health care spending. In addition, governments have become increasingly aware of the evidence that the management and operation of individual hospitals may be inefficient, and that the funding provided to them bears little relationship to the activities that they undertake.

In this chapter we present an overview of the European and Australian interest in and application of DRGs. The countries engaged in DRG projects are characterized by a considerable diversity of arrangements for organizing and funding hospitals that we shall not attempt to summarize here. In all these countries, however, the direct involvement of governments in the financing and in some cases the management of hospitals is greater than in the United States. Nevertheless, it would be misleading to assume that the ability of governments to influence the activities of the hospitals is necessarily stronger than in the United States, especially

---

This chapter describes the collaborative studies of the Health Systems Management Group at Yale University to evaluate the feasibility of implementing DRGs for the management and financing of hospital services in Australia, England, Finland, France, Ireland, Norway, Portugal, Spain, Sweden, and Wales.

where clinical issues are involved. The relatively slow and cautious progress made in changing the funding and management systems to incorporate case-mix measures in some European countries is a reflection of this reality.

In most of the countries considered here a high proportion of the funding made available to hospitals is derived from direct government grants.[2] These payments are normally based on a budget, that is, a forecast of the costs that each hospital expects to incur. As a result, DRG projects have not been designed to create a system of prospective payments with respect to individual patients. Indeed, those people responsible for DRG projects have emphasized that the adoption of a DRG program does not mean that the country intends to introduce the type of payment system used in the United States. Where a major objective has been to use DRGs as part of the funding process—for example, in Portugal, Ireland, and Australia—the measurement of the case mix of each hospital and its costliness relative to other hospitals has loomed as an important component of a global budgeting procedure.[3–5]

A few European countries, notably the Netherlands, oppose the use of DRGs for funding hospitals. Instead, these countries have undertaken DRG studies to improve the internal management of hospitals by moving toward the system of product-line management described in Chapter 4.

THE STANDARDIZATION OF
HOSPITAL DATA SYSTEMS

The creation of DRG systems is based on the availability of specific items of information about each patient discharged from the hospital. The extent to which hospitals are able to provide this information varies widely from country to country. Furthermore, countries differ in the systems used to code the diagnosis and procedure data, in the definitions of some of the key concepts (including which patients are defined as inpatients), and in the quality of the information. All these factors may impede the process of creating and applying DRG systems, especially when DRGs are used to compare hospital utilization between countries. Studies of this kind, and the problems associated with them, are described in Chapter 11.

Several international European organizations are now working to overcome the problems arising from the uncoordinated development of hospital data systems. The Council of Europe has recently recommended that European nations should develop uniform and standardized hospital information systems that include the use of a minimum basic data set (MBDS).[6,7] Further initiatives from international agencies are discussed in a later section of this chapter.

Hospital Data Systems

Each country has developed its own method of collecting data about hospitalized patients in accordance with its national priorities. The factors that influence the methods of collection and the degree of coverage are both cultural and historical. In some countries, notably Britain, nation-wide hospital discharge data have been generated primarily for the purposes of publishing morbidity statistics.[8] In other countries a more restricted coverage of hospitals has produced data designed to yield information about the cost of care. Table 10-1, based on a survey conducted by the Council of Europe, illustrates the great diversity in the ways European countries have organized the collection of hospital patient data, including the extent to which the items of information have been standardized.

It is clear from this table that many countries have projects that are designed to create comprehensive hospital discharge data systems. The extension of standardized data systems to the national level is also increasing.

Table 10-1: European Hospital Discharge Data

Country	Availability of Nationwide Data			Degree of Standardization	
	National	Planned Coverage	Sampling Coverage	Regional	Institute
Austria	No	No	No	Yes	Yes+
Belgium	No	Yes+	No	No	Yes+
Denmark	Yes+	—	—	Yes+	Yes+
Finland	Yes+	—	—	Yes+	Yes+
France	No	Yes+	Yes	No	Yes+
Federal Republic of Germany	No	No	No	Yes+	Yes+
Greece	No	Yes+	No	Yes	Yes+
Ireland	Yes+	—	—	Yes+	Yes+
Italy	No	Yes+	Yes+	Yes+	Yes+
The Netherlands	Yes+	—	—	No	Yes+
Norway	No	Yes+	Yes+	Yes+	Yes+
Portugal	No	Yes+	No	Yes+	Yes+
Spain	No	Yes	No	Yes	Yes+
Sweden	Yes+	—	—	Yes+	Yes+
Switzerland	No	No	Yes+	Yes+	Yes+
United Kingdom	Yes+	—	—	Yes+	Yes+

Key: + = Computerized.

Reprinted from: J.-M. Rodrigues et al., *Computerization of Medical Data in Hospital Services Including University Hospitals* (Strasbourg: Council of Europe, 1988), with permission from the Council of Europe.

Minimum Basic Data Set (MBDS)

The MBDS for use in Europe was introduced at a conference held in Brussels in 1981. This MBDS is designed as the basis for hospital discharge systems, for management and planning purposes, for epidemiological and clinical research, and for international comparisons. Thirteen items have been included in the European MBDS for inpatients undergoing treatment in acute care hospitals:

— Hospital identification
— Patient's number
— Sex
— Age
— Marital status
— Place of residence
— Month and year of admission
— Duration of stay
— Discharge status
— Main diagnosis
— Other diagnoses
— Surgical and obstetric procedures
— Other significant procedures

"Minimum" implied that each hospital should collect not less than these items in a uniform way. Definitions were specified for each item in order to facilitate the collection of comparable data. It was the intention that the MBDS should be obtained for each acute hospital patient discharged in a defined geographical area.

The collection of the MBDS items has expanded rapidly in Europe and by 1986 had embraced ten countries. Proposed uses of DRGs for hospital financing and management have been the stimulus for most of this activity. The situation in 16 European countries in 1985, as established by the Council of Europe survey, is summarized in Table 10-2.

THE YALE DRG PROJECTS

The Health Systems Management Group at Yale University has entered into research contracts with ten European countries and one Australian state in order to develop the capacity in each country for applying DRGs for management and financing purposes. It has also been an important objective of the projects to create data in a suitable form for the making of comparisons of hospital bed utilization and costs between these countries.

The four phases of the Yale projects are:

1. The assessment of the technical feasibility of assigning the country's hospital patient discharge abstracts to DRGs

2. The determination of whether the utilization model defined by the DRGs is adequate to describe the country's hospitalization data

3. The adaptation of the United States DRG-based cost and budgeting model to make it applicable to the country's financial data and hospital setting.

4. The reprogramming of the cost-model software for accounting and budgeting analyses on in-house microcomputers

Phase 1: Technical Feasibility

The technical feasibility phase establishes whether the information required to classify discharges by DRG can be obtained from hospital discharge abstracts and whether it is in the form required by the standard DRG assignment software.The DRG grouper software cannot be used directly with the data available in most European countries since it requires that diseases and procedures be coded according to the *International Classification of Diseases, Ninth Revision, Clinical Modification* (ICD-9-CM). Most European countries use the *International Classification of Diseases, Ninth Revision* (ICD-9) for classifying diseases and a considerable variety of classification schemes to code procedures. Thus, most of the

Table 10-2: Collection of the Minimum Basic Data Set in Europe

Nationwide 1986	*To Commence in 1985*	*Not Nationwide in 1985*
Denmark	Belgium	Austria
Finland	France	Federal Republic of Germany
Ireland	Norway	Greece
The Netherlands	Portugal	Italy*
Sweden		Spain
United Kingdom		Switzerland

*Coverage may vary from year to year.

Reprinted from: J.-M. Rodrigues et al., *Computerization of Medical Data in Hospital Services Including University Hospitals* (Strasbourg: Council of Europe, 1988), with permission from the Council of Europe.

efforts in this phase have been directed toward the development of "mapping" tables for each country's coding systems to convert them to ICD-9-CM. This work has led to the production of mapping tables for all the coding systems in common use in Europe and Australia.

Phase 2: The Applicability of the DRG Model and Definitions

The objective of the second phase is to assess whether the same general relationships among the variables defining DRGs (diagnoses, procedures, age, discharge status) observed in the United States are also found in the country's hospitalization data. Descriptive and regression model analyses are performed to make the assessment, using length of stay as the dependent variable to measure resource utilization.

The descriptive analyses comparing the United States with other countries address four basic issues:

— Whether the DRGs in the other country are relatively homogeneous with respect to length of stay as indicated by the coefficients of variation, and whether there are substantial differences between these coefficients and those found in comparable data from the United States

— Whether the surgical hierarchy, that is, the relative resource intensity of the groups of surgical procedures included in each "major diagnostic category" (MDC) of the DRG system, is similar in the two countries

— Whether the association between diagnostic subcategories within related DRGs and length of stay for medical cases can be characterized in a similar manner in the two countries

— Whether the comorbidities-or-complications variable has a similar effect in increasing the length of stay for related DRGs in the study country and the United States

The calculation of correlation coefficients is the starting point for addressing the last three issues. The correlation coefficients measure the strength of the relationships between the United States length-of-stay values and those from the other country for each DRG within each MDC. Thus, high correlations between the two sets of values, when surgical and medical DRGs are considered separately, provide strong evidence that the influence on resource usage of each of the factors referred to above is similar in the two countries. More detailed analysis, including review by clinicians, may then be required to assess, for example, the appropriateness of the surgical hierarchy and the effects of the comorbidities-or-complications variable.

The adequacy of DRGs may be further assessed by analyzing a country's hospital data at the level of individual patient discharges in the context of a regression model constructed to reflect the underlying structure of the classification scheme. Within each MDC, a statistical model allows one to make inferences regarding the effects of the independent variables (that is, those variables used in the definition of DRGs) on the overall predictive performance of the model. Again, if the sizes of these effects are similar in the United States and the study country, the DRG case-mix classification system is likely to be suitable for use in that country.

Phase 3: Adaptation of the Cost Model

During the third phase the DRG-based cost-finding model is adapted to fit the management structure and accounting and billing methods of the hospitals in the foreign country. Four types of data need to be collected by the hospital staff:

— Patient discharge information

— Patient service information

— Allocation statistics for the overhead initial cost centers

— Financial information

Of critical importance for implementation of the cost model in each country is the availability of information that allows all components of the hospitals' costs for each DRG to be allocated to that DRG. In all the countries considered here there has been as yet no attempt to integrate patient discharge data with financial data reflecting the costs of the individual services provided to patients. To overcome this problem, the cost model provides for the use of weights that reflect the relative cost for each DRG of the main services (nursing, pharmacy, dietary, and so on) associated with patient care. Where data to estimate these weights have not been available for a country, data from the United States have been used.

The cost model establishes the distribution of hospital costs, classified by type, for all DRGs (Chapter 5). Following the review of the results of cost modeling, applications of the information may be further developed to meet the specific needs of each country as determined by the management arrangements of individual hospitals.

In addition, the budgeting component of the cost model may be implemented during this phase. That is, costs and resource needs can be predicted for each hospital using DRG-specific cost information and forecasts of patient volume for each DRG. Basically, this prediction involves running the cost model in reverse, as described in Chapter 5.

Phase 4: Total System Implementation

In the fourth phase the software for the cost model is reprogrammed to run on the microcomputers commonly used in the country. The system is installed and personnel trained so that the software can be used directly without assistance. In addition, analyses and reports are designed in collaboration with the hospitals' staffs to facilitate effective communication between hospital administrators and physicians.

The phases of the Yale projects discussed above represent a useful way of conceptualizing the complex set of activities that are required to validate the process of applying DRGs to the data derived from hospital systems outside the United States, and of implementing the costing and budgeting applications of DRGs in these countries. In practice, some countries that have collaborated with the Yale group have not wished to complete all these phases. In the countries that have not yet decided to use DRGs for funding and budgeting, the projects have included only phases 1 and 2.

Results

The Yale group has completed projects in France, Portugal, Ireland, Norway, Sweden, Finland, Iceland, England, Wales, Spain, and Australia. In each case the results have confirmed that the DRG definitions, in general, are appropriate for use in these countries. Although the hospital discharges studied in these countries revealed that lengths of stay by DRG were usually longer than in the United States, there was nevertheless a strong tendency for the DRGs that were associated with relatively long durations of stay in the United States to display this characteristic in the other countries. Similarly, the DRGs with the shorter lengths of stay in the United States also tended to have shorter stays in the other countries. Thus the values for the correlation coefficients, along with the other studies described above, indicated that similar types of patients were included in the same DRGs in all the countries, including the United States.

Detailed analyses of the results, however, revealed several problems. First, in most of the data sets, because of the need to map from the various coding systems to ICD-9-CM, some DRGs were not represented, or numbers in some DRGs were understated. For example, for the countries where the data have been coded by ICD-9, the absence of a fifth digit in this system meant that no cases were assigned to DRG 27, traumatic stupor and coma with a coma greater than one hour. Similar problems occurred with the mapping of the procedure codes when the classification system used was less specific than the ICD-9-CM procedure codes.

Second, in some countries either certain procedures are not included in the classification of procedures or the code number is not used by medical record coders. For example, several European countries do not code cardiac catheterization, a procedure that is used in conjunction with other procedure and diagnosis codes to define four DRGs in MDC 5, diseases and disorders of the circulatory system.

Third, many of the European countries and Australia tend to treat certain patients in acute care hospitals who would not be found in similar hospitals in the United States. The most important group consists of aged patients with chronic illness problems who in the United States would normally be discharged to a nursing home or to a separate rehabilitation unit. Many of these patients have very long hospital stays that distort the values of the mean and the coefficient of variation of the DRGs to which they are assigned. Chapter 11 discusses the effects of this problem on international comparisons of hospital utilization.

Fourth, several of the countries need to improve the quality of their hospital discharge data. In many countries, including Australia, England, and Wales, data have been collected and published for a considerable period of time, but the information has been little used. In these circumstances it is not surprising that a variety of errors have not been detected. One of the many benefits that accrue from the study of hospital data using DRGs is that it is relatively easy to detect the presence of certain coding and other errors; in three DRGs in particular (468, 469, and 470) the assignment of cases may indicate a coding error. Often these quality-of-data problems are confined to individual hospitals; for a few hospitals included in the Yale projects, for example, more than 20 percent of the records were assigned to DRG 470 because the record did not include sufficient data for assignment to a legitimate DRG.

The detailed analysis of the case mix of the countries studied in the Yale projects does not indicate any reason that DRGs could not be used in these countries. The problems discussed above, however, point to the need for each country to devote further resources to improving the quality of hospital discharge data and to ensuring that all the information required for DRG assignment is present on each record. These problems also indicate a need for further research on the presence of atypical short-stay and long-stay patients in acute care hospitals. The use of ICD-9-CM for the coding of diagnoses, and of a procedure code that contains at least as much detail as the procedures section of ICD-9-CM, would clearly improve the accuracy of DRG assignment in all the countries where this system is not already in use. In addition to the ten European countries listed above that have contracted with the Yale group to test the validity and applicability of DRGs, seven other countries (Austria, Belgium, Denmark, the Federal Republic of Germany, Italy, the Netherlands, and

Switzerland) are also undertaking DRG projects. While these projects have been implemented with local resources, in general the same phases were completed as those identified in the Yale studies.

Progress to Date

The countries that have embarked on DRG studies vary in the progress made with respect to the four phases discussed earlier. Table 10-3 shows the stage each country had completed or initiated at the beginning of 1988. In interpreting this table it is important to bear in mind that the degree of involvement with DRGs of countries listed at a given stage of development varies considerably. The evaluation of the DRG utilization model may have been based on the review of all or most hospital discharges in the country (as in Wales, Finland, and Sweden), or on studies using discharges from a small sample of hospitals (as in Belgium and the Netherlands). To date all the phase 3 and phase 4 developments have been restricted to pilot studies in small samples of hospitals.

The factors that account for the varying levels of involvement with research on DRGs include the availability and comprehensiveness of the patient discharge data, the coding practices and the quality of the data, and the linkage that can be developed between the financial and the patient data. In some countries, moreover, there has been considerable resistance from hospitals and medical staff to the use of DRGs for budgeting and funding purposes. This resistance has led, in a few cases, to a reluctance of governments to support phase 3 and phase 4 studies, since

Table 10-3: Phases Completed or Commenced in DRG Projects, 1988

Phase	Country
4. System implementation	Portugal, France
3. Cost model adaptation	Sweden, Norway, Switzerland, England, Wales, Australia
2. Evaluation of utilization model	Iceland, Belgium, Denmark, Italy, Spain, Korea, Finland, The Netherlands
1. Technical feasibility	Austria, Federal Republic of Germany

Reprinted with permission from: J.-M. Rodrigues, "Overview of European DRG Developments," in *The Management and Financing of Hospital Services: Proceedings of the Second International Conference* (New Haven, CT: Health Systems Management Group, 1988).

these have been perceived as forming the basis for the funding application of DRGs.

OBJECTIVES OF DRG PROJECTS

As was noted earlier, the interest in DRGs of governments in countries outside the United States has stemmed from the desire to improve the methods of funding hospitals, and to provide a basis for increasing the efficiency of hospital management. These objectives are closely related. The proposed changes in the methods used by governments to finance hospitals are designed to provide increased incentives for efficiency. Thus, under an arrangement of this kind, those hospitals with above-average costs, in relation to their case mix as measured by DRGs, would face strong pressures to reduce their costs by becoming more efficient.

Even if DRGs are not used for funding purposes, there is considerable scope for their application within the hospital to improve operating efficiency. Chapter 4 demonstrated that DRGs can form the basis of a system of product-line management in which the components of the costs of caring for patients in a given DRG can be estimated and used for management decision making. DRGs may also be used to form the basis of systems of quality assurance and utilization review (Chapter 2).

The governments of the countries being considered here are usually much more active in planning the development of health services than are governments in the United States. Consequently, it is very important for governments to be able to determine the role and function of each hospital for which they are responsible. The description of the case mix of these hospitals yielded by the assigning of all discharges to DRGs is clearly a major part of the process of establishing precisely the activities currently undertaken by each hospital. This information might then be used to change the roles of the hospitals in the system, as, for example, by concentrating certain types of patients at a certain range of hospitals, and also concentrating the staff and equipment required to treat them. Regionalization policies of this kind have been difficult for governments to implement because they have lacked detailed and meaningful information about the existing case mix of each hospital.

All these potential applications have undoubtedly influenced governments to introduce programs to develop DRGs. At present, however, there are very few examples in these countries of specific uses of DRGs for funding, management, and planning purposes. On the other hand, several governments have indicated recently that they intend to use DRGs to influence the funding of hospitals and for a variety of other applications. These proposals, and the reactions of international agencies to DRGs, are discussed in the following sections.

DRG STUDIES IN SELECTED FOREIGN COUNTRIES

The countries considered here are either those that have pioneered the development of DRGs outside the United States, notably France, or those where very recent government policy pronouncements indicate that major applications of DRGs for funding and other purposes are likely to take place shortly.

France

The first experiments with the use of DRGs in Europe were conducted in France with technical assistance from the Yale group.[9] These studies have served as a prototype for other European developments and for this reason are described here in detail. This description also provides further information about the nature of each of the four phases of a DRG development program.

The initial DRG project, the Project for the Medicalization of Hospital Information Systems (PMSI), was initiated by the French Ministry of Health in 1981, and consisted of the development of a classification scheme applicable to French hospital discharges. The objectives of this project were:

— To experiment with a new system of medical information in short-stay hospitals

— To develop and refine the definition of the French DRGs (*groupes homogènes de malade* or GHMs) using a data base derived from a standard discharge abstract

— To put in place a system for statistical analysis that would operate on existing French computer systems

— To refine hospital accounting capabilities to permit uniform cost reports from different hospitals and then to obtain costs by DRG

— To compare budgets and hospital performance, accounting for different case mixes and different costs of treating the same kinds of patients

This pilot study was completed on a small sample of hospitals in December 1983, and the first version of French GHMs was published in 1986. Upon completion of the French patient classification scheme a new research effort was initiated, involving the development and implementation of a case cost-finding model for French hospitals based on DRGs. The principal objective was to redefine the case cost-finding model originally developed for the United States to make it applicable to French data and hospitals. Data from two hospitals were collected to test the feasibility of implementing the modified model in the French hospital setting. There were both obstacles and positive factors that determined the structure and content of the project. Initial obstacles included:

— The limitations of the hospital information system (at that time there was no generalized, standardized compendium of clinical information on patients in the hospital, a situation that continues today in most French hospitals)
— Delays in the processing of important medical data bases
— A degree of skepticism among health professionals regarding both the quality of what had been achieved and hopes of further, rapid developments

On the other hand, many positive factors influenced the course of this project, such as:

— The expertise acquired by some French hospitals in collecting basic medical, demographic, and administrative data and the implementation of a uniform standardizing procedure
— The French expertise in information sciences developed during the 1960s and 1970s and applied to the economics of health, biostatistics, the classification and codification of diseases, and medical diagnosis and treatment
— The technological developments in information processing that made it possible to have access to multipurpose computers that could undertake the real-time processing of large-scale data bases

The United States cost model was adapted to the French health care and hospital systems. Several adjustments were necessary to account for the difference in the French system. The typical French hospital, for example, is divided into several discrete units or clinical services, each dealing with the care of different kinds of patients and employing its own physicians.

The implementation process for the French cost model involved four phases. The first consisted of the collection of financial and patient data for two hospitals that routinely generated the data required for the cost model. Accounting information and data on activities, linked to both patients and the departmental structure, made it possible to calculate and analyze costs by DRG (GHM) and by function (or cost center) in the two hospitals. Four types of data were used in the project: patient discharge or

RSS *(Résumé de sortie standardisé)*, patient service information, overhead department utilization statistics, and the chart of accounts.

The second phase of the project involved defining the structural layout of the model—the laying out on paper of the cost centers, allocation statistics, and inpatient/non-inpatient costs. In this phase, the hospital's *unités fonctionelles*, or UFs, were grouped into initial cost centers representing similar areas of responsibility. The cost centers were divided into four general types: overhead, non-inpatient, ancillary service, and clinical service cost centers. Costs from all cost centers would ultimately be allocated to patients.

The third phase, data processing, put the data into a form that was readable by the report generation software. The two kinds of data that were to be associated—financial and patient—delineated the two basic types of data processing that were performed. The patient data processing was based on the standardized discharge reports containing the information required for DRG assignment. Ministerial decrees and memoranda required the hospitals to compile the summary reports in accordance with the requisite standards. The RSS ICD-9 information was mapped to ICD-9-CM and processed by the DRG grouper. Then the patient service records and DRG weights were added to the patient record; the result was a data base with statistics by DRG. Finally, the configuration of the cost-model programs was undertaken, as described in Chapter 5.

A further pilot study was subsequently conducted in five hospitals to define the total system of information that will provide input for the model of cost per GHM. The software for cost calculation per GHM came into use on a routine basis in 1987. This software can be used with a large range of computers supporting the Unix operating system and, for that reason, is also compatible with a large number of microcomputers.

French personnel have been trained to transfer the technology for utilization of the cost finding and budgeting system directly to each hospital. It is intended that eventually each hospital in France should be able to determine its costs in detail by DRG.

After the change of government in France in 1986 the implementation of the DRG program slowed down markedly. In particular, no decisions were made about whether DRGs would be used to affect the funding of public hospitals by the Ministry of Health. A new program, begun in 1988, is designed to extend the range of hospitals that are able to provide the basic data required for DRG grouping. The inability (or unwillingness) of many hospitals to provide these data seems to be a major factor at present in limiting progress in the application of DRGs.

Australia

In May 1988 the commonwealth (central) government of Australia announced a five-year program to introduce DRGs for hospital funding, quality assurance, and utilization review. Funding for the program (Aus.$5 million per annum) was included in the commonwealth-state hospital agreements under which the commonwealth government provides monies to the states as part of the national health insurance program (Medicare). The commonwealth government indicated that it would provide funds to state governments and other organizations to conduct studies designed to provide the basis for these applications. The commonwealth government has made it clear that it wishes the states, which are directly responsible for the funding and planning of hospital services, to finance their hospitals using DRGs. The commonwealth also wishes to promote the use of DRGs for quality assurance, utilization review, and other internal management purposes.

Two of the six state governments, with the assistance of the Yale group, have recently completed phases one through three and have commenced work to enable them to use DRGs to influence the allocation of funds to individual hospitals. Another state has published relative-stay indexes for each hospital that use DRGs as the principal method of case-mix standardization.

England and Wales

At the beginning of 1988 the British government commenced a detailed review of the financing and other aspects of the National Health Service (NHS). It is understood that one of the options under serious consideration is the use of DRGs as an element in the creation of an internal market for the services provided by hospitals. It has been proposed, for example, that each district into which the NHS is divided for administrative purposes might pay for the treatment of its residents by the institutions in other districts on a DRG basis.[10] Under these arrangements hospitals could bid competitively to supply services to patients from other districts, by setting a price for each DRG that it had the capacity to provide for.

The NHS has also commenced pilot studies in several hospitals that are designed to introduce a system of resource management. The purpose of this program is to give to clinicians the responsibility for managing the services required to treat specific groups of patients. The information systems being developed to support this process rely heavily on DRGs to categorize patients. This development is proceeding simultaneously with phases 1 through 3 of the DRG studies, with Yale input, in selected regions, in Wales, and in a sample of hospitals.

The final form that the DRG program in Britain will take is not clear at present but there is little doubt that it will embrace a funding component and the extensive use of DRGs for internal management purposes. In the latter regard the British developments recognize the crucial part played by doctors and nurses in making decisions that have very large implications for the total cost of providing hospital and other health services. DRGs are perceived as the appropriate tool for bridging the present gap between the general and financial administration of hospitals and the roles and responsibilities of the medical and nursing staff.

Portugal

At present Portugal has probably made more progress than any other country except the United States in developing the basis for an extensive DRG program and in establishing the details of how DRGs are to be used for funding and other purposes. All hospitals in Portugal have access to a facility for grouping data into DRGs. By the end of 1988 it is planned that each hospital will be able to perform DRG grouping and costing within the institution.[11] This is the result of a three-year program, including the completion of phases 1 through 4 with Yale assistance, during which microcomputer networks were introduced into most hospitals, ICD-9-CM procedure coding was adopted universally, and sufficient data from DRG costings were generated to provide the basis for a hospital payment system.

During 1988 the government paid each hospital an amount equal to 1 percent of its gross expenditure if it supplied DRG data in an electronic format for computer processing. A DRG payment system was introduced in 1989 under which there is a fixed payment for each patient discharged, determined by the DRG cost weight, plus a further amount based on the patient's actual length of stay and a per diem rate. The latter arrangement will reduce, for an interim period, the impact on each hospital of the changeover to DRG funding.

THE ROLE OF INTERNATIONAL AGENCIES

The World Health Organization

At an October 1987 planning meeting sponsored by the World Health Organization (WHO) regional office for Europe the progress in the development of DRGs for payment purposes in European countries was reviewed. In the paper that reported on the proceedings of the conference the following points were made:

— The DRG classification of patients provides a common basis for cooperation and discussion between the major disciplines engaged in health care delivery.

— The DRG system had been adopted in preference to other patient classification systems in the projects of most participating countries. A standard measure was therefore available for comparing hospital activity across European countries.

— New approaches to health care financing and budgeting based on DRGs are being developed and implemented. However, widespread applications of DRGs will occur only if incentives are attached to their use.

— Use of patient classification systems should be extended to cover the entire care process, including ambulatory, psychiatric, chronic, and geriatric care.

— The achievement of the goals of the Health for All by the Year 2000 program could be furthered by health planning based on DRGs—for example, by the establishment of output targets for DRGs that are accorded social priority.

— Cost and activity profiles by DRG provide the basis for the measurement of performance and efficiency at all levels of hospital systems.[12]

The WHO report pointed to the need for the provision of detailed, high-quality cost information at the hospital, department, and physician level. It suggested, however, that initial work on hospital costs by DRG could be based on the work already undertaken on the determination of cost weights in other European countries or in the United States. The report called for agreement on the definitions of the categories of hospital costs to be included in DRG costings; such agreement is needed for further development of case-mix cost information—for example, for comparison of costs across countries.

Finally, the pressing need was noted for the standardization of coding systems and methods in Europe, especially for procedures. The hope was expressed that when WHO introduces ICD-10 the requirements of European DRG projects would be taken into account.

The Council of Europe

In 1985 the Council of Europe, which has 21 member states, sponsored a study of the computerization of medical data in hospital services. The study gave considerable emphasis to a review and formulation of recommendations about DRG developments in Europe. Its report recommended that member states should conduct pilot projects designed to evaluate the application of DRGs for financing, planning, and measurement of efficiency and quality of care; compare case mix and cost by DRG between hospitals in order to analyze the sources of variation; adopt a uniform coding system for diagnoses and procedures, and ultimately for case-mix classification; and conduct educational programs on the DRG system at the academic and professional levels.[13]

The European Economic Community

The European Economic Community (EEC) has given high priority to the development of a strong and competitive health technology industry, and also wishes to promote a European internal market in the provision of health services. To further these aims, the EEC in 1988 launched a project, Advanced Informatics in Medicine (AIM), which provides funds, with support from the private sector, for research and development activities in this area. It is expected that AIM will sponsor research designed to produce a standardized set of clinical and economic data for health institutions and services, including uniform diagnosis and procedure-coding systems. Other research and development activities directly related to the measurement of case mix are also likely to be supported under the AIM program.

Patient Classification Systems/Europe

At a meeting in Lisbon in 1987 the decision was made to establish an organization consisting of government, hospital, university, and other personnel engaged in DRG and related studies. Representatives from 15 countries, including Australia and the United States, currently constitute the membership of Patient Classification Systems/Europe (PCS/E). The principal aim of PCS/E is the exchange of information about research on DRGs and the development of case-mix-based methods of funding and managing hospitals. In addition, the network of members of PCS/E may have a very important role to play in coordinating and integrating across international boundaries the large number of DRG-based studies that are currently being implemented.

CONCLUSION

It is clear from this review of developments and applications in Europe and Australia that DRGs have become firmly established in many developed countries as the standard method of categorizing the case mix of acute care hospitals. It is also evident that the applications of DRGs for funding, planning, and internal-management purposes are escalating rapidly in response to a common set of problems in all these countries, including the perceived inadequacies in implementing these activities under the existing arrangements.

Strong government support for DRG studies in most of the countries covered here, along with the official endorsement of such international agencies as WHO, the Council of Europe, and the European Economic Community, suggests that we may be on the threshold of a new phase in DRG development in which their widespread use becomes a routine aspect of health services finance and management.

ACKNOWLEDGMENTS

We would like to thank Joe Scuteri, Stephen Duckett, and Beth Reid (Australia); John Catterall, Ian Mills, Hugh Sanderson, and Tim Scott (England); Mats Brommels (Finland); Fabrice Boulay, François Delafosse, Daniel Gautier, Jean de Kervasdoue, and Jean-Marie Rodrigues (France); Miriam Wiley (Ireland); I. H. Monrad Aas (Norway); Margarita Bentes, Don Hindle, Don Holloway, Augusto Mantas, and João Urbano (Portugal); Merce Casas i Galofre (Spain); Stefan Hakansson and Eric Paulson (Sweden); and John Wyn Owen and Mic Webb (Wales) for their efforts in evaluating the feasibility of implementing DRGs for the management and financing of hospital services in their respective countries.

REFERENCES

1. J.-M. Rodrigues, "Overview of European DRG Developments," in *The Management and Financing of Hospital Services: Proceedings of the Second International Conference* (New Haven, CT: Yale University, 1988).
2. W. A. Glaser, *Paying the Hospital: The Organization, Dynamics, and Effects of Differing Financial Arrangements* (San Francisco: Jossey-Bass Publishers, 1987).
3. J. Urbano and D. Hindle, "Grupos de Diagnosticos Homogeneos: DRGs in Portugal," in *The Management and Financing of Hospital Services: Proceedings of the Second International Conference on DRGs* (New Haven, CT: Yale University, 1988).
4. M. M. Wiley, "The Management and Financing of Hospital Services: Ireland," in *The Management and Financing of Hospital Services: Proceedings of the Second International Conference on DRGs* (New Haven, CT: Yale University, 1988).
5. G. R. Palmer, "The Management and Financing of Hospitals in Australia," *Australian Economic Review* (third quarter 1986): 60–72.
6. F. H. Roger, *The Minimum Basic Data Set for Hospital Statistics in the EEC* (Luxembourg: Commission of the European Communities, 1981).
7. J.-M. Rodrigues et al., *Computerization of Medical Data in Hospital Services Including University Hospitals* (Strasbourg: Council of Europe, 1988).

8. L. J. Kozak, R. Andersen, and O. W. Anderson, *The Status of Hospital Discharge Data in Six Countries*, National Center for Health Statistics (NCHS) publication no. 80-1354 (Hyattsville, MD: NCHS, U.S. Department of Health, Education, and Welfare, 1980).

9. J.-M. Rodrigues et al., "Le Projet de Médicalisation du Système d'Information: Méthode, définition, organisation," *Gestion hospitalières* no. 224 (March 1983).

10. National Association of Health Authorities (NAHA), *Financing the National Health Service* (London: NAHA, 1988).

11. Urbano and Hindle, "Grupos de Diagnosticos."

12. World Health Organization (WHO) Regional Office for Europe, *Report on the Development of DRGs in Europe* (Geneva: WHO, 1987).

13. Rodrigues, "Overview of European DRG Developments."

11

Using DRGs for International Comparisons

George R. Palmer and Jean L. Freeman

For many years, statistics have been available that point to substantial variations in the utilization of health services between different countries and between different regions within the same country.[1-3] Similarly, total expenditure on health services, whether expressed per capita or as a percentage of gross domestic product, varies widely between countries, even when this comparison is restricted to countries at broadly comparable levels of economic development.[4-6] However, it is difficult to interpret these data, partly because of the lack of comparability of the material on utilization, and partly because of the absence of adequate detail on the components of both utilization and expenditure. Thus, aggregate measures of hospital bed utilization, and hence of hospital costs, often cannot be compared between countries because of greatly varying definitions of what types of institutions are covered by the term *hospital*. In addition, the differences between countries in the disease and procedure coding systems discussed in the previous chapter create considerable accuracy problems in determining hospital discharge rates on a diagnosis- or procedure-specific basis.

With the development of DRGs a uniform descriptive framework for studying hospital utilization and costs is available. DRGs provide a comprehensive summary of the varied reasons for hospitalization and of the complexity of the cases each hospital treats. As a framework for describing the products of a hospital—classes of patients with similar expected patterns of resource use—DRGs facilitate meaningful comparisons of hospital activity and performance, which provide a basis for further analysis and interpretation.[7,8]

DRGs allow specific comparisons to be made across health systems, demonstrating differences in treatment and length of stay for patients with similar diagnoses or procedures, and differences in hospital utilization rates based on country or region. This feature of DRGs is exemplified in one of the studies discussed below, which demonstrated a substantial difference in the rates of cesarean section performed in the United States and Australia. The United States performed this operation at a rate of 30 per 10,000 of population, compared with 13 per 10,000 in Australia. These studies also demonstrated considerable differences in the length of stay associated with this procedure—12.1 days in France, 9.6 days in Sweden and Australia, 9 days in Portugal, and 6 days in the United States.

Comparing the characteristics of health care systems in different countries can enhance our understanding of the problems individual countries face and the possibilities for changing policies and practices. Through an international comparison of hospital utilization and costs, a country can evaluate its own health care system's performance in relation to that of other countries using alternative approaches to patient care, management, and financing.

Studies documenting large geographic variations in hospital use by DRG within and among countries have important implications for the control of health care expenditures. They allow us to compare practices at a very detailed level. Just as an individual surgeon might be surprised to find that his or her practices are quite different from those of the surgeon in the next operating room, so might health service policymakers and governments be surprised to discover substantial differences in patient management and the costs of care from those in an adjoining country. These comparisons may be regarded as examples of hospital utilization review data for which the country becomes the unit of analysis.

Interest in international comparisons is also stimulated by the conviction held by many health planners that the utilization and cost of acute care hospitals are too high in relation to alternative patterns of resource allocation in the health sector. Many policy and planning initiatives over the last 10 to 15 years have stemmed, at least in part, from this belief, including rationalization programs designed to reduce the number of acute hospital beds (Australia) and prospective payment arrangements for hospitals (United States).

THE YALE HOSPITAL DATA BASE: WORK IN PROGRESS

As a result of the European and Australian studies described in the previous chapter, together with the other DRG development and refinement projects described elsewhere in this book, the Health Systems Management Group of Yale University has acquired hospital discharge data from 12 countries, including comprehensive details of the case mix of several hundred individual hospitals. This has afforded a unique opportunity to examine variations among countries, and among the same types of hospitals in each of those countries, in a range of factors associated with hospital utilization and costs.

The work of analyzing this data base is still at a relatively early stage. To date, comparisons of the principal length-of-stay characteristics (arithmetic mean, geometric mean, and coefficient of variation) are available in a standard format for most of the countries (to be published in the near future). Work is also in progress to calculate age-standardized discharge rates, per thousand of population, by DRG for each data set where there is a comprehensive coverage of hospitals in defined geographical regions for which the characteristics of the population can be determined. Subsequent analyses will examine the case-mix characteristics of teaching hospitals, their relationship to regionalization policies, and the data that have been acquired on costs by DRG.

One of the most important outcomes of the work completed to date is the increase in understanding of the differences among countries both in the ways certain types of patients are cared for and in how hospital services are organized. An understanding of these differences is an essential first step in overcoming the problems or controlling for their effects, in making valid comparisons, and in interpreting the results in a meaningful way.

In this chapter we report a selection of the comparison results in which the principal focus is variations in length of stay. A few preliminary comparisons of discharge rates by DRG are also included. In addition we examine some of the conclusions, with possible policy and planning implications, that may be drawn from these results.

PROBLEMS WITH INTERNATIONAL COMPARISONS

A number of difficulties arise in comparing hospital utilization across countries.[9] These problems are the result of different definitions of hospitals, inpatients, and hospital discharges, and also differences in the collection and coding of the data elements required for DRG assignment.

The most frequent problem in international comparisons of hospital systems is that the term *hospital* is applied to a wide range of institutions, treating very different types of patients.[10] In Britain and Australia there is a group of geriatric hospitals that care mainly for aged, chronically ill patients. In both countries these institutions are part of the general, government-funded hospital system. The types of patients treated, however, are usually very similar to those found in nursing homes in the United States. The inclusion of these institutions in comparative hospital utilization statistics violates the principle that like should be compared with like.

A variant of this problem is the tendency in most hospital systems for acute care hospitals to care for varying proportions of long-stay, chronically ill patients or those who are undergoing lengthy rehabilitation programs. Studies comparing length-of-stay characteristics must take into account this lack of comparability of data from different hospital systems.

A further important issue is the fuzziness that has developed in many countries in the distinction between an inpatient and an outpatient. With an increased emphasis on the efficient use of hospital resources, patients undergoing minor surgery do not stay in the hospital overnight. Whether these cases are defined as inpatients or not appears to vary widely from country to country, with at least some of this variation being associated with the way in which hospitals are financed.

In the United States, where third parties, governments, or health insurance organizations pay hospitals for treating individual patients, strict rules have emerged that define the cases to be classed as inpatients. On the other hand, as we noted in the previous chapter, the typical arrangement in the hospital systems of Europe and Australia is that governments subsidize hospitals on the basis of an estimate of their total financial requirements. In these circumstances much less attention is given by governments to individual patients, and to precise definitions of the categories of patients. Often the hospitals are left to determine which patients shall be called inpatients and which shall be called outpatients or ambulatory patients.

In some countries (for example, Sweden) the hospital department is treated as the basic unit; a transfer from one department to another in the same hospital counts as a discharge followed by a new admission. In comparison with the usual treatment of internal transfers, whereby they are not counted as discharges, this procedure will yield a larger number of recorded discharges and shorter recorded lengths of stay.

The section of Chapter 10 dealing with European coding and data systems exemplifies some of the difficulties that arise because of the need to map from one coding system to another before discharges can be allocated to DRGs, and international comparisons undertaken. Some DRGs may not be represented when mapped data are used for grouping, and some other DRGs may be underestimated or overestimated as a consequence.

RESOLUTION OF PROBLEMS

Some of these problems are relatively easy to resolve. Most of the important policy questions about hospitals are associated with the acute, short-stay institutions that are the most expensive and in which the great majority of patients are treated. In the United States a short-stay hospital is defined for official purposes as one that has a mean length of stay of less than 30 days. Since an important part of our purpose was to compare other countries with the United States, we have excluded from the data base all those institutions in other countries with a mean length of stay of 30 days or more. Similarly, the problem of intrahospital transfers was dealt with by combining the data for the separate episodes for each patient who was reported as being discharged and admitted to the same hospital over a brief time period.

The problems created by long-stay, nursing-home-type patients and short-stay, quasi outpatients are more difficult to deal with, both in principle and in practice. On the one hand, these patients form part of the total reported utilization and inpatient cost of short-stay hospitals. The recognition of their presence is required if the variations in these factors are to be explained. It may be argued, in the context of explanatory models of hospital behavior, that the use of acute hospitals by some of these patients may reflect excess capacity in the system. On the other hand, the inclusion of these types of patients in the analysis complicates considerably the examination of the results on a DRG basis. It should be noted that the DRG system is not designed to measure the characteristics of either of these types of patients.

In general, in the international comparisons reported on here, the long-stay and short-stay patients have been included, partly because of the difficulties in clearly identifying them in all data bases, and partly because of the interest in exploring the wider aspects of hospital utilization referred to above. Further work is required on this issue, which also has considerable implications for the case-mix funding of hospitals in many countries.

SPECIFIC ISSUES THAT CAN BE ADDRESSED
BY INTERNATIONAL COMPARISONS

It is of particular interest to compare recent United States statistics on hospital bed utilization with those of other countries with alternative approaches to the management and financing of hospital services. These comparisons provide answers to such questions as: How are beds used in countries where explicit rationing is used as a method of cost control? Does the United States continue to have higher rates of elective surgery than other countries? In relation to similar institutions in other countries, do United States hospitals tend to treat a more complex mix of patients? Do United States hospitals tend to treat a higher or lower proportion of

DRGs amenable to outpatient substitutions? If United States hospitals have managed to decrease length of stay without evidence of sacrificing quality, is there room for such gains in efficiency in other countries? How long are stays in other countries compared to those experienced by patients for similar conditions in the United States? Finally, what are the implications of these differences for practicing clinicians, hospital managers, health planners, and persons responsible for formulating health policy?

Numerous studies have explored the reasons why hospital bed utilization may vary both within and between countries.[11–13] While many of these studies are concerned with individual procedures and diagnoses, the conclusions reached may still be applicable to the overall utilization of inpatient services. The following propositions summarize the views on hospitalization that have gained a measure of acceptance among health services researchers and planners, but probably not among clinicians:

— Hospitalization is often one of many possible options for patient treatment; the relationship between hospital or other treatment and improved health status is uncertain for a wide range of health problems.

— Hospitalization decisions made by physicians can be influenced by a wide range of factors unrelated to the clinical condition of the patient.

— The supply of hospital beds and physicians, accepted practices within the medical community, the monetary or status rewards to the physician, and the net cost to the patient may have a substantial influence on the rate of hospitalization.

— The factors influencing hospitalization vary widely both within and between countries.

These propositions must still be regarded as hypotheses, needing further verification, about the determinants of hospital bed utilization. Studies on a DRG-specific basis, using data from a range of countries, have an important role to play in testing these hypotheses and in adding an additional dimension to studies with similar objectives conducted within individual countries. We illustrate this general approach below in a comparison of hospital usage for the United States and Australia.

The following tables illustrate the differences in mean length of stay between several countries for similar patient groups. Although they are based on preliminary analysis, these initial comparisons demonstrate that there is considerable variability in mean length of stay across countries as well as differences in discharge rates, all of which suggest that different models of bed utilization are operating under these health care systems.

One major feature of the preliminary analyses was the presence of longer hospital stays for the European countries, which persisted across a broad range of DRGs. Table 11-1 compares the mean length of stay for selected United States and French hospitals. Overall, durations of French hospitals were between one and one-half to two times as long as those in United States hospitals. This difference is illustrated for selected major operating room procedures that were chosen because of their high frequency and because they represent different organ systems.

Table 11-2 compares the mean lengths of stay of high-volume DRGs associated with minor operating room procedures, some of which have a high potential for outpatient substitution. The data for these procedures also indicate a difference of one and one-half to two times in mean length of stay. An even greater difference, of the order of threefold, was found for lens procedures.

Tables 11-3 and 11-4 present similar information for selected Portuguese hospitals, Stockholm County (Sweden) hospitals, and United States hospitals for 1984. The mean lengths of stay in Portuguese hospitals are of the same order as those in French hospitals, whereas lengths of stay in Stockholm hospitals fall somewhere between those of the United States and those of other European countries.

Table 11-1: Mean Length-of-Stay Comparisons, Major Operating Room Procedures, Selected French and U.S. Hospitals, 1980

| | Selected French | | All U.S. | |
	No.*	Mean LOS	No.*	Mean LOS
Uncomplicated appendectomy	3,639	8.0	211,698	4.5
Complicated hysterectomy	97	23.6	90,739	10.4
Uncomplicated hysterectomy	622	14.3	524,790	7.6
Cholecystectomy without C.D.E., complicated	405	24.7	116,672	12.6
Cholecystectomy without C.D.E., uncomplicated	760	15.5	236,124	8.6
Cesarean section, uncomplicated	1,086	12.1	499,978	6.0
Major small and large bowel procedures, complicated	375	27.5	119,030	20.5
Major small and large bowel procedures, uncomplicated	243	19.1	72,266	13.2

*Discharges with LOS ≥ 100 days are excluded.
Source: G. R. Palmer, J. L. Freeman, R. B. Fetter, and M. Mador, "International Comparisons of Hospital Usage: A Study of Nine Countries," Health Systems Management Group, Yale University, New Haven, 1988.

Table 11-2: Mean Length-of-Stay Comparisons, Minor Operating Room Procedures, Selected French and U.S. Hospitals, 1980

	Selected French		*All U.S.*	
	No.*	*Mean LOS*	No.*	*Mean LOS*
Lens procedures	627	11.3	431,127	3.6
Breast biopsy and local excision for nonmalignancy	389	5.6	193,066	2.8
Dilatation and curettage, except for malignancy	804	4.0	479,081	2.3
Knee procedures, uncomplicated	331	9.9	240,240	5.0
Hand procedures, except ganglion	297	4.7	151,154	3.1

*Discharges with LOS ≥ 100 days are excluded.
Source: G. R. Palmer, J. L. Freeman, R. B. Fetter, and M. Mador, "International Comparisons of Hospital Usage: A Study of Nine Countries," Health Systems Management Group, Yale University, New Haven, 1988.

Table 11-3: Mean Length-of-Stay Comparisons, Major Operating Room Procedures, Selected Portugese, Swedish, and U.S. Hospitals

	Selected Portugese (1983–84)		*Stockholm County (1984)*		*All U.S. (1984)*	
	No.*	*Mean LOS*	No.*	*Mean LOS*	No.*	*Mean LOS*
Uncomplicated appendectomy	941	7.2	1,637	4.0	198,438	3.9
Complicated hysterectomy	54	23.6	142	16.2	113,972	8.9
Uncomplicated hysterectomy	941	14.2	1,093	10.5	510,300	6.6
Cholecystectomy without C.D.E., complicated	163	26.8	263	14.5	153,364	9.9
Cholecystectomy without C.D.E., uncomplicated	353	21.6	1,052	7.9	225,183	6.6
Cesarean section, uncomplicated	1,314	9.0	1,115	9.6	694,769	5.4
Major small and large bowel procedures, complicated	166	23.5	561	25.8	159,364	17.7
Major small and large bowel procedures, uncomplicated	190	21.7	563	18.8	69,728	11.6

*Discharges with LOS ≥ 100 days are excluded.
Source: G. R. Palmer, J. L. Freeman, R. B. Fetter, and M. Mador, "International Comparisons of Hospital Usage: A Study of Nine Countries," Health Systems Management Group, Yale University, New Haven, 1988.

Table 11-4: Mean Length-of-Stay Comparisons, Minor Operating Room Procedures, Selected Portugese, Swedish, and U.S. Hospitals

	Selected Portugese (1983–84)		Stockholm County (1984)		All U.S. (1984)	
	No.*	Mean LOS	No.*	Mean LOS	No.*	Mean LOS
Lens procedures	380	13.1	2,373	4.0	477,525	2.4
Breast biopsy and local excision for nonmalignancy	186	7.6	67	4.0	90,099	2.6
Dilatation and curettage, except for malignancy	1,028	2.4	2,852	3.0	157,149	2.2
Knee procedures, uncomplicated	76	15.6	731	5.6	184,071	3.6
Hand procedures, except ganglion	129	12.3	452	3.1	103,959	3.1

*Discharges with LOS ≥ 100 days are excluded.
Source: G. R. Palmer, J. L. Freeman, R. B. Fetter, and M. Mador, "International Comparisons of Hospital Usage: A Study of Nine Countries," Health Systems Management Group, Yale University, New Haven, 1988.

COMPARISON OF HOSPITAL UTILIZATION IN AUSTRALIA AND THE UNITED STATES

Tables 11-5 through 11-8 present the results of a comparison between mean lengths of stay and discharge rates per 10,000 of population in three states of Australia (Victoria, New South Wales, and South Australia) and the United States for high-volume DRGs that showed substantial variation between the two countries. These data are used to illustrate how the pattern of hospital bed utilization on a DRG basis provide additional evidence regarding the hypotheses discussed above.

In comparing Australia and the United States, one major difference that needs to be emphasized is the number of acute care beds in relation to the population. In 1985, there were 5.9 acute care beds per 1,000 people in Australia; the United States figure in 1984 was 4.3. The precise ways in which Australia's greater volume of beds causes higher utilization, and the impact of high bed volume on the types of patients treated, may have important policy and planning implications. One possibility is that the greater availability of beds leads to a disproportionately large increase in the admission of patients with problems of lesser severity.

The precise reasons for these differences cannot be determined without more detailed study of, for example, the diagnoses and procedures included in each DRG and of clinical management practices.

Table 11-5: Hospital Discharges by Selected DRG: Mean Length of Stay (Days), U.S. Short-Stay Hospitals, 1984, and Victoria, 1984–85, South Australia, 1985 and New South Wales, 1984, Recognized Public Hospitals; Untrimmed Data (U.S. stays shorter)

DRG		U.S.	Victoria	South Australia	New South Wales
12	DEGENERATIVE NERVOUS SYSTEM DISORDERS	12.6	22.4	26.6	26.4
14	SPECIFIC CEREBROVASCULAR DISORDERS EXCEPT TIA	11.9	23.0	20.4	23.8
39	LENS PROCEDURES	2.4	5.7	5.8	6.8
60	TONSILLECTOMY &/OR ADENOIDECTOMY AGE 0–17	1.6	2.6	2.5	2.9
89	SIMPLE PNEUMONIA & PLEURISY AGE ≥ 70 &/OR CC	9.0	15.1	11.9	13.4
130	PERIPHERAL VASCULAR DISORDERS AGE ≥ 70 &/OR CC	7.7	15.4	11.4	15.7
298	NUTRITIONAL & MISC METABOLIC DISORDERS AGE 0–17	4.3	8.4	5.3	5.3
371	CESAREAN SECTION W/O CC	5.4	10.0	9.8	9.5
372	VAGINAL DELIVERY W COMPLICATING DIAGNOSES	3.7	7.0	8.2	7.0
373	VAGINAL DELIVERY W/O COMPLICATING DIAGNOSES	2.7	6.4	5.7	5.7
382	FALSE LABOR	1.3	2.8	1.6	2.6
384	OTHER ANTEPARTUM DIAGNOSES W/O MEDICAL COMPLICATIONS	2.6	6.0	4.4	7.0
388	PREMATURITY W/O MAJOR PROBLEMS	7.2	20.1	13.3	14.3
429	ORGANIC DISTURBANCES & MENTAL RETARDATION	10.6	35.4	103.8	27.6
467	OTHER FACTORS INFLUENCING HEALTH STATUS	4.5	7.8	9.9	3.5

Sources: National Center for Health Statistics, National Hospital Discharge Survey, Computer Tape, Washington, DC, NCHS, 1984; computer tapes of hospital discharge data supplied by the Health Commission of Victoria, the Health Commission of South Australia, and the New South Wales Department of Health.

Table 11-6: Hospital Discharges by Selected DRG: Mean Length of Stay (Days), U.S. Short-Stay Hospitals, 1984, and Victoria, 1984–85, South Australia, 1985 and New South Wales, 1984, Recognized Public Hospitals; Untrimmed Data (U.S. stays longer)

DRG		Mean Length of Stay (Days)			
		U.S.	Victoria	South Australia	New South Wales
71	LARYNGOTRACHEITIS	3.2	2.2	2.0	2.3
183	ESOPHAGITIS, GASTROENT & MISC DIGEST DIS AGE 18–69 W/O CC	3.9	2.5	2.5	2.8
270	OTHER SKIN, SUBCUT TISS & BREAST O.R. PROC AGE <70 W/O CC	3.5	2.0	2.3	2.3
275	MALIGNANT BREAST DISORDERS AGE <70 W/O CC	5.2	2.9	4.2	7.4
332	OTHER KIDNEY & URINARY TRACT DIAGNOSES AGE 18–69 W/O CC	4.2	2.5	2.9	4.6
351	STERILIZATION, MALE	3.5	1.0	1.2	1.1
410	CHEMOTHERAPY	3.1	1.3	2.6	1.8
430	PSYCHOSES	15.6	9.7	16.1	18.2
461	O.R. PROC W DIAGNOSES OF OTHER CONTACT W HEALTH SERVICES	6.4	2.3	4.2	1.8
462	REHABILITATION	31.1	12.8	15.8	22.6

Sources: National Center for Health Statistics, National Hospital Discharge Survey, Computer Tape, Washington, DC, NCHS, 1984; computer tapes of hospital discharge data supplied by the Health Commission of Victoria, the Health Commission of South Australia, and the New South Wales Department of Health.

Table 11-7: Hospital Discharges by Selected DRG: Number of Discharges per 10,000 of Population, U.S. Short-Stay Hospitals, 1984, and Victoria, 1984–85, South Australia, 1985 and New South Wales, 1984, Recognized Public Hospitals; Untrimmed Data (U.S. rates lower)

DRG	Number of Discharges per 10,000 of Population			
	U.S.	Victoria	South Australia	New South Wales
26 SEIZURE & HEADACHE AGE 0–17	2.56	5.40	8.36	8.30
40 EXTRAOCULAR PROCEDURES EXCEPT ORBIT AGE ≥18	1.89	3.63	2.75	3.50
41 EXTRAOCULAR PROCEDURES EXCEPT ORBIT AGE 0–17	1.19	3.64	4.55	2.36
62 MYRINGOTOMY AGE 0–17	1.53	4.91	8.61	3.36
71 LARYNGOTRACHEITIS	1.02	4.98	9.65	5.23
72 NASAL TRAUMA & DEFORMITY	0.72	3.16	3.17	2.95
119 VEIN LIGATION & STRIPPING	2.00	4.33	3.84	4.01
143 CHEST PAIN	2.57	7.55	18.20	12.01
187 DENTAL EXTRACTIONS & RESTORATIONS	2.35	8.34	17.44	7.85
252 FX, SPRN, STRN, & DISL FOREARM, HAND, FOOT AGE 0–17	1.74	5.38	7.89	7.96
255 FX, SPRN, STRN, & DISL OF UP ARM, LOW LEG EX FOOT AGE 0–17	1.63	2.93	6.91	4.22
269 OTHER SKIN, SUBCUT TISS & BREAST O.R. PROC AGE ≥70 &/OR CC	1.65	2.65	2.22	3.91
270 OTHER SKIN, SUBCUT TISS & BREAST O.R. PROC AGE <70 W/O CC	4.68	15.81	11.08	24.03
275 MALIGNANT BREAST DISORDERS AGE <70 W/O CC	0.93	4.23	0.96	0.93

282	TRAUMA TO THE SKIN, SUBCUT TISS & BREAST AGE 0–17	1.65	2.60	3.51	3.70
284	MINOR SKIN DISORDERS AGE <70 W/O CC	2.04	3.37	8.34	4.82
317	RENAL FAILURE W DIALYSIS	—	33.41	100.11	57.29
332	OTHER KIDNEY & URINARY TRACT DIAGNOSES AGE 18–69 W/O CC	1.77	4.84	2.87	3.14
340	TESTES PROCEDURES, NON-MALIGNANT AGE 0–17	1.55	3.26	3.64	3.10
343	CIRCUMCISION AGE 0–17	0.86	3.40	3.94	4.08
351	STERILIZATION, MALE	0.06	4.58	5.71	3.16
359	TUBAL INTERRUPTION FOR NON-MALIGNANCY	2.69	4.02	3.10	7.80
360	VAGINA, CERVIX, VULVA PROCEDURES	3.47	12.17	7.35	11.57
361	LAPAROSCOPY & ENDOSCOPY (FEMALE) EXCEPT TUBAL INTERRUPTION	4.74	10.09	8.20	8.75
362	LAPAROSCOPIC TUBAL INTERRUPTION	2.48	6.21	8.05	0.79
364	D&C, CONIZATION EXCEPT FOR MALIGNANCY	8.78	18.66	18.92	17.92
381	ABORTION W D&C	10.78	21.65	33.93	20.40
396	RED BLOOD CELL DISORDERS AGE 0–17	1.17	2.46	0.51	1.46
404	LYMPHOMA OR LEUKEMIA AGE 18–69 W/O CC	2.43	6.05	4.57	4.26
410	CHEMOTHERAPY	0.34	4.66	10.85	3.59
461	O.R PROC W DIAGNOSES OF OTHER CONTACT W HEALTH SERVICES	0.04	5.40	4.20	5.58
462	REHABILITATION	1.53	5.48	0.18	0.44
467	OTHER FACTORS INFLUENCING HEALTH STATUS	10.11	51.33	47.53	16.41

Sources: National Center for Health Statistics, National Hospital Discharge Survey, Computer Tape, Washington, DC, NCHS, 1984; computer tapes of hospital discharge data supplied by the Health Commission of Victoria, the Health Commission of South Australia, and the New South Wales Department of Health.

Table 11-8: Hospital Discharges by Selected DRG: Number of Discharges per 10,000 of Population, U.S. Short-Stay Hospitals, 1984, and Victoria, 1984–85, South Australia, 1985 and New South Wales, 1984, Recognized Public Hospitals; Untrimmed Data (U.S. rates higher)

DRG		Number of Discharges per 10,000 of Population			
		U.S.	Victoria	South Australia	New South Wales
39	LENS PROCEDURES	20.35	7.10	6.61	7.73
89	SIMPLE PNEUMONIA & PLEURISY AGE ≥70 &/OR CC	19.91	5.63	7.53	5.94
91	SIMPLE PNEUMONIA & PLEURISY AGE 0–17	9.15	2.22	4.82	3.86
132	ATHEROSCLEROSIS AGE ≥70 &/OR CC	16.26	2.85	6.74	5.82
134	HYPERTENSION	12.23	3.11	5.07	6.16
138	CARDIAC ARRHYTHMIA & CONDUCTION DISORDERS AGE ≥70 &/OR CC	11.72	3.44	4.90	5.07
174	G.I. HEMORRHAGE AGE ≥70 &/OR CC	9.18	2.86	3.73	3.52
197	TOTAL CHOLECYSTECTOMY W/O C.D.E. AGE ≥70 &/OR CC	6.46	2.64	2.70	2.39
243	MEDICAL BACK PROBLEMS	40.80	14.05	26.97	23.90
294	DIABETES AGE ≥36	16.25	6.72	6.90	7.46
296	NUTRITIONAL & MISC METABOLIC DISORDERS AGE ≥70 &/OR CC	10.98	1.51	2.81	1.81
320	KIDNEY & URINARY TRACT INFECTIONS AGE >70 &/OR CC	9.41	2.44	2.91	3.05
355	NONRADICAL HYSTERECTOMY AGE <70 W/O CC	21.63	7.32	7.47	7.69
371	CESAREAN SECTION W/O CC	30.07	12.87	14.98	16.10
389	FULL TERM NEONATE W MAJOR PROBLEMS	12.57	3.78	3.93	3.59
390	NEONATES W OTHER SIGNIFICANT PROBLEMS	14.32	3.50	3.76	3.97
430	PSYCHOSES	21.46	4.96	7.36	8.86
438	ALCOHOL & SUBSTANCE-INDUCED ORGANIC MENTAL SYNDROME	15.20	2.56	—	6.33

Sources: National Center for Health Statistics, National Hospital Discharge Survey, Computer Tape, Washington, DC, NCHS, 1984; computer tapes of hospital discharge data supplied by the Health Commission of Victoria, the Health Commission of South Australia, and the New South Wales Department of Health.

Nevertheless, the results of the comparison, along with other information, provide a basis for drawing several conclusions about international variations in patient management and other factors likely to influence hospital bed utilization. The results showed a much longer mean length of stay in Australian hospitals for DRGs known to be associated with chronically ill, aged patients. Much of the difference was eliminated when outliers (cases with very high length-of-stay values) were removed from the data. On the other hand, very short stays were found in Australia for patients undergoing minor surgical procedures. These latter results are likely to reflect the presence in the Australian data of many day-surgery cases who would not be treated in a hospital in the United States, or not admitted as inpatients. Discharge rates per 10,000 of population were markedly higher in the United States for several major elective surgical procedures and for a number of very-high-volume medical DRGs.

The comparisons presented reveal several potential sources of inefficiency in the delivery of hospital services. Apart from the waste of scarce resources, these inefficiencies may also affect the quality of care. It is evident that there is a greater tendency in Australia, as compared with the United States, to use acute care hospital facilities for long-term chronically ill patients. Most likely, this process generates higher costs. In the case of long-stay patients, specialized nursing home facilities may be able to provide services more efficiently while providing higher-quality care through more appropriate services.

The DRG-specific data presented here show that certain elective surgical procedures and several medical diagnostic categories in the United States are associated with high rates of inpatient services. The data also support the finding of past studies that "excessive" provision of services is apparently more expensive in the United States than in Australia, since the United States has a concentration of services in the higher-cost DRGs. Thus, the comparisons provide a partial explanation of why the costs per capita for providing hospital services are much greater in the United States than in Australia.

The results of comparing utilization rates in Australia and the United States appear consistent with the hypothesis that when beds are available they will tend to be used (Roemer's law).[14] The greater number of beds in Australia has resulted in an increased tendency to admit patients with less serious problems. The extension of the methods used in this study to other countries should provide further evidence of the relationship between bed capacity and the decision to admit patients with conditions of varying degrees of severity. The results also suggest that greater control over admission and discharge practices could promote greater efficiency and possibly higher quality of care in both countries.

CONCLUSION

International comparisons will become increasingly valuable as DRG data are refined and extended, and as more detailed analysis of these data are conducted. International comparisons can be used by health planners and hospitals to assess differences in health delivery that may ultimately lead to a more efficient and effective system of health care. There is widespread belief in most countries that many desirable policy changes, such as the development of primary health care systems, can be funded only after an increase in efficiency in the provision of hospital inpatient care.

ACKNOWLEDGMENTS

We would like to thank Robert Mullin, Christine Ferrigno, and Beth Reid for technical assistance in the mapping of diagnosis and procedure codes of various countries to ICD-9-CM to allow assignment of DRGs, and Martin Mador and Robert Newbold for computer programming.

REFERENCES

1. J. Bunker, "A Comparison of Operations and Surgeons in England and Wales," *New England Journal of Medicine* 282 (1970): 135–44.
2. J. Wennberg et al., "Professional Uncertainty and the Problem of Supplier-Induced Demand," *Social Science and Medicine* 16 (1982): 811–24.
3. K. McPherson et al., "Small Area Variations in the Use of Common Surgical Procedures," *New England Journal of Medicine* 307 (1982): 1310–14.
4. Organisation for Economic Cooperation and Development (OECD), *Measuring Health Care, 1960–1983* (Paris: OECD, 1985).
5. Organisation for Economic Cooperation and Development (OECD), *Financing and Delivering Health Care* (Paris: OECD, 1987).
6. G. J. Schieber and J. P. Poullier, "International Health Spending and Utilization Trends," *Health Affairs* 7, no. 4 (1988): 105–12.
7. G. R. Palmer and J. L. Freeman, "Comparisons of Hospital Bed Utilization in Australia and the United States Using DRGs," *Quality Review Bulletin* 13, no. 7 (1987): 256–61.
8. G. R. Palmer, "International Comparisons of Hospital Usage and Costs Based on DRGs," in *The Management and Financing of Hospital Services: Proceedings of the Second International Conference on DRGs* (New Haven, CT: Yale University, 1988).
9. L. J. Kozak, R. Andersen, and O. W. Anderson, *The Status of Hospital Discharge Data in Six Countries* (National Center for Health Statistics [NCHS] publication no. [PHS] 80–1354; Hyattsville, MD: NCHS, U.S. Department of Health, Education, and Welfare, 1980).
10. W. A. Glaser, *Paying the Hospital: The Organization, Dynamics, and Effects of Differing Financial Arrangements* (San Francisco: Jossey-Bass Publishers, 1987).
11. Wennberg et al., "Professional Uncertainty."

12. W. McClure, "Toward Development and Application of a Quantitative Theory of Hospital Utilization," *Inquiry* 19 (1982): 117–35.
13. McPherson et al., "Small Area Variations."
14. M. I. Roemer, "Bed Supply and Hospital Utilization: A Natural Experiment," *Hospitals* 35 (1961): 36–42.

Part V

DRG Analogues for Ambulatory
Care and Long-Term Care

12

The AVG System for Ambulatory Care

Karen C. Schneider, Jeffrey L. Lichtenstein, Jean L.
Freeman, Robert C. Newbold, Robert B. Fetter, Louis
Gottlieb, Philip J. Leaf, and Carol S. Portlock

National health expenditures in the United States in 1986 were $458 billion, or 10.9 percent of the gross national product. The average annual rate of increase since 1965 has been 12.1 percent.[1] Considerable attempts have been made to control these spiraling costs, particularly over the last decade. A major effort began in 1983 with the introduction of Medicare's Prospective Payment System (PPS), based on payment by diagnosis-related group (DRG).

Interest in managing the cost of health care is now increasingly turning to the ambulatory care area. Ambulatory care visits have increased in a way that parallels the growth of the national health spending. In 1984 almost 1.2 billion ambulatory care visits were made.[2] Most of these visits were to physicians' offices. Twenty-three percent of them occurred in emergency rooms or hospital outpatient departments.[3]

The application of diagnosis-related groups as both a payment system and a management tool for short-stay hospitals has sparked interest in expanding the concept of product definition to ambulatory care services. Here the products are the sets of services provided to patients during their visits to physicians' offices, emergency rooms, hospital

Adapted from "Ambulatory Visit Groups: An Outpatient Classification System," *The Journal of Ambulatory Care Management*, Vol. 11, No. 3, pp. 1–12, with permission of Aspen Publishers, Inc., © August 1988.

This chapter describes the work of "Development of an Ambulatory Patient Classification System" final report of grants nos. 18-P-98361/1-01 and 18-C-98361/1-02 between the Health Care Financing Administration (HCFA) and Yale University: Robert B. Fetter, principal investigator; John Petrie, project officer; December 1987.

outpatient departments, health clinics, and surgical centers. Work at Yale University toward defining the products of ambulatory care began in 1978 under a contract with the Social Security Administration. This research led to a classification of patient encounters in the ambulatory care setting that was distributed to the public in 1980.[4] There were 154 classes or groups of visits, based on such variables as age, presenting problem, principal diagnosis, visit status (old or new patient with an old or new problem), referred (yes or no), and use of psychotherapy.

The first revision of these ambulatory visit groups (AVGs) was produced under a contract with the Health Care Financing Administration that began in September 1983. The present chapter discusses this new AVG system, which classifies outpatient encounters between patients and physicians into groups that are hypothesized to have similar types and amounts of resources consumed. Each AVG identifies a different type of encounter that can be considered a different product of the ambulatory health care system.

A number of patient classification systems have been devised specifically for ambulatory care.[5-13] Those that were of particular importance in the development of the revised AVGs were the diagnosis clusters of Schneeweiss and colleagues at the University of Washington in Seattle and the Reason for Visit Classification (RVC) developed by Schneider and associates.[10,12]

The diagnosis clusters were groups of diagnostic codes designed to facilitate the analysis of ambulatory care data. The West Coast team originally derived 92 diagnosis clusters from the 1977 and 1978 National Ambulatory Medical Care Survey (NAMCS) data.[14,15] The clusters covered 86 percent of the 1,734 distinct diagnoses that were coded according to the *Eighth Revision, International Classification of Diseases, Adapted for Use in the United States* (ICDA-8).[16] The original clusters were expanded to 100 in 1986 with use of 2,858 diagnoses from the 1980 and 1981 NAMCS data.[17,18] These diagnoses were coded according to the *International Classification of Diseases, Ninth Revision, Clinical Modification* (ICD-9-CM).[19]

Schneider and associates developed a method for categorizing a patient's complaints, problems, or reasons for seeking ambulatory care that utilized seven modules: symptom; disease; diagnostic, screening, and preventive; treatment; injuries and adverse effects; test results; and administrative.[20] The emphasis in the RVC system is on the patient's perspective on the reason for seeking care. This system has been used by NAMCS since 1977.

The objectives of the study to revise the AVGs were based on the early experience with AVGs[21] and on methods recently developed to describe ambulatory care.[22,23] The objectives were:

— To base the system on ICD-9-CM and the *CPT 1985: Physicians' Current Procedural Terminology, Fourth Edition* (CPT-4), currently the most widely used coding conventions in the ambulatory setting[24]

— To examine measures of resource use in addition to physician time

— To develop distinct groups for ambulatory surgery and other procedures

— To construct group definitions to facilitate a linkage with the DRGs

The first AVG project used ICDA-8, which is now out-of-date. The subsequent project used ICD-9-CM to categorize diagnoses. While there are other coding schemes for diagnoses and ICD-9-CM has some limitations, ICD-9-CM was chosen because (1) it has become the standard for diagnosis coding, (2) the DRGs used it, (3) most insurers use it, and (4) most of the data bases acquired for the project employed ICD-9-CM diagnosis codes.

CPT-4 was chosen for procedures. For outpatient care CPT-4 is the standard. Most physicians' offices use CPT-4 to describe procedures for billing purposes. Medicare has required the use of CPT-4 in the coding of hospital outpatient surgery since 1987 and in the coding of laboratory services since 1984. This requirement was to be extended to radiology and other diagnostic services in 1988 and 1989, respectively.

The first AVG project focused exclusively on physician time as a measure of resource consumption. It relied on the 1975–76 NAMCS, which contains data about visits to physicians who are primarily involved in office-based practices.[25] The new project used additional measures of resource use, such as selected ancillary services, relative value units (RVUs), and charges.

Ambulatory surgery was not considered in previous work, but the performance of a procedure has such important implications for resource consumption that it cannot be ignored in a comprehensive ambulatory classification system. Therefore, significant ambulatory procedures were used as independent variables in defining many of the AVGs.

The final project objective was to define the groups in a manner that would allow the use of medical care to be tracked across ambulatory and inpatient settings. Accordingly, the AVG medical clusters were created to be as consistent as possible with the DRG major diagnostic categories.

A number of guidelines were followed in the development of the revised AVGs. Some of them arose from the Yale DRG project;[26] others were based on the work of Pettengill and Vertrees.[27] These guiding principles are listed below and described more fully in the succeeding paragraphs:

— Use variables that are easy to collect and measure.
— Limit variables to those descriptive of the patient, the purpose of the visit, the status of the visit (new or established patient), and significant procedures, if any, performed.
— Create a manageable number of groups.
— Construct groups that are clinically interpretable.
— Focus on the principal diagnosis.
— Organize major categories to correspond with body systems.

Since data collection in ambulatory care facilities is not as advanced as it is in hospitals, AVGs must be sensitive to the ease with which variables are collected and measured. The variables used must describe the patient, the purpose of the visit, the status of the visit, and the procedures performed during the visit. In particular, age, sex, reason for visit, diagnosis, whether the patient was new or established, and procedure were utilized in the creation of AVGs.

The usefulness of a classification system decreases when the number of groups gets too large. The AVGs, like the DRGs, number in the hundreds rather than the thousands.[28,29] This number allows a reasonable amount of homogeneity within each group as well as enough cases within each group to make meaningful case-mix comparisons.[30]

As with the DRGs, AVGs need to be clinically interpretable. Physician consultants were involved in the development of the revised AVGs to ensure that they are interpretable by and acceptable to physicians. The major categories of diagnoses roughly correspond to organ system and to physician specialty, as do the major diagnostic categories of the DRGs. Patients within an AVG have a "family resemblance" to one another. Their disease processes are similar and the diagnostic and therapeutic resources required for their care are similar. Furthermore, they tend to be treated by the same kinds of doctors.

CONSTRUCTION OF AMBULATORY VISIT GROUPS

The AVG classification scheme is visit based. A single encounter is the basic building block of ambulatory care. Before larger or more complex units of service were considered, it was necessary to define these basic building blocks. Therefore, even in areas that are traditionally thought of as episode based, such as pregnancy or surgical care, AVGs have been defined in terms of single encounters or visits. In the future, visits can be linked together to define episodes of care.[31] Some experience in using AVGs will provide the background for a solid effort at examining utilization by episode in the ambulatory care setting and eventually to constructing an episodic definition of health care delivery that is independent of facility or setting.

Ambulatory visit groups are concerned with the professional services of physicians in ambulatory settings. The AVG system classifies visits to all physicians except pathologists, radiologists, and anesthesiologists. NAMCS, the major source of data for the project, considered physicians in these specialties to be out of scope.[32] This project has done the same.

The following variables are required to define AVGs: principal diagnosis (by ICD-9-CM), procedure (by CPT-4), age, sex, and status of the visit (new patient or established patient). In addition, five AVGs require visit disposition or supplementary reasons for visit that are not normally collected in outpatient data systems. Descriptions of these variables are included in the AVG definitions manual.[33]

An overview of the ambulatory classification scheme is shown in Figure 12-1. On the basis of the principal diagnosis, each visit was classified into one of 18 body-system categories or into a "preventive," "administrative," or "other" therapeutic category. These are the major ambulatory diagnostic categories (MADCs). The scheme next branched according to whether or not a significant ambulatory procedure or service was performed during the visit. If such a procedure was performed, the visit was classified into one of the procedure AVGs; otherwise, it belonged to a medical AVG. A key variable in the definition of the medical AVGs was the status of the visit (whether the patient was new or established). The visits were then classified into groups of diagnoses or clusters that were analogous for new patients and for established patients. On occasion, other variables were of importance in defining the medical AVGs. These included age, sex, visit disposition, and a complaint of chest pain.

For the most part, the 285 medical and 285 procedure AVGs were created as described above; however, there were several exceptions. These involved encounters for malignancies, preventive and administrative purposes, pediatric conditions, and mental disorders.

Major Ambulatory Diagnostic Categories

AVG formation began with aggregating ICD-9-CM diagnosis codes into MADCs (Table 12-1). The MADCs are analogous to the 23 major diagnostic categories (MDCs) that were used in the DRG classification. Individual

Figure 12-1: Overview of Ambulatory Visit Group Classification Scheme

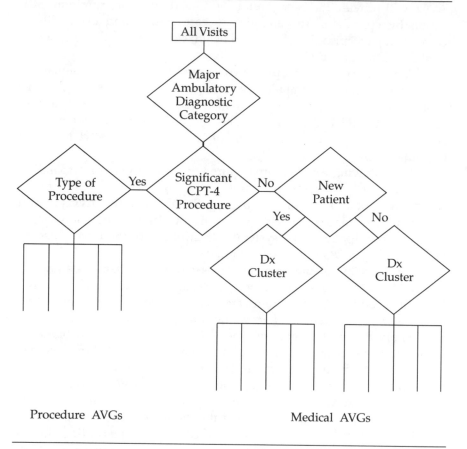

Source: Robert B. Fetter, "Development of an Ambulatory Patient Classification System."

MDCs, for the most part, correspond to major body systems, such as the nervous system or the musculoskeletal system.

In general, there is a one-to-one correspondence between MADCs and MDCs. There are, however, two major differences between the AVG categories and the DRG categories. First, in the AVG system several MDCs were combined. For example, MDC 6, diseases and disorders of the digestive system, and MDC 7, diseases and disorders of the hepatobiliary system and pancreas, were combined to form MADC 6, digestive and hepatobiliary systems and pancreas.

Second, in the DRGs, malignancies were generally included with the body system or MDC that the disease affected. In the inpatient setting, the

Table 12-1: Major Ambulatory Diagnostic Categories (MADCs)

	MADC No.	Corresponding MDC No.
Visits related to a specific body system		
Nervous system	1	1
Eye	2	2
Ear, nose, throat, and respiratory system	3	3&4
Circulatory system	5	5
Digestive and hepatobiliary system and pancreas	6	6&7
Musculoskeletal system and connective tissue	8	8
Skin	9	9
Endocrine, nutritional, and metabolic diseases and disorders	10	10
Kidney and urinary tract	11	11
Male reproductive system	12	12
Female reproductive system	13	13
Pregnancy, childbirth, and the puerperium	14	14
Newborns and neonates	15	15
Blood and immune system	16	16
Malignancy (excluding carcinoma of skin) and myeloproliferative diseases	17	17*
Systematic infectious and parasitic diseases	18	18
Mental diseases and disorders and substance abuse	19	19&20
Injuries, poisonings, and toxic effects of drugs	21	21&22
Visits not related to a specific body system		
Preventive, administrative, and other therapeutic encounters	23	23

*MDC 17 contains poorly differentiated neoplasms. All other neoplasms in the DRGs are included in the appropriate body systems.

Source: Robert B. Fetter, "Development of an Ambulatory Patient Classification System."

most significant part of cancer treatment, in terms of resource use, is usually a surgical procedure. The resources used for a particular surgical procedure are similar whether or not the patient has cancer. In the ambulatory care setting, however, radiation therapy and chemotherapy predominate. The treatment is less differentiated according to body system than it is according to such considerations as the kind of chemotherapeutic agent. Therefore, for the AVGs all malignant diseases with the exception of most skin cancer were included in one MADC. (Malignant melanoma was included in the malignancy MADC.)

Most MADCs pertain to a specific body system. MADC 23 (preventive, administrative, and other therapeutic encounters) is the one exception. These visits are of a more generalized nature, such as a routine physical examination, well-child care, vaccinations, and medical counseling.

Procedure AVGs

The procedure AVGs represent aggregations of significant ambulatory procedures. A significant ambulatory procedure or service is defined as a CPT-4 procedure or service that is relatively resource intensive, is generally scheduled in advance, constitutes the main reason for the visit, and can be performed safely with no overnight stay in the hospital. It may be performed in a physician's office or it may require either a full surgical unit or an invasive radiographic unit.

Procedures that are done exclusively by diagnostic radiologists, pathologists, or anesthesiologists were considered out of scope. Radiological or pathological procedures that might commonly be performed by other physicians were included, however. For example, cardiac imaging by ultrasound is often done by cardiologists as well as radiologists. Therefore, it is included as a significant ambulatory procedure.

Procedures that are done exclusively in the inpatient setting, such as craniotomies, were also excluded. A liberal view was taken in designating procedures that could be performed on an ambulatory basis. A procedure was considered a significant ambulatory procedure if, in some circumstances, it might be appropriately performed as an outpatient procedure. This does not imply that it should be done in all or even most cases as an ambulatory procedure. By and large, the designations corresponded to a proposed list of covered surgical procedures for ambulatory surgical centers that was provided by the Health Care Financing Administration.[34]

Physician consultants and project staff reviewed the list of significant ambulatory CPT-4 procedures for each MADC and formed procedure categories. For example, sigmoidoscopy and colonoscopy were categorized into MADC 6, digestive and hepatobiliary systems and pancreas. However, some ambulatory procedures or services can be assigned to more than one MADC. For example, transurethral resection of the prostate might be performed for a patient with a diagnosis of benign prostatic hypertrophy that would be classified in MADC 12, male reproductive system, or for patients with obstructive uropathy that could be classified in MADC 11, kidney and urinary tract.

Procedure Hierarchy. On occasion, more than one significant ambulatory procedure might be performed at a single visit. When this occurs, patients are classified according to the procedure hierarchy described more fully in the AVG definitions manual.[35] The procedure hierarchy is a ranking of procedures within an MADC in descending order of resource intensity.

This ranking was developed by examining RVUs and charges for each significant ambulatory procedure. The RVUs used were produced by Relative Value Studies, Incorporated, in Denver, Colorado.[36] The charges were obtained from a data base of 60 million Medicare visits in Florida in 1983.

Procedures for Malignancy. The ambulatory classification system handled procedures for MADC 17, malignancy and myeloproliferative diseases, somewhat differently than most of the other MADCs. An office visit for chemotherapy was considered a significant ambulatory procedure. CPT-4 codes were used to distinguish simple, complex, and very complex chemotherapies. A new category not defined by existing CPT-4 codes was established and called the "initial visit for chemotherapy." Paradoxically, this is a visit where chemotherapy is generally not administered. Instead, it is a visit to explain what will be involved in the chemotherapy (including expected benefits and risks), and to obtain informed consent. Because there is no existing CPT-4 code to capture this type of visit, a checkoff box on an encounter form will need to be used to assign patients to this AVG. Other significant procedures in this MADC include radiation therapy, vascular access installation, lumbar and ventricular puncture, bone marrow aspiration, and administration of blood products.

Many other significant ambulatory procedures could be done for patients with malignant neoplasms. For most ambulatory care patients, these are biopsies. The resource use for a biopsy, however, is similar whether the original lesion was malignant or benign. Therefore, biopsies and other surgical procedures for patients with malignant neoplasms were reclassified into the MADC most appropriate for the procedure, and from there into the appropriate procedure AVG. For example, a breast biopsy done for a patient with a malignancy would be reclassified into the breast procedure AVG within the female reproductive MADC. A colonoscopic polypectomy for a malignant polyp would be reclassified into a colonoscopy AVG in the digestive system MADC. MADC 17 procedures that reclassify MADC number are listed in the definitions manual.[37]

Medical AVGs

Considerable clinical review and an analysis of NAMCS data using multivariable regression procedures were required to create the medical AVGs. Almost all of them are defined only on the basis of the principal diagnosis and the status of the visit (new or established patient). The patient's sex must also be noted. For patients with no significant procedure, the first step in classifying the visit into a medical AVG is to partition according to the status of the visit. The next step is to categorize the visit into one of 153 medical clusters or clinically meaningful groups of ICD-9-CM diagnoses on the basis of the principal diagnosis. All of the over 10,000 ICD-9-CM diagnosis codes were grouped into 153 medical clusters that are fully described in the final report for this project.[38]

"Hypertension" and "respiratory signs and symptoms" are examples of medical clusters. The hypertension cluster consists of 16 diagnosis codes indicating different kinds of hypertension. The respiratory signs and symptoms cluster has 14 diagnoses, including hyperventilation, hemoptysis, cough, and painful respiration.

Medical clusters are analogous for new and established patients. For example, MADC 12, male reproductive system, contains eight medical AVGs. Four represent new patients and four represent established patients. They are: (1) new patient, prostatic disease; (2) new patient, sexually transmitted disease, male; (3) new patient, testicular and related disease; (4) new patient, other male reproductive disorders; (5) old patient, prostatic disease; (6) old patient, sexually transmitted disease, male; (7) old patient, testicular and related diseases; and (8) old patient, other male reproductive disorders.

Three subgroups of the medical AVGs deserve special comment: preventive and administrative AVGs; pediatric AVGs; and mental diseases and disorders and substance abuse AVGs.

Preventive, Administrative, and Other AVGs

If a visit is not related to a specific body system on the basis of the principal diagnosis, it is classified into MADC 23, preventive, administrative, and other therapeutic encounters. This MADC contains five categories of ICD-9-CM codes, which are shown in Figure 12-2: prevention, treatment, medicolegal problems, administrative visits, and other. Each of these is further broken down. Prevention, for example, includes the five subcategories of physical examination, well-child care, screening and surveillance, prophylactic measures, and other prevention. The subcategories are not further divided by new or established patient and therefore form the final groups or AVGs. Treatment AVGs are social problem counseling, medical counseling, rehabilitation, surgical aftercare, injections and medications, and desensitization to allergens. Medicolegal-problem AVGs include rape, battered child, and psychiatric exam. Administrative-visit AVGs are partially physical and partially administrative encounter. There is one final AVG designated "other."

Pediatric AVGs. With the exception of the visits for battered children noted above, ambulatory visits for pediatric conditions are partitioned

Figure 12-2: Preventive, Administrative, and Other Therapeutic Encounters (MADC 23)

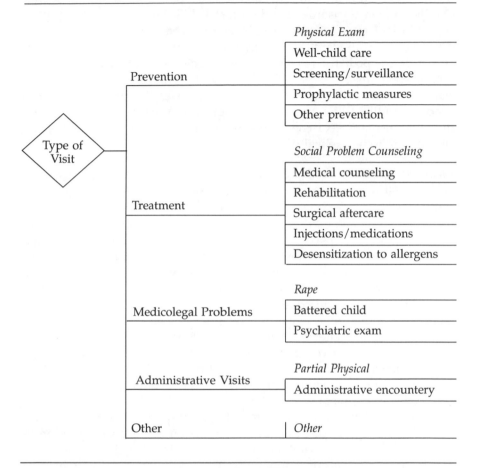

		Physical Exam
		Well-child care
	Prevention	Screening/surveillance
		Prophylactic measures
		Other prevention
Type of Visit		*Social Problem Counseling*
		Medical counseling
		Rehabilitation
	Treatment	Surgical aftercare
		Injections/medications
		Desensitization to allergens
		Rape
	Medicolegal Problems	Battered child
		Psychiatric exam
		Partial Physical
	Administrative Visits	Administrative encountery
	Other	*Other*

Source: Robert B. Fetter, "Development of an Ambulatory Patient Classification System."

into new-patient and old-patient visits and then into pediatric clusters. Pediatric clusters were created for special groups of pediatric patients who were considered to be different from other patients in an MADC. Pediatric clusters consist of patients who require relatively intense resources and whose medical care tends to be specialized and often regionalized into special hospital outpatient clinics. The following clusters were developed: normal newborn; complicated neonate; multiple and congenital anomalies; pediatric neurologic disease; pediatric ear, nose, and throat

(ENT) conditions; pediatric respiratory disease; pediatric cardiovascular disease; pediatric musculoskeletal disease; pediatric failure to thrive; childhood mental disorders; and battered children.

Most of the pediatric groups were based entirely on ICD-9-CM diagnosis codes, regardless of age. For example, cystic fibrosis was included in the pediatric respiratory disease cluster because an individual with cystic fibrosis will probably be treated by the same group of physicians throughout life. However, in several cases the patient's age was used in addition to diagnosis to define groups. Age less than 18 was used to define pediatric ENT conditions, pediatric cardiovascular disease, and pediatric musculoskeletal disease.

Mental Diseases and Disorders AVGs and Substance Abuse AVGs. Resource use for a visit in psychiatry is less dependent on diagnosis than are other physician specialties. AVGs for mental conditions and substance abuse were therefore handled differently. Six AVGs were developed to categorize the activities of psychiatrists. The first is the comprehensive evaluation, which is the initial interview. Two AVGs describe the different kinds of individual therapy: (1) supportive therapy, which is generally short in duration, and (2) extensive therapy, which often lasts 40 minutes to an hour. Another AVG describes group therapy. There is also a group for medication monitoring, which is a fairly brief visit for adjusting dosage and checking side effects. (The patient's blood level of a drug may be measured, his or her compliance with a drug regimen may be checked, and the patient may be asked about particular problems.) Last, an AVG was created for unscheduled crises. These visits often take place in the emergency department.

Psychiatrists are not the only types of physicians that care for patients with mental diseases and disorders and substance abuse problems. Visits by these patients to physicians in specialties other than psychiatry were classified into eight AVGs based first on whether the patient was a new patient or an established patient, and then on four diagnosis clusters. The four clusters are (1) childhood mental disorders; (2) sexual disorders; (3) alcohol and drug problems; and (4) other mental disturbances. The distinction between therapy by a psychiatrist and by a nonpsychiatric physician was based on whether or not a psychiatric CPT-4 procedure code was used to describe the visit.

CONCLUSION

AVGs were developed as a patient classification system for visits to physicians in the ambulatory setting. The system is intended to serve as a basis for the management and payment of outpatient services. The initial AVG project defined visits that are similar in resource consumption and in clinical meaningfulness. The present study extends and updates the AVGs by constructing a revised system that uses current coding conventions; is appropriate for various measures of resource use, including physician time; is clinically coherent; and can be linked to the DRGs. In addition, the revised AVGs describe visits both with and without significant ambulatory procedures.

Although the revised AVGs represent a significant advance over the earlier version, they still have several limitations. First, the scope of the system is limited to visits to physicians in office-based practice, excluding pathologists, radiologists, and anesthesiologists. The revised AVGs may, however, prove useful for describing the activities of other health professionals, such as nurse practitioners, physicians' associates, social workers, and physical therapists. Their utility for other providers of care needs further evaluation.

Second, unlike the DRGs, the AVG classification system does not partition the diagnostic and procedure categories into complicated and uncomplicated cases. The reason is that no consistent pattern was found in variables, such as additional diagnoses or age, that were expected to increase the physician's time. This issue has not, however, been investigated intensively. Further research is needed to determine, for example, whether specific sets of comorbidities and complications have an effect within the diagnostic and procedure categories.

There may be a problem with the definitions of new and established patients when AVGs are used in diverse settings. A new patient was defined in the revised AVGs as a patient who had not been treated or evaluated by the physician or practice in five years. An established patient was a patient who was not a new patient. All emergency department patients were considered new patients. Lion, Malbon, and Bergman raise concerns about the appropriateness of these definitions for hospital clinics and multispecialty clinic practices.[39]

The revised AVGs require further evaluation in a wide variety of ambulatory care facilities. Some evaluations have been conducted with data from HMOs, hospital outpatient departments, freestanding health centers, and emergency departments.[40–42] Since the medical AVGs were constructed on the basis of physician time, more research is needed to examine these AVGs with other measures of resource use.

The 570 medical and procedure AVGs—product definitions for ambulatory care—do seem to provide the most promising tool currently available for managing the full range of ambulatory care services and for playing an important role in the payment for such services.

ACKNOWLEDGMENTS

We are especially grateful to Hsiao-Hsing Lo for programming support, and to Donald Brand, Jeanette Ryan, and Theresa Langer for their assistance with the data analysis throughout the project.

REFERENCES

1. Division of National Cost Estimates, Office of the Actuary, Health Care Financing Administration, "National Health Expenditures, 1986–2000," *Health Care Financing Review* 8 (1987): 1–36.
2. National Center for Health Statistics, U.S. Public Health Service, and Ries, P. W., "Current Estimates from the National Health Interview Survey, United States, 1984," *Vital and Health Statistics*, series 10, no. 156 (U.S. Department of Health and Human Services publication no. [PHS] 86-1584; Washington, D.C.: U.S. Government Printing Office, July 1986).
3. American Hospital Association, *Hospital Statistics, 1985 Edition* (Chicago: American Hospital Association, 1985).
4. R. B. Fetter, R. F. Averill, J. L. Lichtenstein, and J. L. Freeman, "Ambulatory Visit Groups: A Framework for Measuring Productivity in Ambulatory Care," *Health Services Research* 19 (1984): 415–37.
5. World Organization of National Colleges, Academies and Academic Associations of General Practitioners/Family Physicians, *International Classification of Health Problems in Primary Care (1979 Revision)* (London: Oxford University Press, 1979).
6. H. L. Tindall, L. Culpepper, J. Froom, R. A. Henderson, A. D. Richards, W. W. Rosser, and H. T. Wiegert, "The NAPCRG Process Classification for Primary Care," *The Journal of Family Practice* 12 (1981): 309–18.
7. M. R. Greenlick, A. V. Hurtado, C. R. Pope, E. W. Saward, and S. S. Yoshioka, "Determinants of Medical Care Utilization," *Health Services Research* 3 (1968): 296–315.
8. A. V. Hurtado and M. R. Greenlick, "A Disease Classification System for Analysis of Medical Care Utilization, with a Note on Symptom Classification," *Health Services Research* 6 (1971): 235–50.
9. D. M. Steinwachs and A. I. Mushlin, "The Johns Hopkins Ambulatory-Care Coding Scheme," *Health Services Research* 13 (1978): 36–49.
10. R. Schneeweiss, R. A. Rosenblatt, D. C. Cherkin, C. R. Kirkwood, and G. Hart, "Diagnosis Clusters: A New Tool for Analyzing the Content of Ambulatory Medical Care," *Medical Care* 21 (1983): 105–22.
11. R. Schneeweiss, D. C. Cherkin, L. G. Hart, D. A. Revicki, L. J. Wollstadt, M. J. Stephenson, J. Froom, E. V. Dunn, H. L. Tindall, and R. A. Rosenblatt, "Diagnosis Clusters Adapted for ICD-9-CM and ICHPPC-2," *Journal of Family Practice* 22 (1986): 69–72.
12. D. Schneider, L. Appleton, and T. McLemore, "A Reason for Visit Classification for Ambulatory Care," *Vital and Health Statistics* (National Center for Health Statistics, U.S. Public Health Service) series 2, no. 78 (Department of Health, Education, and Welfare publication no. [PHS] 79-1352; Washington, D.C.: U.S. Government Printing Office, February 1979).
13. P. M. Tenan, H. H. Fillmore, B. Caress, W. P. Kelly, H. Nelson, D. Graziano, and S. C. Johnson, "PACs: Classifying Ambulatory Care Patients and Services for

Clinical and Financial Management," *Journal of Ambulatory Care Management* 11 (1988): 36–53.

14. National Center for Health Statistics, U.S. Public Health Service, "National Ambulatory Medical Care Survey, 1977 Summary," *Vital and Health Statistics,* series 13, no. 44 (Department of Health, Education, and Welfare publication no. [PHS] 80-1795; Washington, D.C.: U.S. Government Printing Office, 1980).

15. National Center for Health Statistics, "National Ambulatory Medical Care Survey, 1978 Summary," advance data from *Vital and Health Statistics,* no. 60 (Department of Health, Education, and Welfare publication no. [PHS] 80-1250; Washington, D.C.: U.S. Government Printing Office, 1980).

16. National Center for Health Statistics, *Eighth Revision, International Classification of Diseases, Adapted for Use in the United States,* volume 2 (publication no. 1693; Washington, D.C.: U.S. Government Printing Office, 1968).

17. National Center for Health Statistics, National Ambulatory Medical Care Survey public use data tapes, 1980 (Hyattsville, MD: U.S. Public Health Service, 1980).

18. National Center for Health Statistics, National Ambulatory Medical Care Survey public use data tapes, 1981. (Hyattsville, MD: U.S. Public Health Service, 1981).

19. Commission on Professional and Hospital Activities, *International Classification of Diseases, Ninth Revision, Clinical Modification* (Ann Arbor, MI: Commission on Professional and Hospital Activities, 1978).

20. Schneider, Appleton, and McLemore, "A Reason for Visit Classification."

21. Fetter et al., "Ambulatory Visit Groups: A Framework."

22. Schneeweiss et al., "Diagnosis Clusters."

23. Schneider, Appleton, and McLemore, "A Reason for Visit Classification."

24. American Medical Association, *CPT 1985: Physicians' Current Procedural Terminology, Fourth Edition* (Chicago: American Medical Association, 1984).

25. National Center for Health Statistics, "National Ambulatory Medical Care Survey: Background and Methodology, United States, 1967–72," *Vital and Health Statistics,* series 2, no. 61 (Department of Health, Education, and Welfare publication no. [HRA] 74-1335; Washington, D.C.: U.S. Government Printing Office, 1974).

26. R. B. Fetter, *The New ICD-9-CM Diagnosis Related Groups Classification Scheme* (Health Care Financing Administration publication no. 03167; Washington, D.C.: U.S. Government Printing Office, 1983).

27. J. Pettengill and J. Vertrees, "Reliability and Validity in Hospital Case-Mix Measurement," *Health Care Financing Review* 4 (1982): 101–28.

28. Ibid.

29. R. B. Fetter, Y. Shin, J. L. Freeman, R. F. Averill, and J. D. Thompson, "Case Mix Definition by Diagnosis Related Groups," *Medical Care* 18 (supplement; 1980).

30. Pettengill and Vertrees, "Reliability and Validity."

31. Office of Technology Assessment, U.S. Congress, *Payment for Physician Services: Strategies for Medicare* (publication no. OTA-H-294; Washington, D.C.: U.S. Government Printing Office, February 1986).

32. National Center for Health Statistics, "National Ambulatory Medical Care Survey, 1979 Summary," *Vital and Health Statistics,* series 13, no. 66 (Department of Health, Education, and Welfare publication no. [PHS] 82-1727; Washington, D.C.: U.S. Government Printing Office, 1982).

33. K. C. Schneider, J. L. Lichtenstein, R. B. Fetter, J. L. Freeman, and R. C. Newbold, *The New ICD-9-CM Ambulatory Visit Groups Classification Scheme: Definitions Manual* (New Haven, CT: Yale University, 1986).

34. Health Care Financing Administration, *List of Covered Surgical Procedures for Ambulatory Surgical Centers* (final notice draft, August 1, 1985).
35. Schneider et al., *The New ICD-9-CM Ambulatory Visit Groups Classification Scheme: Definitions Manual.*
36. Relative Value Studies, Inc. (Denver), *Relative Values for Physicians* (New York: McGraw-Hill Book Company, 1984).
37. Schneider et al., *The New ICD-9-CM Ambulatory Visit Groups Classification Scheme: Definitions Manual.*
38. R. B. Fetter, K. Schneider, J. Lichtenstein, J. Freeman, D. Brand, et al., *Development of an Ambulatory Classification System* (final report of Health Care Financing Administration grants nos. 18-P-98361/1-01 and 18-C-98361/1-02; New Haven, CT: Health Systems Management Group, School of Organization and Management, Yale University, 1987).
39. J. Lion, A. Malbon, and A. Bergman, "Ambulatory Visit Groups: Implications for Hospital Outpatient Departments," *Journal of Ambulatory Care Management* 10 (1987): 56–69.
40. Fetter et al., *Development of an Ambulatory Classification System.*
41. Lion, Malbon, and Bergman, "Ambulatory Visit Groups."
42. J. Lion, M. Henderson, A. Bergman, and A. Malbon, "Ambulatory Visit Groups: How They Perform for Oncology Outpatient Departments," *Journal of Cancer Program Management* 2 (1987): 22–33.

13

The PDG System for Long-Term Care

Donald A. Brand, Helen L. Smits, Leo M. Cooney, Jr.,
Karen C. Schneider, Christopher M. Murtaugh, and
Robert B. Fetter

The adjustment of prices to reflect the care needs of patients in long-term care began more than ten years before DRGs were introduced for prospective pricing in hospitals. Since 1969, Illinois has adjusted payments to nursing homes on the basis of residents' characteristics.[1] Like other early state payment systems that followed it, the Illinois scheme was not based on a statistically developed classification system resembling DRGs. Instead, patient characteristics and services believed to be associated with cost were identified and priced in a relatively informal manner.

By the late 1970s, other states had become interested in adding a case-mix component to their pricing systems. Their interest arose in response to budgetary pressures and problems in placing the most dependent patients. Several states currently use patient characteristics in determining their payment for operating costs; other states are in the process of developing systems.[2,3] A major experiment in nursing home payment, which included increased payments for more dependent patients, was completed in San Diego County in the early 1980s.[4]

The implementation of case-mix payment systems has suffered from a paucity of research on which to base pricing. Direct measurement of the care provided to nursing home residents is expensive. In addition, many individuals remain in a nursing home too long to permit an accurate

Adapted from "Resource Utilization Groups: Validation and Refinement of a Case Mix System for Long Term Care Reimbursement," (final report, grant no. 18-C-98499/1-01, between the Health Care Financing Administration (HCFA) and Yale University, Robert B. Fetter, principal investigator; Marni Hall, project officer; April 1986 [revised December 1986]). The views and opinions expressed in this chapter are the contractor's and no endorsement by HCFA is intended or should be inferred.

description of their care needs on the basis of a single assessment. This problem represents one of the most interesting and challenging questions concerning case-mix measures for long-term care: How often must a patient be assessed if the patient's requirements in a nursing home are to be described accurately?

In 1981, Cameron and associates developed a classification scheme based on the need for nursing services (according to expert opinion) and the need for ancillary services (according to measured costs).[5] Because the dependent variable was based in part on expert opinion, rather than on actual measurements, the validity and generalizability of the system are open to question. Also in 1981, Fries and Cooney developed a long-term care patient classification scheme based on data from a Connecticut professional standards review organization and from the Battelle Human Affairs Research Centers. They called their patient classes "resource utilization groups." Several alternative forms of this scheme were presented in their final report.[6,7]

In the following sections, we describe the "patient dependency group" (PDG) classification system developed by the Health Systems Management Group at Yale University as an outgrowth of the resource Utilization Groups of Fries and Cooney.[8,9] The PDG system is based on simple, easily measurable patient characteristics. The system has been tested on data sets other than the one used for its development. To determine how often patients' care needs should be assessed, the PDG system was used to measure the rate of change of patients' dependency status in a nursing home over time.

THE PDG MODEL

A patient classification scheme, if it is to be used for payment, must recognize differences in the care requirements of different classes of patients. In a nursing home, the greatest single expense is nursing care, which includes the services of registered nurses, licensed practical nurses, and nurses' aides. In developing the PDG model, our goal was to identify patient characteristics that are good predictors of the amount of nursing care required.

Derivation

Data Source. Data collected by the Battelle Human Affairs Research Centers during 1974 and 1977 were used to derive the patient dependency groups that constitute the PDG model. The 1974 data contained 1,615 observations on residents from 12 facilities; the 1977 data contained 1,245 observations from 16 facilities. The investigators described these facilities as a representative sample of nursing homes.[10] Since there were no major alterations in the Battelle data collection instrument between 1974 and 1977, the two years were combined for the present analysis, providing a total of 2,860 observations.

An "observation" consisted of a description of a patient's behavior, mental status, and level of dependency, as well as a measurement of the quantity of nursing services received over the 48 hours preceding the data collection. The patient's *behavior and mental status* were described by indicating whether the patient was unresponsive or withdrawn, was disoriented, wandered, was verbally or physically abusive, or was depressed. The patient's *level of dependency* was indicated by recording the presence of selected chronic diseases thought to be related to dependency, such as chronic brain syndrome, senility, or diseases of the nervous system (for example, Parkinson's disease, multiple sclerosis, epilepsy); the presence of a toileting device (such as a catheter); the amount of help required (if any) with bathing, transferring (getting into or out of a bed or chair), dressing, and feeding; and control of bowel and bladder function. The *quantity of nursing services* was indicated by recording the amount of time spent with the patient by licensed practical nurses and registered nurses, as well as the amount of time spent by nurses' aides and orderlies. Both times were recorded in minutes.

Analysis. Since our goal was to identify predictors of total nursing resources, we created a variable that combined the time spent by nurses and by nurses' aides. According to the 1977 National Nursing Home survey,[11] the ratio of a nurse's salary to an aide's salary was 1.69. We therefore constructed a composite variable, WTIME (for weighted time), using the formula WTIME = aide time + (1.69 × nurse time), where all times are expressed in minutes per 24-hour period.

To allow pooling of data across facilities, it was necessary first to convert time measurements from minutes to a standardized unit. This was essential because nursing staff-to-patient ratios differed considerably from facility to facility. Nursing staffs in facilities with higher ratios would be expected to spend more time with all patients, since more time would be available to them. To correct for this type of variation, we identified a "reference group" of patients in each facility, calculated the average WTIME of patients in the reference group, called the resulting quantity a "unit of service," and expressed the nursing care received by any given patient as a multiple of this unit of service.

It was arbitrarily decided that the reference group (labeled "PDG 1") would be composed of patients with the lightest care needs. An operational definition of the reference group was established as follows: a patient belonged to the reference group if he or she required no help dressing or transferring, required no help or limited help eating, and was continent. One activity of daily living—bathing—was not considered, because assistance with bathing is often required as a matter of institutional policy regardless of a patient's actual need for that assistance.[12]

Half the observations in the Battelle data base were used for the development of the PDG model, the remaining half being reserved for the validation phase. Before the data base was divided, certain observations had to be excluded. Of the 2,860 observations from 1974 and 1977 combined, 288 were excluded because of irresolvable errors on the data tape. In addition, data from several facilities were eliminated because the numbers of patients in their respective reference groups were inadequate to allow reliable estimates of the average WTIME. (We required at least 12 cases in the reference group, or 6 cases after dividing the data base.) We eliminated 503 observations from 9 facilities for this reason, leaving 2,069 observations from 18 facilities.

These 2,069 observations were divided into two subsets by assigning every other observation to the first subset and the remainder to the second. This procedure yielded 1,034 and 1,035 observations, respectively.

The statistical package AUTOGRP was applied to the 1,034 observations in the first subset.[13] AUTOGRP was used to identify independent variables that best accounted for the observed variability of the dependent variable (amount of nursing care). Nursing care was expressed in units of service, as defined earlier.

AUTOGRP employs a version of the Automated Interaction Detector (AID) statistical method of Sonquist and Morgan.[14] AUTOGRP partitions a data base into groups, using independent variables, to achieve increased homogeneity of the resultant groups with respect to the dependent variable. The parent population is divided and subdivided in a manner that maximizes variance reduction of the dependent variable. The AUTOGRP analysis considered each of the behavioral and dependency variables, listed earlier, as candidates for partitioning. The partitioning was continued as long as additional splits reduced the overall variance by at least 1 percent and the resultant groups contained at least 25 cases each.

Results. The AUTOGRP analysis selected seven variables during the partitioning process: level of help required to dress, level of help required to eat, level of help required to transfer, control of bowel function, control of bladder function, level of orientation, and degree of wandering. The last two variables were disqualified because of ambiguities in the pertinent questions and because the high degree of subjectivity of these items would probably make them unacceptable as a basis for payment. The AUTOGRP analysis was therefore reapplied, disallowing level of orientation and degree of wandering as independent variables. This analysis led to a five-group PDG model, based on five variables, which achieved a variance reduction of 35.2 percent. After validating this five-group model on the second subset of 1,035 observations (see "Validation" section below), data from the two subsets were recombined to generate the model parameters (mean units of service for each PDG) as accurately as possible.

A representation of the five-category PDG model is shown as a tree structure in Figure 13-1. The order of the branching criteria in the figure differs slightly from that produced by the AUTOGRP analysis. This adjustment was made because it yielded a visual representation that is easier to remember and apply. The figure shows the criteria for classifying patients into the different PDGs, as well as the number of patients and mean units of service in each category. Mean service utilization ranges from 1.00 in PDG 1 (the reference group) to 3.72 in PDG 5. (Median units of service range from 0.83 in PDG 1 to 3.39 in PDG 5.)

The patient characteristics that define the PDG model are simple and reasonably objective: level of help required to eat, level of help required to dress, level of help required to transfer, and control of bowel and bladder function. (Table 13-1 shows the coding for each of these items.) If used for a payment scheme, these characteristics could easily be audited by an independent reviewer.

Validation

The validity of a classification such as the PDG scheme may be defined as its ability to describe and predict resource use accurately in populations other than the one from which the classification was derived. A review of existing long-term care data bases yielded only one data base other than Battelle that contained direct measures of patient dependency as well as nursing contact time on a patient-by-patient basis. This was a data base assembled in New York State by Anderman, Schneider, Fries, and colleagues.[15] Two populations were therefore available for direct testing of the PDG model: the second Battelle subset, containing 1,035 observations that were not used in the initial model development, and the data from New York State. In addition to these two direct tests, the model was tested indirectly with use of data from the National Health Corporation and from the National Center for Health Services Research by constructing surrogate dependent variables and observing whether the surrogate measures were consistent with patients' PDG assignments.[16,17]

Battelle. The PDG model derived from the first Battelle subset (1,034 observations) achieved a 35.2 percent reduction in the variance of the dependent variable. When this model was applied to the second Battelle subset (1,035 observations), the variance reduction was 31.2 percent. This

Figure 13-1: Desciption of the Five-Catagory Patient Dependency Group (PDG) Model

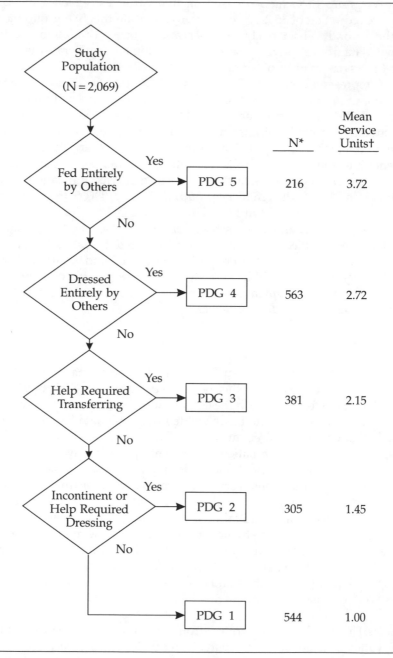

Table 13-1: Coding of Five Variables Used in the Patient Dependency Group (PDG) Model

Variable	Codes	Comments
Dressing	1 = Dresses without help 2 = Dresses with some help 3 = Dressed entirely by others 9 = Missing value	
Feeding	1 = Eats without help 2 = Eats with some help 3 = Spoon fed by others 4 = Fed by tube 9 = Missing value or fed parenterally	Almost all of the individuals who have a code of "9" were fed parenterally. It is not possible, however to distinguish these individuals from those who have missing values.
Transferring	1 = Transfers without help 2 = Transfers with some help 3 = Transferred only by others 4 = Bedfast 9 = Missing value	1974 data are derived from a question which included information about whether or not the patient had an ostomy.
Bowel function	1 = • Cares for self at toilet completely, no incontinence (1), or • Impactions (2), or • Cares for self at toilet completely, no incontinence (1), or • Needs to be reminded, or needs help in cleaning, or has rare (weekly at most) accidents (2), or • Frequent wetting only (3), or • No control of bladder (6)	1977 data are from a single question concerning independence in toileting, and bowel and bladder continence.

Continued

Table 13-1: Continued

Variable	Codes		Comments
	2 = • Involuntary loss (3), or • Frequent soiling only (4), or • Frequent wetting and soiling (5), or • No control of bowels (7), or • No control of bowels and bladder (8)	1974 ⎫ 1977 ⎬	1974 data are derived from a question which included information concerning whether or not the patient had an ostomy, indwelling catheter or "external device."
	9 = Missing value		
Bladder function	1 = • No problem (1), or • Cares for self at toilet completely, no incontinence (1), or • Needs to be reminded, or needs help cleaning, or has rare (weekly at most) accidents (2), or • Frequent soiling only (4), or • No control of bowels (7)	1974 ⎫ 1977 ⎬	1977 data are from a single question concerning independence in toileting, and bowel and bladder continence.
	2 = • Involuntary loss (3), or • Other impairment (4), or • Frequent wetting only (3), or • Frequent wetting and soiling (5), or • No control of bladder (6), or • No control of bowels and bladder (8)	1974 ⎫ 1977 ⎬	
	9 = Missing value or retention (= 2, 1974 database)		

Source: Robert B. Fetter, "Resource Utilization Groups: Validation and Refinement of a Case Mix System for Long-Term Care Reimbursement."

result—that the model's explanatory power was nearly as great in the test series as in the model-building series—provided the first level of validation.

New York State. A more stringent test of a predictive model involves applying it to an entirely new, independent data base. The New York State data base was used for this purpose. Data were collected from 52 facilities that volunteered to participate and were chosen as representative according to geographic location, bed size, ownership (profit versus voluntary), sponsorship (hospital-based versus freestanding), and level of care (many levels versus a single level of care). After three facilities were excluded because of incomplete data and an additional ten facilities were excluded because they had fewer than six patients in the reference group, 2,277 observations from 39 facilities remained.

Table 13-2 shows the results of using the PDG model to classify these 2,277 cases. This classification achieved a 21.0 percent variance reduction, as compared with 35.2 percent for the entire Battelle data base (that is, subsets 1 and 2 combined). The range of resource use across groups was smaller in New York State than in Battelle (1.00–2.50 in New York State versus 1.00–3.72 in Battelle). In spite of these differences, the

Table 13-2: Distribution of Cases and Mean Services Units* by Patient Dependency Group in the Battelle, New York State, National Health Corporation (NHC), and National Center for Health Services Research (NCHSR) Data Bases

						Data Base					
	Battelle			New York State			NHC			NCHSR†	
PDG	No.	%	Mean Service Units	No.	%	Mean Service Units	No.	%	Mean Service Units	No.	%
1	544	27.1	1.00	84	3.7	1.00	815	10.1	1.00	375	9.5
2	305	15.2	1.45	241	10.6	1.26	1,166	14.4	1.62	458	11.7
3	381	18.9	2.15	380	16.7	1.82	1,927	23.8	2.22	1,226	31.2
4	563	28.0	2.72	525	23.0	2.00	2,154	26.6	2.75	1,169	29.8
5	216	10.8	3.72	1,047	46.0	2.50	2,033	25.1	3.99	702	17.9
Total	2,009‡	100.0		2,277	100.0		8,095	100.0		3,930	100.0

*See text for explanation.
†Mean service units not computed for NCHSR data base.
‡60 observations with missing data excluded.
Source: Robert B. Fetter, "Resource Utilization Groups: Validation and Refinement of a Case Mix System for Long-Term Care Reimbursement."

groups appear to be reasonable in the sense that the rank ordering of the five PDGs is the same in the two populations.

A possible explanation for the smaller range of utilization across PDGs in New York State is that New York's relatively stringent regulatory requirements may result in a high fixed, minimum time devoted to each patient in activities such as record keeping. Such a result would diminish the difference in time spent with the least dependent versus the most dependent patients.

National Health Corporation. The PDG model was validated indirectly through use of data collected by the National Health Corporation (NHC). NHC owns nursing homes located primarily in the southeastern states. It has been operating a computerized patient assessment system since 1976.[18] Data are collected at the time of admission, at specific times during the patient's stay, and at discharge.[19] A total of 8,095 observations from 65 nursing homes were used for this evaluation, including admission evaluations of patients admitted during the first three months of 1983 and continued-stay evaluations of patients admitted before 1983 and not discharged until 1983 or later.

The NHC data include a variable called "management minutes" that is assigned to each resident in the NHC system on the basis of an algorithm developed through expert opinion. Each observation contained the licensed (registered nurse and licensed practical nurse) and unlicensed (aide) management minutes for a 24-hour period.

Management minutes were used as surrogates for observed nurse time and aide time by weighting the nurse management minutes by 1.69, the ratio of nurse-to-aide salaries that was used in developing the PDG model. "Units of service" were derived from the weighted management minutes in a manner analogous to what was done with the Battelle data, except that the analysis was not done facility-by-facility. The heaviest-care group in the NHC population had 3.99 times the average service utilization of the lightest-care group, compared with 3.72 times in the Battelle population (Table 13-2).

National Center for Health Services Research. A second indirect test of the PDG model made use of data collected by the National Center for Health Services Research (NCHSR) in 36 skilled nursing facilities in San Diego County, California, between November 1980 and April 1983.[20] The NCHSR data included measurements of individual events in nursing home care, such as bathing and feeding, but did not measure the total time used by individual residents.

These data were used to test the PDG model indirectly by examination of the variables shown by other investigators to be associated with cost.[21-25] If variables previously shown to be associated with high costs proved also to be associated with greater patient dependency according to the PDG model, this result would provide evidence in support of the model. In that case, the relatively simple PDG system would have captured many diverse elements of cost as a result of the relationships among the dependency measures used to create PDGs and other factors contributing to the cost of care.

Two types of variables cited by other investigators were used for validation: patient characteristics and special treatments and services. Patient characteristics included bathing, toileting, walking, wheeling, behavior patterns, disturbance of mood, mobility, and orientation. Special treatments and services included special skin care, decubitus care, intravenous therapy, oxygen therapy, intake and output, tracheostomy care, sterile dressing, suctioning, multiple injections, vital signs evaluation, observation and assessment, and restraints (for both safety and control).

A total of 3,930 nursing home residents admitted during an 18-month study period were used for this analysis. An admission assessment of each resident provided the necessary data. Data from subsequent admissions of the same resident were excluded. (Approximately 18 percent of the admission cohort had multiple admissions.) Table 13-2 shows the distribution of patients among the five PDGs.

NCHSR data were examined by two-way tables, and chi-square statistics were computed to determine whether each of the above variables was associated with PDG membership. Seven of eight patient characteristics and four of thirteen special treatments and services showed a significant relationship to the PDG (Table 13-3).

The association of PDG membership with behavior and mental status factors and additional dependency measures in a direction that confirms the model is further evidence that PDGs are good indicators of the level of basic nursing care required. It is more difficult, however, to come to a conclusion about how well PDGs capture the need for skilled nursing services. Six of the thirteen special treatments and services evaluated occurred so infrequently in the NCHSR validation data base that statistical testing could not be performed. Three other special treatments and services (special skin care, oxygen therapy, and sterile dressing) were not associated with PDG membership. A larger study of nursing home patients receiving skilled services is needed. If PDG membership is found to be associated with most special treatments and services, then it may be possible to use one set of PDG rates for individuals needing only basic nursing care and another, higher, set of PDG rates for individuals requiring skilled nursing services. If PDG membership is not associated with most of these services, then another mechanism of reimbursement for needed special treatments and services must be found.

Table 13-3: Association between Patient Characteristics and Patient Dependency Group (PDG) Membership and between Special Treatments and Services and PDG Membership in the National Center for Health Services Research Data Base

	p *Value**
Patient characteristics	
Bathing	<0.0001
Toileting	<0.0001
Continence, bowel	<0.0001
Continence, bladder	<0.0001
Walking	<0.0001
Wheeling	—
Behavior patterns	<0.0001
Disturbance of mood	<0.0001
Mobility	<0.0001
Orientation	<0.0001
Special treatments and services	
Special skin care	NS
Decubitus	<0.0001
Intravenous tube	—
Oxygen therapy	NS
Tracheostomy care	—
Intake and output	0.0036
Sterile dressing	NS
Suctioning	—
Multiple injections	—
Vital signs evaluation	0.0019
Observation and assessment	0.0033
Restraints (safety)	—
Resraints (control)	—

*For association between given variable and a patient's PDG.
NS = not significant ($p > 0.05$).
Source: Robert B. Fetter, "Resource Utilization Groups: Validation and Refinement of a Case Mix System for Long-Term Care Reimbursement."

CHANGE IN PATIENT DEPENDENCY OVER TIME: THE FACILITY

If a nursing home is paid a per diem rate for each patient in the home, that rate should reflect the average level of nursing care required by the patients in the home. The average level of care depends on the proportion of patients in each of the five PDGs, that is, on the facility's case mix. The greater the proportion of more dependent patients, the greater should be the per diem rate of payment.

If a facility's case mix changes appreciably over a short time, then the case mix would need to be measured frequently and the payment rate adjusted accordingly. If the case mix remains relatively stable over an extended period, less frequent (for example, yearly) measurements would be adequate. To determine the degree of stability of case mix, we devised a case-mix index and used it to measure the case mix in each NHC facility at the end of each quarter of 1982. The results were then used to compare a yearly schedule of case-mix measurement with a quarterly one and to consider the relative merits of the different schedules as a basis for setting the per diem payment rate.

Methods

For a given facility, we defined a case-mix index as follows:

$$c = (1/k) \sum_{i=1}^{k} w_i$$

where w_i = the PDG weight for patient i, and k is the total number of patients in the facility. The case-mix index describes the average nursing service requirement of a patient at the facility, one unit of service being defined as the average nursing time for the least dependent patients.

To estimate the magnitude of change in the case-mix index from quarter to quarter, we computed the index on the last day of each quarter at each facility in the 1982 NHC data base. Each patient who was a resident of a given facility on the last day of the quarter was assigned a PDG weight based on his or her most recent review. The case-mix index for this facility, this quarter, was then computed as the average PDG weight for this group of patients.

If C_1, C_2, C_3, and C_4 represent the case-mix index values at a given facility in quarters 1 through 4, respectively, the cumulative error introduced by measuring the case mix only once a year, rather than every quarter, would be given by:

$$\text{Percentage error} = \frac{[(C_4 - C_1) + (C_4 - C_2) + (C_4 - C_3) + (C_4 - C_4)]}{(C_1 + C_2 + C_3 + C_4)}$$

Results

Figure 13-2 shows the distribution, for 49 NHC facilities, of percentage errors due to measuring the case mix only once a year. Ninety-five percent of the facilities had percentage errors that fell between -5.9 percent and 4.9 percent. The median magnitude (absolute value) of error was 1.8 percent.

Figure 13-2: Percentage Errors in Case-Mix Index Due to Annual Measurement*

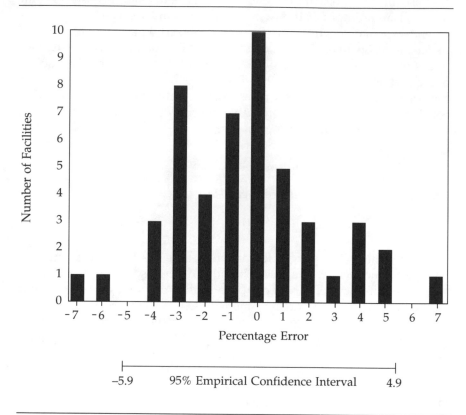

*N = 49 NHC facilities analyzed; see text for details.
    Source: Robert B. Fetter, "Resource Utilization Groups: Validation and Refinement of a Case Mix System for Long-Term Care Reimbursement."

Implications. The above result indicates that measuring the case mix at a facility once a year, rather than every quarter, would underestimate or overestimate the case-mix index by roughly 2 percent, this error rarely (less than 5 percent of the time) exceeding 5–6 percent. In other words, the case-mix index varies relatively little over the course of a year, and an annual review of patients at each facility would probably be adequate.

    The median magnitude of percentage error and 95 percent empirical confidence interval may be converted to dollars to determine the practical effect of alternative case-mix measurement policies. If, for example, reimbursable costs at a given facility based on the "true" case mix (measured quarterly) were $1 million over a year, then reimbursement based on an annual measurement of case mix would result in a median underpayment or overpayment of $18,000 for the year (0.018 × $1 million). The 95 percent empirical confidence interval for the payment error would be − $59,000 to $49,000.

Because level of dependency was assessed only once in a quarter for many patients in the NHC data base, we could not assess intraquarter variations in case mix over time: three months was the finest division of the time scale. It may be worthwhile in a future study to assess patients more frequently and apply the above case-mix analysis, substituting month or week for quarter and quarter for year.

CHANGE IN PATIENT DEPENDENCY OVER TIME: THE INDIVIDUAL

The previous section demonstrated that the average level of patient dependency, or case mix, in a given facility varies little over the course of a year. It is possible, nevertheless, that individual patients might meander considerably among the various PDGs, the individuals' movements being hidden in the averages. Predicting nursing care requirements of individual patients could be helpful to the managers of nursing homes in organizing their nursing services.

Methods

To describe changes in an individual patient's level of dependency, transition probability matrices were constructed with use of the NHC data base (spanning the period from January 1, 1982, through December 31, 1983), which was divided into eight quarters for analysis. These matrices indicate the probability of entry into a given PDG at the time of admission to a nursing home (Table 13-4) and the probability of transition from one PDG to another between quarters and of death or discharge from a PDG during a quarter (Table 13-5).

Two types of analysis were carried out: admission and transition. In the admission analysis, the study sample consisted of all patients admitted to a nursing home between January 1, 1982, and December 31, 1983. In the transition analysis, the sample was composed of patients who were residents of a nursing home on the last day of a given quarter. The second sample provided a series of eight "snapshots" of a nursing home's resident population.

Table 13-4: Patient Dependency at the Time of Admission to a Nursing Home, According to the Location of the Patient Immediately Prior to Admission*

Location Prior to Admission	Patient Dependency Group (PDG) upon Admission					
	1	2	3	4	5	Total
Home	215 (12)	356 (21)	669 (39)	305 (18)	179 (10)	1,724 (100)
Hospital	532 (4)	825 (6)	4,657 (36)	3,088 (24)	4,001 (30)	13,103 (100)
Nursing home	53 (6)	99 (11)	347 (38)	204 (22)	209 (23)	912 (100)
Other†	63 (14)	105 (24)	152 (34)	68 (15)	56 (13)	444 (100)
Total	863 (5)	1,385 (9)	5,825 (36)	3,665 (23)	4,445 (27)	16,183 (100)

*Based on 16,183 nursing home admissions in the 1982–83 NHC data base. Table gives number and, in parentheses, percentage of patients in each dependency group.
†Includes specialty hospital, residential care facility, hospice, and community-based service.
Source: Robert B. Fetter, "Resource Utilization Groups: Validation and Refinement of a Case Mix System for Long-Term Care Reimbursement."

Table 13-5: Patient Dependency in the Immediately Succeeding Quarter as a Function of the Patient's Dependency in the Present Quarter*

Present Quarter PDG	Succeeding Quarter Patient Dependency Group (PDG)					Discharge or Death	Total
	1	2	3	4	5		
1	3,511 (63.43)	751 (13.57)	209 (3.78)	58 (1.05)	21 (0.38)	985 (17.79)	5,535 (100.00)
2	718 (10.15)	4,151 (58.69)	712 (10.07)	428 (6.05)	83 (1.17)	981 (13.87)	7,073 (100.00)
3	234 (2.23)	775 (7.38)	5,152 (49.04)	1,379 (13.13)	236 (2.25)	2,729 (25.98)	10,505 (100.00)
4	41 (0.33)	265 (2.13)	1,002 (8.05)	8,109 (65.18)	1,235 (9.93)	1,789 (14.38)	12,441 (100.00)
5	5 (0.04)	32 (0.28)	122 (1.05)	837 (7.22)	6,597 (56.91)	3,999 (34.50)	11,592 (100.00)
Total	4,509 (9.56)	5,974 (12.67)	7,197 (15.27)	10,811 (22.93)	8,172 (17.33)	10,483 (22.24)	47,146 (100.00)

*Based on 47,146 observations (quarter-to-quarter transitions) in 17,025 patients in the 1982–83 NHC data base. Table gives number and, in parentheses, percentage of transitions in each status category.
Source: Robert B. Fetter, "Resource Utilization Groups: Validation and Refinement of a Case Mix System for Long-Term Care Reimbursement."

Results

Sixty-five NHC facilities were included in the two-year study sample. There were 16,183 admissions to the 65 facilities and 17,025 patients, who generated 47,146 observations for the transition analysis. (The number of admissions differs from the number of patients because not all admitted patients were nursing home residents on the last day of some quarter, because some patients in the data base were admitted to a nursing home prior to January 1, 1982, and because some patients were admitted more than once during the two-year period.)

Admissions. Table 13-4 displays the admission probability matrix, which gives the likelihood that a patient will exhibit a particular level of dependency upon admission to a nursing home as a function of the patient's location immediately prior to admission. PDG 3 was the most likely level of dependency on admission, accounting for 36 percent of all patients. Eighty-six percent of admissions initially required moderate to high levels of care (PDGs 3, 4, and 5).

Transitions. Table 13-5 displays the transition probability matrix, which gives the likelihood of transition from one PDG to another and the likelihood of death or discharge from a nursing home. The table shows that patients are more likely to remain at the same level of dependency than to change levels from one quarter to the next. The probability of remaining at the same level ranged from 49 percent in patients belonging to PDG 3 to 65 percent in patients belonging to PDG 4. The relative likelihood of becoming more dependent, becoming less dependent, or leaving a nursing home between quarters varied greatly from PDG to PDG, as might be expected. For example, among 4,995 patients in PDG 5 who changed status from one quarter to the next, 80 percent of the changes were accounted for by death (47 percent [2,367/4,995]) or discharge (33 percent [1,632/4,995]), and 72 percent (1,172/1,632) of the discharges consisted of patients who were transferred to a hospital (Tables 13-5 and 13-6). In contrast, among 2,922 patients in PDG 2 who changed status, only 2 percent (47/2,922) died and only 199 of the 934 discharged patients (21 percent) were transferred to a hospital. The majority of the patients in PDG 2 who changed status (66 percent [1,941/2,922]) remained in the nursing home at a higher or lower level of dependency.

From the transition probabilities (Table 13-5) we calculated the expected length of time a patient would remain in a nursing home as a function of the patient's level of dependency on admission (Table 13-7).[26]

Table 13-6: Level of Dependency upon Discharge from a Nursing Home by Type of Disposition*

Disposition	Patient Dependency Group (PDG) upon Discharge					Total
	1	2	3	4	5	
Home	671 (21.2)	551 (17.4)	1,374 (43.4)	381 (12.0)	191 (6.0)	3,168 (100.0)
Hospital	130 (4.6)	199 (7.0)	682 (24.0)	661 (23.2)	1,172 (41.2)	2,844 (100.0)
Nursing home	92 (7.7)	141 (11.8)	410 (34.4)	309 (25.9)	241 (20.2)	1,193 (100.0)
Death	17 (0.6)	47 (1.6)	191 (6.3)	392 (13.0)	2,367 (78.5)	3,014 (100.0)
Other	75 (28.4)	43 (16.3)	72 (27.3)	46 (17.4)	28 (10.6)	264 (100.0)
Total	985 (9.4)	981 (9.4)	2,729 (26.0)	1,789 (17.1)	3,999 (38.1)	10,483 (100.0)

*Based on 10,483 patients who were discharged from, or died in, a nursing home in the 1982–83 NHC data base. Table gives number and, in parentheses, percentage of patients in each patient dependency group for each disposition category.
Source: Robert B. Fetter, "Resource Utilization Groups: Validation and Refinement of a Case Mix System for Long-Term Care Reimbursement."

Table 13-7: Expected Length of Time in Each Patient Dependency Group (PDG) According to the Patient's PDG on Admission

PDG on Admission	PDG during Stay in Nursing Home (Length of Time in Quarters*)					
	1	2	3	4	5	Total
1	3.10	1.14	0.55	0.56	0.23	5.58
2	0.87	2.89	0.79	0.91	0.35	5.81
3	0.31	0.57	2.28	1.07	0.40	4.63
4	0.17	0.34	0.63	3.35	0.83	5.32
5	0.04	0.09	0.17	0.60	2.57	3.47

*One quarter = 3 months.

Source: Robert B. Fetter, "Resource Utilization Groups: Validation and Refinement of a Case Mix System for Long-Term Care Reimbursement."

For example, patients admitted to a nursing home at dependency level (PDG) 2 spent, on average, 0.87 quarters in PDG 1, 2.89 quarters in PDG 2, 0.79 quarters in PDG 3, 0.91 quarters in PDG 4, and 0.35 quarters in PDG 5, or a total of 5.81 quarters (slightly under a year and a half) in the facility.

Implications

The expected-time data in Table 13-7 provide the basis for predicting the total nursing resources required to care for a patient during his or her entire stay in a nursing home as a function of the patient's level of dependency on admission. If a payment system disbursed an amount proportional to each patient's level of dependency, then it would become a straightforward matter for a facility to predict the total revenue a given patient would generate, on average, and, analogously, for a payer to predict the amount it would be required to pay.

Assume, for the sake of argument, that the per diem payment rate for a patient in PDG 1 were set at $40 ($3650 per quarter), and that payment rates for patients in PDGs 2, 3, 4, and 5 were set at higher levels proportional to the associated mean service units of Figure 13-1. In that case, a patient admitted to a nursing home at PDG level 1 would generate $30,347 in expected revenues ($3650 [(1.00 × 3.10) + (1.45 × 1.14) + (2.15 × 0.55) + (2.72 × 0.56) + (3.72 × 0.23)]) during an expected overall stay of 509 days (5.58 quarters × 91.25 days per quarter). The average per diem revenue for such a patient would therefore be $59.62 ($30,347/509 days). Similar expected revenues for patients admitted to a nursing home at each level of dependency are shown in Table 13-8. This information

Table 13-8: Expected Total Revenues, per Diem Revenues, and Lengths of Stay for Patients Admitted to a Nursing Home at Each Level of Dependency, Assuming the per Diem Payment for the Least Dependent Patients (Patient Dependency Group 1) Were Set at $40

PDG on Admission	Expected Total Revenues ($)	Expected per Diem Revenues ($)	Expected Length of Stay (Days)
1	30,347	59.62	509
2	38,457	72.56	530
3	38,095	90.27	422
4	51,892	106.99	485
5	42,809	135.04	317

Source: Robert B. Fetter, "Resource Utilization Groups: Validation and Refinement of a Case Mix System for Long-Term Care Reimbursement."

should be useful to both facilities and payers for planning, budgeting, and cash flow projections.

ADMINISTRATIVE FEASIBILITY

In developing a payment system for acute hospital care, policymakers decided to use existing standardized coding of medical illnesses and procedures even though this coding presented some inherent problems and inconsistencies. The widespread use of the coding method far outweighed the inherent limitations of the system.

In long-term care, unfortunately, no single set of dependency measures is collected and reported by all nursing homes. Consequently, variables to be used for payment must be selected de novo from the vast array of dependency measures described in the research literature. In making this choice, standard measures of reliability and validity are not sufficient for determining the administrative feasibility of a case-mix payment system. A system must also meet the following criteria:

— Necessary data must be relatively economical to obtain.

— Measurements must be capable of verification through audit.

— Measures must be unambiguous, that is, there must be a general consensus about the meaning of terms.

Economy of Measurement

Two factors determine the cost of obtaining a measurement: the number of elements to be measured and the amount of time required to carry out a measurement. Because the PDG system uses only five characteristics—dressing, feeding, transferring, and bowel and bladder continence—the system would be economical to operate. Three of the characteristics—dressing, feeding, and transferring—can be measured in a short time. For an individual not familiar with the patient, acquiring these data may require episodic observation over several hours. The intervening time, however, could be used to observe other residents in the same institution.

Each individual element other than bowel and bladder continence can be determined by a brief observation carried on at an appropriate time. In the case of feeding, for example, an observer could collect data on many patients during a single meal. An individual observer visiting an institution for the first time and relying on primary observation rather than the chart could obtain accurate measurements on most elements for a number of residents in a single working day. Bowel and bladder continence are exceptions, since episodic incontinence may occur but not be observed during a single eight-hour period. For these two items chart review supplemented by patient interview would probably be necessary.

The PDG elements, in short, are economical from an administrative point of view. They are considerably less costly to collect, both from the standpoint of the institution and from that of the agency making payment, than most of the data sets currently in use in state-based case-mix systems for Medicaid.

AUDIT VERIFICATION

Ideally, a case-mix payment system for long-term care should be administered by the facility and verified by audit. Such an arrangement is less costly than a system requiring the payer to collect all data. This holds particularly for Medicare, since the small number of patients in some institutions would make frequent on-site visits to evaluate new patients excessively costly even if the actual data collection period were brief.

Clarity of Data Elements

Data elements that can be viewed differently by different observers are not suitable as a basis for payment. The elements proposed for the PDGs are clear and simple. They have been used extensively in a wide variety of settings for various purposes. Since the PDG variables can be obtained from direct observation rather than chart review, it would be difficult for an institution to manipulate the data source to increase payments. Because so few elements are included, careful documentation of borderline decisions could be prepared and made available in the adjudication of difficult cases.

CONCLUSIONS

Patient dependency groups provide a simple, understandable system for the classification of long-term care residents. The items used for classification are objective and can be measured or validated by personnel visiting a nursing home for a brief period. This fact is important in reimbursement schemes where an institution reports patient dependency and auditing is essential.

The PDG scheme was demonstrated in data bases other than the one from which it was developed. The model fit reasonably well in data, recently collected in New York State, in which the dependent variable was measured.

The system was also indirectly validated through use of "management minutes," a constructed measure of resource use calculated for all residents in nursing homes owned by the National Health Corporation. Management minutes were originally based on expert opinion and have the drawbacks of any such scheme. However, they have been widely used across a variety of institutions to organize and plan staffing. After patients in the NHC data base were classified into the five PDGs, the relative weights derived from management minutes were found to be quite close to those identified in our model.

Finally, PDGs were indirectly validated through data collected for the nursing home payment experiment of the National Center for Health Services Research (NCHSR). Seven of eight patient characteristics selected for study because they had been shown to be related to cost (bathing, toileting, walking, wheeling, behavior patterns, disturbance of mood, mobility, and orientation) were associated with PDG membership in a direction that confirmed our model. One item—wheeling—could not be analyzed because data were insufficient. When a group of thirteen special treatments and services from the NCHSR data was tested against the PDGs, significant association was found for four of the items (decubitus, intake and output, vital signs evaluation, and observation and assessment). The remaining nine variables (special skin care, intravenous therapy, oxygen therapy, tracheostomy care, sterile dressing, suctioning, multiple injections, and restraints for safety and control) were not associated with PDG ($p > 0.05$) or did not occur frequently enough to permit analysis.

The PDG classification scheme in its current form does not account for the services provided by licensed or registered physical therapists. In a payment system based on PDGs, a supplementary payment for rehabilitation services is likely to be necessary. The results of preliminary research conducted at Yale to identify patient characteristics associated with need for different amounts of rehabilitation services has been reported elsewhere.[27]

The facilities in the NHC sample demonstrated relatively modest change in their case mix over time, as measured by the PDG model. Annual rather than quarterly revisions of case mix indices would tend to underestimate or overestimate case mix by only 2 percent. The error would rarely (less than 5 percent of the time) exceed 5 to 6 percent. This suggests that an annual revision of the case-mix index, perhaps with an appeal mechanism for institutions that believe that their index has changed, would be sufficient for an equitable reimbursement system.

A single annual measurement of case mix that could be altered only through an appeal mechanism would provide interesting incentives: to admit light-care patients and vigorously pursue rehabilitation early in the year but to begin admitting heavier-care patients toward the end of the year. If the timing of measurements were staggered so that, for example, 25 percent of all facilities were reassessed every quarter, the payment system could provide a simple, straightforward method under which at least some institutions would tend to find heavier care residents attractive.

The analysis of patient dependency over time illustrates the mechanisms leading to the relatively stable case mix for each facility. Although patients do change from one dependency level to another, they tend to change relatively slowly. The patient's PDG status at the end of one quarter is a strong predictor of PDG status at the next quarter. In addition, change that does occur tends to be slight. In PDG 2, for example, 59 percent of all patients are still in PDG 2 the next quarter while 10 percent are in PDG 1 and another 10 percent in PDG 3. Relatively few patients move to nonadjacent PDGs.

The PDG model captures differences in the basic care needs of most nursing home patients. Although individual patients move among the different PDGs over time, a facility's aggregate case mix appears to change little. PDGs are economical to measure, can be verified by audit rather than chart review, and depend on variables that are reasonably clear and unambiguous. The PDG model can therefore provide the basis for an administratively feasible case-mix payment system.

ACKNOWLEDGMENTS

We would like to thank Brant Fries and Mark Meiners for conducting analyses during the validation phase and for serving on the advisory panel, Judy Powell and William Weissert for serving on the panel, Rebecca DerSimonian for statistical advice, Theresa Langer for technical assistance, and Hsiao-Hsing Lo and Robert Newbold for computer programming.

REFERENCES

1. T. Walsh, "Patient-Related Reimbursement for Long-Term Care," in *Reform and Regulation in Long-Term Care,* ed. V. Laporte and J. Ruben (New York: Frederick A. Praeger, Publishers, 1979).
2. S. Foley, M. Zahn, R. Schlenker, and J. Johnson, *An Analysis of Long-Term Care Payment Systems: Case Mix Measures and Medicaid Nursing Home Payment Rate Determination in West Virginia, Ohio, and Maryland* (Study paper 1; Denver: Center for Health Services Research, University of Colorado Health Sciences Center, March 1984).
3. D. Schneider, B. E. Fries, W. Foley, M. Desmond, and W. J. Gormley. "Case Mix Measurement for Nursing Home Payment: Resource Utilization Groups (RUG-II)," *Health Care Financing Review* (supplement; 1988): 39–52.
4. M. Meiners, P. Thornburn, P. Roddy, and B. Jones, *Nursing Home Admissions: The Results of an Incentive Reimbursement Experiment* (Research report, Long-Term Care Studies Program, National Center for Health Services Research and Health Care Technology Assessment, publication no. [PHS] 86-3397; Washington, D.C.: U.S. Government Printing Office, October 1985).
5. J. Cameron, "Case-Mix and Resource Use in Long-Term Care," *Medical Care* 23 (1985): 296–309.
6. B. Fries and L. Cooney, "Resource Utilization Groups," *Medical Care* 23, no. 2 (1985): 110–22.
7. L. Cooney and B. Fries, "Validation and Use of Resource Utilization Groups as a Case-Mix Measure for Long-Term Care," *Medical Care* 23, no. 2 (1985): 123–32.
8. Fries and Cooney, "Resource Utilization Groups."
9. Cooney and Fries, "Validation and Use of Resource Utilization Groups."
10. K. McCaffree, J. Baker, and E. Perrin, *Long Term Care Case Mix, Employee Time, and Costs* (National Center for Health Services research contract no. HRA-230-76-0285, Battelle Human Affairs Research Centers, February 28, 1979).
11. J. VanNostrand, A. Zappolo, E. Hing, B. Bloom, B. Hirsch, and D. Foley, "The National Nursing Home Survey, 1977: Summary for the United States," *Vital and Health Statistics,* series 13, no. 43 (U.S. Department of Health, Education, and Welfare publication no. [PHS] 79-1794; Washington, D.C.: U.S. Government Printing Office, July 1979).
12. S. Katz, A. B. Ford, R. W. Moskowitz, B. A. Jackson, and M. W. Jaffee. "Studies of Illness in the Aged: The Index of ADL," *Journal of the American Medical Association* 185 (1963): 914–19.
13. R. Mills, R. Fetter, D. Riedel, and R. Averill, "AUTOGRP: An Interactive Computer System for the Analysis of Health Care Data," *Medical Care* 14 (1976): 603–15.
14. J. Sonquist and J. Morgan, *The Detection of Interaction Effects* (Ann Arbor, MI: Institute for Social Research, The University of Michigan, 1964).
15. Schneider et al., "Case Mix Measurement for Nursing Home Payment."
16. C. Adams and J. Williams, *Patient Assessment Computerized* (Murfreesboro, TN: National Health Corporation, 1980).

17. Meiners et al., *Nursing Home Admissions.*
18. Adams and Williams, *Patient Assessment Computerized.*
19. J. Powell, "Completing the Form Manual," in *Patient Assessment Computerized* (Murfreesboro, TN: National Health Corporation, March 1982).
20. Meiners et al., *Nursing Home Admissions.*
21. McCaffree, Baker, and Perrin, *Long Term Care Case Mix, Employee Time, and Costs.*
22. K. McCaffree, S. Winn, and C. Bennett, *Cost Data Reporting System for Nursing Home Care* (National Center for Health Services research grants nos. HS 01114-01A1 and ES 01115-01A1, Battelle Human Affairs Research Centers, October 1, 1976 [revised March 1977]).
23. J. Cameron and R. Knauf, *Long Term Care Facilities Study* (California Department of Health Services contract no. 80-64671, December 14, 1981).
24. W. Weissert, W. Scanlon, T. Wan, and D. Skinner, "Care for the Chronically Ill: Nursing Home Incentive Payment Experiment," *Health Care Financing Review* 5 (Winter 1983): 41–49.
25. Foley et al., *An Analysis of Long-Term Care Payment Systems.*
26. S. Lee, L. Moore, and B. Taylor, *Management Science* (Dubuque, IA: Wm. C. Brown Company, 1981), 401–4.
27. C. M. Murtaugh, L. M. Cooney, R. R. DerSimonian, H. L. Smits, and R. B. Fetter, "Nursing Home Reimbursement and the Allocation of Rehabilitation Therapy Resources," *Health Services Research* 23, no. 4 (1988): 468–93.

Index

Acute Physiology and Chronic Health
 Evaluation, 58
Acute Physiology and Chronic Health
 Evaluation II, 62–63
Additional diagnoses: class
 interactions, 70–71; exceptions, 71,
 73–75; medical classes, 73; and
 resource use, 66–68; surgery, 70, 73
Adjacent DRGs (ADRGs), 64, 73
Advanced Informatics in Medicine,
 268
Allocation of costs from direct cost
 centers to DRGs: actual cost, 118–
 19; cost to charge ratio, 118;
 relative value units, 119; standard
 cost, 119; weighted length of stay,
 118
Ambulatory care: growth, 242
Ambulatory visit groups: ambulatory
 surgery, 293; ancillary services, 293;
 charges, 293; construction, 294–98;
 development, 292; guidelines for
 revising, 293–94; malignancy, 299;
 medical, 299–300; medical clusters,
 300; medical clusters consistent
 with DRGs, 293; mental diseases
 and disorders, and substance
 abuse, 302; pediatric clusters, 301;
 physicians' professional services,
 295; physician time as measure of
 resource consumption, 293;
 preventive, administrative, and
 other, 300; procedure hierarchy,
 298–99; procedures, 298–302;
 psychiatrists, 302; relative value

units, 293; variables definition, 295;
 visit-based classification scheme
 construction, 294–95
American Hospital Association, 149;
 cost-finding study of nursing
 service and education, 151–52;
 Medicare nursing differential in
 reimbursement, 152–53; PPS
 evaluation, 238
American Nurses' Association, 122;
 nursing costs study, 153; nursing
 intensity in DRGs, 136
APACHE. See Acute Physiology and
 Chronic Health Evaluation
Australia: comparison with U.S.
 utilization, 279–84; definition of
 hospital, 273; DRG studies, 265;
 length of stay, 285
Austria: Yale DRG projects, 259
AUTOGRP: statistical package, 310
Automated Interaction Detector, 310
AVG. See Ambulatory visit groups
Aydelotte, M. K., 129

Battelle Human Affairs Research
 Centers: long-term care patient
 classification scheme, 308; patient
 dependency group model
 validation, 311, 315
Belgium: Yale DRG projects, 259
Bergman, A., 303
Blue Cross: prospective primary
 payment methods, 242

About the Editors

Robert B. Fetter, D.B.A., is Harold H. Hines, Jr., Professor Emeritus of Health Care Management, Yale University. He has served as a consultant to DuPont, McKinsey, the World Health Organization, and 3M Health Information Systems, and is a director of Health Systems International and of the Dead River Company. He is a fellow of the Academy of Management and of the Decision Sciences Institute. In recent years Dr. Fetter has been active in research on health services, was one of the founders of the Center for Health Studies at Yale, and was director of the Health Systems Management Group at the Yale School of Organization and Management until his retirement in 1989.

Donald A. Brand, Ph.D., is a senior researcher, Research and Development, United HealthCare Corporation, Minneapolis. Previously, he was a senior research scientist and the associate director for research, Health Systems Management Group, School of Organization and Management, Yale University. He also has served as assistant director of the Yale Trauma Program, Department of Surgery, and has taught in the Yale School of Public Health. His research interests include medical decision making, clinical data bases, expert systems, clinical epidemiology, and patient classification systems. He has directed a number of multicenter studies to evaluate and improve patient care in emergency rooms.

Dianne Gamache, B.S., worked at Yale University for fourteen years in various positions, including assistant editor of the journal *Medical Care*, assistant with the Health Systems Management Group, and most recently as manager of Executive Education at the School of Management. She is now a freelance editor.